"Bravo! This book is a powerful instrument for improving mental health. The contributors teach you how to navigate, resist, and change mental health institutions and policies. I highly recommend this outstanding book to educators, practitioners, researchers, students, and to members of the public interested in mental health."

Lillian Comas-Díaz, PhD, *Clinical Professor, George Washington University Department of Psychiatry and Behavioral Sciences, and Author,* Multicultural Care, A Clinician's Guide to Cultural Competence

"The time is right for this truth-driven, liberating book that guides readers in an exploration of race-related clinical, research, and leadership struggles that many BIPOC individuals experience. This interdisciplinary group of renown scholars ingeniously frame the issues, reminding all of the collective strength of BIPOC populations. This anthology has something for everyone."

Ramona Denby-Brinson, PhD, ACSW, LMSW, *Dean and Professor, University of North Carolina at Chapel Hill School of Social Work*

"An invaluable guide for anyone considering a career in behavioral health, confronting discrimination in their discipline or workplace, or seeking a more inclusive society. Personal histories, thoughtful reflections, and practical suggestions provide useful options for how to thrive in unfair systems. Covers diverse career-development stages, positionality combinations, and behavioral health disciplines."

Roberto Lewis-Fernández, MD, MTS, *Professor of Clinical Psychiatry at Columbia University, Director of the New York State Center of Excellence for Cultural Competence and the Hispanic Treatment Program, Research Area Leader for Anxiety, Mood, Eating, and Related Disorders at the New York State Psychiatric Institute, and editor of the* DSM-5 Handbook on the Cultural Formulation Interview

"This book compiles the wisdom of esteemed leaders, healers, and ground-breaking scholars who understand firsthand the barriers and the values that graduate students and early career professionals must balance and address to evolve our respective fields. The authors provide a wealth of mentorship and guidance essential for social work and psychology."

Helen H. Hsu, PsyD, *President, American Psychological Association Division 45 (Society for the Study of Race, Culture, and Ethnicity) and Director of Outreach, Stanford University Counseling and Psychological Services*

"Important and timely. Drs. Lausell Bryant and Chang takes us on a journey to learn from the experience of racial and ethnic professionals about how to navigate and change the exclusionary and repressive effects of white academic institutions, policies, and health and human services delivery systems. It is a call for a larger praxis of social change and transformation of the very conditions that promote such a state of affairs."

Rosa M. Gil, DSW, *President & CEO, Comunilife Inc.*

"Drs. Chang and Bryant have given us a brilliant book that provides a rare opportunity to learn from some of the most influential scholars of our time. The authors merge rigorous research and their lived experiences to give us a timely view of multiculturalism in action. A truly joyful read!"

Gayle Skawen:nio Morse, PhD, *Professor and Licensed Psychologist and editor,* Applying Multiculturalism: An Ecological Approach to the APA Guidelines and Understanding Indigenous Perspectives: Visions, Dreams, and Hallucinations

"*Transforming Careers in Mental Health for BIPOC* is an inspiring and infuriating book. Inspiring, as a wide-ranging number of highly successful BIPOC leaders and academics tell their stories of struggle, perseverance, and triumph with humbling insight and hard-earned wisdom that so many others can learn from. And, yes, infuriating because after 40 years of various calls for more diversity, equity, and inclusion, the underlying systems of oppression and marginalization in higher education and human services remain almost unchanged. Anyone who thinks otherwise needs to read this book. Maybe twice."

Steve Burghardt, MSW, PhD, *Professor of Social Work, Silberman School of Social Work – Hunter College, CUNY*

"Dr. Doris F. Chang and Dr. Linda Lausell Bryant have gathered a distinguished group of BIPOC scholars to provide advice and their personal experiences on how to navigate, resist, and transform mental health systems, policies, and organizations. This book gives strategies for transformational change and healing at a systems level."

Debra M. Kawahara, PhD, *Associate Dean of Academic Affairs and Distinguished Professor, California School of Professional Psychology, Editor-in-Chief of Women & Therapy and Executive Director of the Illumination of Mindfulness Institute*

"*Transforming Careers in Mental Health for BIPOC* offers revolutionary insights from leading BIPOC clinicians, administrators, and educators on how to transform mental health practice, policy, and education as well as the academy itself, demonstrating how we can all build careers that are fulfilling and liberating. With heartfelt reflections from innovators who have learned through their own courageous and often painful experiences, this is a veritable guidebook for generations of BIPOC scholars to come and an inspiring resource for creating justice in healing and education."

Kamilah Majied, PhD, LCSW, *author of* Joyfully Just: Black Wisdom and Buddhist Insights for Liberated Living; *Professor, mental health therapist, contemplative inclusivity and equity consultant*

"The clinical expertise and organizational and lived experiences of the BIPOC authors described in this unique text represents an undeniable opportunity to advance the delivery of behavioral health services in the United States."

Vincent Guilamo-Ramos, PhD, MPH, LCSW, PMHNP-BC,
Director of the Institute for Policy Solutions, Johns Hopkins School of Nursing

Transforming Careers in Mental Health for BIPOC

This book provides targeted advice to Black, Indigenous, and People of Color (BIPOC) in the mental health professions on how to navigate, resist, and transform institutions and policies that were not designed for them.

A diverse team of BIPOC leaders reveal their experiences of race-related stress and how they draw on cultural strengths and anti-oppressive frameworks to create more inclusive, equitable, and culturally affirming approaches to mental health training, research, and practice. This book illustrates how it is possible for BIPOC students and professionals to have a career that is more sustainable, allows authenticity to emerge, and sparks transformative change in clients, students, organizations, and society. It addresses the unique professional development needs of BIPOC individuals across different career stages and professional roles. Covering topics such as how to respond to microaggressions from patients, become a media contributor, or step into organizational leadership, each core chapter includes a discussion of the pertinent literature, culturally grounded theories, personal reflections, and actionable strategies for community healing and social change.

This essential guide will inspire trainees, practitioners, educators, and administrators in the fields of social work, psychology, counseling, psychiatry, education, and public health, to envision a path toward a more culturally affirming and transformative career.

Doris F. Chang, PhD is a licensed clinical psychologist, Associate Professor at New York University Silver School of Social Work, USA, and Co-Founder/Chief Clinical Officer at Unmute, a BIPOC-centered mental health start-up.

Linda Lausell Bryant, PhD, MSW is a social worker, Clinical Professor and Associate Dean for Academic Affairs at New York University Silver School of Social Work, USA.

Transforming Careers in Mental Health for BIPOC

Strategies to Promote Healing and Social Change

EDITED BY DORIS F. CHANG AND LINDA LAUSELL BRYANT

Routledge
Taylor & Francis Group
NEW YORK AND LONDON

ISBN: 978-1-032-31445-7 (hbk)
ISBN: 978-1-032-31446-4 (pbk)
ISBN: 978-1-003-30979-6 (ebk)

DOI: 10.4324/9781003309796

Typeset in Dante and Avenir
by Apex CoVantage, LLC

For my family: Jon, Eli, and Reed, who remind me to be grateful for today; and for my students, who give me hope for tomorrow (DFC).

For Marshall and Jasmine Yesenia, who hold me up with their love (LLB).

Contents

List of Contributors

Hector Y. Adames is a neuropsychologist and full Professor at The Chicago School, College of Professional Psychology, USA. He is the co-founder of the IC-RACE Lab (Immigration, Critical Race, and Cultural Equity Lab) and has co-authored several books, including *Speaking the Unspoken*; *Succeeding as a Therapist*; *Cultural Foundations and Interventions in Latinx Mental Health*; and *Decolonial Psychology*.

Briana Bivens is a postdoctoral research associate at Rutgers, The State University of New Jersey, USA. Informed by her background in educational theory and multi-issue community organizing, Briana's interdisciplinary scholarship explores community-based education, child and family care policy, and care and sustainability in transformative, justice-oriented social movements.

Linda Lausell Bryant is Associate Dean for Academic Affairs and Clinical Professor at New York University's Silver School of Social Work, USA. She directs the Adaptive Leadership in Human Services Institute at Silver and her work is informed by three decades of senior management experience in child, youth, and family agencies.

Doris F. Chang is a practicing clinical psychologist and Associate Professor at New York University's Silver School of Social Work, USA. Her research on Asian Americans and other BIPOC examines how sociocultural and structural factors impact psychological health and interrracial dynamics, and seeks to develop culturally affirming interventions that integrate mindfulness and other contemplative traditions.

Nayeli Y. Chavez-Dueñas is a full Professor at The Chicago School, College of Professional Psychology, USA, where she coordinates the graduate concentration in Latinx Mental Health. She is co-founder of the IC-RACE Lab (Immigration, Critical Race, and Cultural Equity Lab) and has authored several books and therapeutic approaches, including HEART (Healing Ethno and Racial Trauma).

Terrance Coffie is a social worker and adjunct faculty at the Silver School of Social Work, New York University, USA. As a formerly incarcerated person, he has committed himself to creating social and political change within the criminal justice system. He is founder and CEO of The Social Justice Network and host of the podcast, *It's Coffie Time.*

Kevin Cokley is the University Diversity and Social Transformation Professor, and Professor and Associate Chair of Diversity Initiatives in the Department of Psychology, University of Michigan, Ann Arbor, USA. He studies the psychosocial experiences of African American students and students of color, the impostor phenomenon, and its relationship to mental health and academic outcomes.

E. J. R. David is a full Professor in the Clinical-Community Psychology PhD Program at University of Alaska, Anchorage, USA. He also directs the Alaska Native Community Advancement in Psychology (ANCAP) Program, and co-chairs the Division on Filipino Americans (DoFA) of the Asian American Psychological Association.

Milo Dodson is a licensed counseling psychologist in California, USA and serves as Senior Manager for Diversity and Inclusion and Community Outreach for Belkin International, Inc. An advocate for service-based leadership, he has directed hip-hop artist Common's Dreamers and Believers Summer Youth Camp for nearly six years, and volunteers for organizations such as Colin Kaepernick's Know Your Rights Camp.

Ramani Durvasula is a licensed clinical psychologist, Professor Emerita of Psychology at California State University, Los Angeles, USA, and founder/CEO of LUNA Education, Training, and Consulting. She is also host of the podcast *Navigating Narcissism*, author of numerous books on narcissism and its impact on relationships, and creator of the popular YouTube channel, "Doctor Ramani."

Bryana French is an Associate Professor in the Graduate School of Professional Psychology at the University of St. Thomas, USA. Her work focuses on racial and sexual trauma and recovery among BIPOC adults, and has been recognized with awards from the American Psychological Association, the

National Multicultural Conference and Summit, and the Association of Black Psychologists.

Robyn L. Gobin is a licensed clinical psychologist and Associate Professor at the University of Illinois, Urbana-Champaign, USA. She is also a mindfulness and self-compassion teacher, trauma therapy trainer, self-care consultant, and author of *The Self-Care Prescription* among other books.

Joseph P. Gone is a clinical-community psychologist and Professor of Anthropology and of Global Health and Social Medicine at Harvard University, USA. He has collaborated with American Indian and other Indigenous communities for nearly 30 years to re-envision conventional mental health services for advancing Indigenous well-being. He is an enrolled member of the *Aaniiih*-Gros Ventre Tribal Nation of Montana.

Gordon Nagayama Hall is an Emeritus Professor at the University of Oregon, USA. He was President of the American Psychological Association Society for the Psychological Study of Ethnic Minority Issues and editor of *Cultural Diversity and Ethnic Minority Psychology*. He is developing Mind Boba, an NIMH-funded problem-solving therapy app for Asian Americans (https://trifoia.com/mindboba/).

Kenneth V. Hardy is the President of the Eikenberg Academy for Social Justice and Director of the Eikenberg Institute for Relationships. He is also Professor of Family Therapy at Drexel University in Philadelphia, Pennsylvania, USA. He is a frequent workshop presenter, trainer, and consultant on the topics of cultural and racial diversity, trauma, and oppression.

Ran Hu is an Assistant Professor at The Ohio State University, College of Social Work, USA. Informed by her transnational work with (im)migrant women in the sex industry, Ran's scholarship explores and addresses intersecting social-structural and epistemic inequities that contribute to violence against sex workers, human trafficking, and gender-based violence.

Larke Nahme Huang is a licensed clinical-community psychologist, Senior Advisor in the Office of the Assistant Secretary for Mental Health and Substance Use, and Director of the Office of Behavioral Health Equity at the Substance Abuse and Mental Health Services Administration in the Department of Health and Human Services, USA.

Karen Jackson-Weaver has been an academic leader in global higher education for over two decades. Prior to her current Vice Presidency at New York University, USA, she was a Dean-in-Residence and Visiting Scholar at the Blavatnik School of Government at Oxford University, and a former Academic Dean at Princeton and Harvard Universities.

Kirk "Jae" James is Clinical Assistant Professor and Director of the DSW program at NYU Silver School of Social Work, USA. He is Chair of the Diversity, Race, Oppression, and Privilege (DROP) curriculum area and is on the editorial board of *Abolitionist Perspectives in Social Work*. Jae has authored numerous academic articles and book chapters on mass incarceration, abolition praxis, and liberatory pedagogy.

Linda P. Juang is a Professor of Inclusive Education at the University of Potsdam, Germany. Her research focuses on what families and schools can do to provide nurturing environments that allow young people to be affirmed, valued, and supported for who they are.

Sophia Williams Kapten is a practicing licensed clinical psychologist at Therapists of New York, USA. She has held clinical training positions at Mount Sinai, Beth Israel, New York Presbyterian, Columbia University Irving Medical Center, Montefiore Medical Center, The New School's Counseling Center, and Kings County Hospital.

Maryam Kia-Keating is a licensed clinical psychologist and Professor at the University of California, Santa Barbara, USA, where she directs the Trauma & Adversity, Resilience & Prevention (TARP) research lab. She is also a children's media consultant, co-creator of the HEROES family resilience program, and the founder of Reach and Shine.

Grace S. Kim is a Clinical Associate Professor and Chair of the Counseling Psychology and Applied Human Development department at Boston University, USA. Her research focuses on social justice education and Asian American Psychology. She explores effectively teaching diversity and social justice, and wellness for Asian Americans, centering their struggles for liberation, social agency, and solidarity with other marginalized groups.

Eunjung Lee is a Professor and Endowed Chair in Mental Health & Health at the Factor-Inwentash Faculty of Social Work at the University of Toronto, Canada. Using critical theories in language, discourse and power, her research focuses on everyday interactions and power dynamics in cross-cultural psychotherapy.

Jioni A. Lewis is an Associate Professor and Co-Training Director of the Counseling Psychology Doctoral Program at the University of Maryland, College Park, USA. She is a leading expert on gendered racism, radical healing, and Black women's health. She is a Fellow of the American Psychological Association and is an award-winning researcher, teacher, and social justice advocate.

Sandra Mattar is a Clinical Associate Professor at the Boston University School of Medicine, USA. She is Director of Training at the Immigrant and Refugee Health Center at Boston Medical Center. Her clinical and research interests focus on psychological trauma; immigrant and refugee mental health; multicultural and international psychology; and mindfulness and spirituality.

Amanda Mays is a practicing clinical social worker and a Founding Partner at MCM Collaborative, a group psychotherapy practice in New York City that centers BIPOC and LGBTQIA+ communities. She has taught at NYU's Silver School of Social Work. Her work integrates anti-oppressive principles to elevate affirmative identity and community formation.

Iris Yi Miao is a postdoctoral fellow in clinical neuropsychology at the Medical College of Wisconsin. She has held numerous leadership positions including at the Asian Neuropsychological Association. Her clinical and research interests span multicultural neuropsychological assessment, various neuropsychological syndromes, and cognitive rehabilitation.

Helen Neville is a counseling psychology researcher and Professor of Educational Psychology and African American Studies at the University of Illinois at Urbana-Champaign, USA. She has held numerous national leadership positions and her research on race, racism, and healing among Black Americans and other People of Color has been published widely.

Jeannette Pai-Espinosa, President of Justice and Joy National Collaborative, has led the 140-year-old organization through its reinvention process since 2007. Today, it is an intergenerational gender and racial justice advocacy and organizing non-profit. Prior experience includes partnership in a social change agency and leadership roles in human/civil rights and higher education.

Brean'a Parker is an Assistant Professor in the Counseling and Counselor Education program at North Carolina State University. Brean'a's research interests include examining narratives of interpersonal violence within Black and marginalized communities, cultural healing praxis toward wellness for survivors of violence and trauma and social justice embodiment for counseling students within counselor education programs.

Jeffrey Proulx is Assistant Professor of Behavioral and Social Sciences (Research) and Assistant Professor of Psychiatry and Human Behavior (Research) at Brown University. Bridging Native American and African-American traditional contemplative and healing practices and mainstream mindfulness practices, his research examines how mindfulness affects resilience and well-being across a person's developmental trajectory.

Anneliese Singh (she / they) serves as Chief Diversity Officer / Associate Provost for Diversity and Faculty Development and is a Professor in the schools of social work and psychology at Tulane University. Anneliese's research and community organizing explores racial healing, justice and liberation, South Asian counseling, trans and nonbinary communities, and EDI (equity, diversity, and inclusion) and antiracism initiatives in various settings.

Lisa B. Spanierman is Professor of counseling and counseling psychology and Associate Dean of Academic Personnel at Arizona State University, USA. Her research focuses on white racial attitudes and racial microaggressions. She has published more than 80 articles and book chapters and is a Fellow of the American Psychological Association.

Derek H. Suite is a board-certified psychiatrist, founder of Full Circle Health, and Associate Adjunct Professor at Teachers College, Columbia University, USA. He is the consulting team psychiatrist to the New York Knicks, New York Rangers, and New York Jets and consults for Major League Soccer on restorative practices and cultural sensitivity.

Karen L. Suyemoto is Professor of Clinical Psychology and Asian American Studies at the University of Massachusetts, Boston. Her teaching, research, and consultations focus on processes of racism and resistance against oppression for People of Color and white people, and organizational change to promote anti-racism and social justice in the academy and psychological practice.

Tolulola Taiwo-Hanna is a research coordinator, course instructor, and a PhD student at the University of Toronto, Canada. Some of Tolu's research interests include social work practice with diverse populations, trauma and mental health, racism and racial microaggressions in human service organizations, organizational development, and social work leadership.

Nari Yoo is a PhD candidate at New York University, Silver School of Social Work, USA. Her research focuses on the mental health, behavioral health, and well-being of racial / ethnic minorities and immigrants in both the United States and Asian contexts.

Xiang Zhou is a licensed psychologist and Assistant Professor of Counseling Psychology at Purdue University, USA. His research interests include health disparity, parenting and family systems approach, as well as culturally adapted counseling interventions, particularly among Asian and Asian American diaspora communities.

Acknowledgements

We would like to thank our students, past and present, for being our teachers and co-learners, and for reminding us of why this work is so important. We are grateful for colleagues at the NYU Silver School of Social Work for valuing us and our mission. To our chapter contributors, we invited you to contribute to this project because of your achievements and impact on the field and for the love ethic that infuses your work. We thank each of you for sharing your full humanity and wisdom with us, and for continuing to inspire us with your words and actions. We extend a special thanks to Lisa Spanierman for your contribution to our chapter for white racial justice allies, and your friendship and support for this project.

I, Doris, thank my partner Jon and our two incredible boys for their unwavering patience and support during the many late nights and weekends spent working on this book. Eli and Reed, I am so proud to be your mother. I hope that this book contributes toward building a more just and equitable world for you to live in. I also thank my parents Ben and Helen Chang, for your sacrifices and support, and for encouraging me to pursue my dreams, even when they take me far from home. My siblings Diana and Danny and my extended family have been a stable source of love, advice, and care, vacations and cultural rituals (Thanksgivingkah, anyone?). I feel so lucky to have you all in my life.

I am deeply grateful to my community of BIPOC colleagues and collaborators, friends and white allies for validating my experiences and for helping me to feel less alone in the struggle. Special thanks to the BIPOC-centered spaces that have been a professional refuge for me at various times

xxiixxii   Acknowledgements

in my lifein my life, including the American Psychological Association Society for the Psychological Study of Culture, Ethnicity, and Race, and the Asian American Psychological Association. My OG mentors Stanley Sue, David T. Takeuchi, Byron and Mary-Jo DelVecchio Good, and Roberto Lewis-Fernandez set the bar super high while remaining so down to earth, in the best possible way. I am especially grateful to Fabienne Doucet, Karen Suyemoto, Lisa Rubin, Sumie Okazaki and the rest of our Kimchi Slappers group chat, Lisa Savage, Jeffrey Povero, Claudia Ghigliotty, and Millie Benson for being there for me over the years. You have made me laugh when all I wanted to do is cry, inspired me with your brilliance, and made me feel like everything was going to be okay. I could not have done this without you all.

I, Linda, give thanks and to my ancestors beginning with my grandparents, Candita and Gilberto Rosado, who came from Puerto Rico as young adults with barely a dollar in their pockets but a fistful of dreams. I honor my parents, Damian and Josephine Lausell. Dad, you were a scholar, even though you only had an 8th grade education, and Mom, you were a striver who always believed in me. *Yo soy la realización de tus sueños. Tus sacrificios no fueron en vano.* Thank you to my brother Dae, for your unconditional love.

I give so much thanks and love to my husband, Marshall and our children, all of whom are committed to the pursuit of justice and equity. Marshall, we are blessed with this beautiful, blended family: Jasmine Yesenia, Sara, Little Alice, Antoine, Dyami, Gabriel and Gideon, as well as our daughters-in-love Zawadi, Kim, and Dee Dee, and our grandchildren, Dakari, Zaire, Alex, and Nova. Jasmine Yesenia, thank you for your understanding during the many hours of working on this book.

Thanks to Steve Burghardt and Pat Beresford for their staunch support and my tribe of lifetime sister-friends, Lynne, Marcy, Lakshmi, Bernie, Candi, Darcel, Deidre, Arlene, Susan, and Bonita. Your love and support keep me together. Thank you MaryAnne, for your support and for delighting in me.

Thank you to every fellow BIPOC changemaker. Let us raise the bar for us and future generations. Survival is a means, not an end. Let us be the change as whole, healthy, united people. Together we can roll the proverbial rock up the hill, even demolish it, or flatten the hill. Ain't no stopping us!

Finally, we thank Sarah Rae and the team at Routledge/Taylor and Francis for championing this book and for your editorial support. We also thank Eugenia Puglisi for your administrative help.

This book is dedicated to those trailblazers on whose shoulders we stand and to all prior, current, and future mental health professionals working for healing, liberation, and justice.

Introduction

Doris F. Chang and Linda Lausell Bryant

Like a flower in the mud, the idea for this book blossomed in 2020, during a moment of crisis. As two women of color in the mental health field – an Asian American clinical psychologist and an Afro-Latina social worker, both faculty colleagues in a school of social work – we were overwhelmed and grieving, fearful and furious about the racial injustices and collective traumas of the COVID-19 pandemic. As US-based scholars and practitioners focused on mitigating the effects of racism and other forms of oppression, we recognized the resulting surge in white supremacy, anti-Blackness, anti-Asian[1] hate and xenophobia as a historical pattern. Yet, we still were not prepared for the devastation to our communities, nor for the ways we would be called into service.

In the Global North, minoritized people of the Global Majority – including Black, Indigenous, Asian, Pacific Islanders, Middle Eastern, North African, and Latine individuals in the United States – were becoming infected with the virus and dying at a disproportionate rate (Mude et al., 2021; Rubin-Miller et al., 2020). Racial inequities in employment, housing, and healthcare drove racial disparities in COVID-19 exposure, treatment, and mortality rates

---

1 Throughout this book, we capitalize racial categories for groups from the Global Majority (e.g., Black, Asian, Indigenous, and so on) given their shared history and culture. However, departing from APA Style 7 but following recent shifts in media conventions (e.g., 2020 Associated Press Stylebook), we do not capitalize white. This also reflects our efforts to decenter whiteness in our discussion of mental health training, education, and practices.

DOI: 10.4324/9781003309796-1

(Yearby & Mohapatra, 2020), reproducing the structural violence of pre-pandemic society on a larger scale. On one end of the societal continuum were the most privileged, who leveraged their connections and resources to access lifesaving vaccines, treatments, and country houses for remote work, significantly reducing their risks of exposure and death. At the other end of the continuum, a disproportionate number of Black, Indigenous, and People of Color (BIPOC) were trapped in crowded living conditions and unsafe neighborhoods, unemployed or working "essential" jobs that put them in harm's way, with limited access to adequate dependent care and medical services (Dickinson et al., 2021; Robertson & Gebeloff, 2020). As two BIPOC mental health professionals and faculty members, we fell somewhere in the middle. And against the backdrop of this evolving health crisis, our communities faced rising anti-Asian and anti-immigrant prejudice, police killings of unarmed Black Americans, and discrimination on our streets, online, and in the workplace, increasing our stress burden as well as our workload (Chae et al., 2021; Hswen et al., 2021; Li & Lartey, 2023).

In the months that followed – as we toggled between spaces of advantage and vulnerability – we found ourselves moved, and increasingly asked, to use our mental health training and expertise to respond to the crisis. Like so many other BIPOC in the mental health professions, we marched in the streets, gave media interviews, created public education campaigns, facilitated healing circles, conducted antiracism trainings, and wrote grants to study the effects of the pandemic on BIPOC communities, all on top of our regular job duties, remote teaching, and increased personal caregiving responsibilities (Cho et al., 2022; Mogro-Wilson et al., 2022). We were answering the call . . . and paying the price (Hermann & Neale-McFall, 2020).

Our personal experiences were supported by studies documenting how the COVID-19 pandemic intensified pre-existing racial and gendered disparities in academia. Black, Indigenous, and Women of Color (BIWOC) faculty were expected to provide emotional labor, as caretakers and counselors, roles that were not expected of male faculty and neither financially compensated nor valued in the tenure and promotion system (Cho et al., 2022; Mitchell & Hesli, 2013). Drawing on Anzaldua's borderlands framework, Cho et al. (2022) used *testimonio* and *plática* methodologies to explore how the pandemic encroached on boundaries between the BIWOC authors' professional and individual intersectional identities, extending institutional and structural violence into the sacred space of the home. A common theme was "how these notions of care, commitment, and responsibility were weaponized against us to elicit additional work and labor from us" (p. 734), resulting in feelings of guilt, exhaustion, and burnout. Not surprisingly, Black female academics and mothers (regardless of race) experienced greater declines in productivity compared to white male academics during the pandemic years (Staniscuaski et al., 2021). These conditions have set the stage to potentially widen the pre-pandemic racial and gendered disparities in teaching and service, funding awards, and rates of promotion and tenure in academia (Chaudhary et al., 2020; Chen et al., 2022; Lin & Kennette, 2022; Wood et al., n.d.).

Growing political, legal, and cultural challenges to diversity, equity, and inclusion (DEI) have further increased the vulnerability of BIPOC engaged in mental health research, teaching, and practice. In 2020, following the summer of what became a global Movement for Black Lives, former President Donald Trump issued Executive Order 13950, which sought to prohibit federal agencies and contractors from teaching so-called "divisive concepts" such as white privilege, systematic racism, and critical race theory (CRT). Although President Biden reversed EO 13950 and instituted a new order that required all federal agencies to prioritize and create opportunities for historically underserved communities, more than 777 anti-CRT efforts have been introduced at the local, state, and federal levels (UCLA School of Law, Critical Race Studies Program, n.d.). As of November 2023, anti-CRT measures have been adopted in 41 states, affecting the public institutions where BIPOC scholars, students, and clinicians teach, train, and work. Furthermore, the US Supreme Court, dominated by a conservative majority as of 2022, has already issued a number of decisions – including overturning both affirmative action in college admissions and women's rights to an abortion – that have disrupted decades of progress toward a more racially just and equitable society.

Confronting these challenges to our cherished values and facing an uncertain future, we felt an urge to seek refuge in community, to connect with historical reminders of our brilliance and resistance, to give ourselves permission to rest, and to reaffirm our roles as agents of change. The idea for this book was born.

Gathering Our Strength, Planting Seeds for Transformation

As the pandemic and the racial reckoning of 2020–2021 (and subsequent backlash) reminded us, mental health professionals are uniquely positioned to address social suffering. We are trained to foster insight and healing in classrooms and therapy offices, provide social services to those caught in oppressive systems, and develop theory, interventions, and policy to address a range of social ills. BIPOC social workers, psychologists, counselors, and psychiatrists also have particular insights into the systemic barriers to health and well-being faced by BIPOC communities, as well as the systemic changes that are needed. And yet, because BIPOC mental health professionals are themselves vulnerable to the racism and white supremacy that pervade their disciplines, their cultural insights and ways of knowing are often devalued or appropriated by others. It is not enough to just show up for our clients and our students. As Buchanan et al. (2021) note, "Changing systemic racism requires multi-systemic change" (p. 1097).

Although social justice-oriented research and practice approaches predate the pandemic (e.g., Ferguson, 2007; Metzl & Hansen, 2014), increased media attention on the brutalizing effects of anti-Black racism and structural oppression has led to urgent calls for antiracist, decolonizing, and anti-oppressive approaches to mental health research, training, and practice. Since 2021, numerous models and guidelines for transforming the mental health disciplines have appeared in the flagship journals of psychology (Buchanan et al., 2021; Neville et al., 2021), social work (Friedline et al., 2023; Goings et al., 2023), and psychiatry (Cénat, 2020; Shim, 2021). For example, the Public Psychology for Liberation (PPL) training model seeks to "directly address the anti-Blackness, racial oppression, and myth of [w]hite supremacy that are embedded in society, often fed by psychological theories and research, and built uncritically, into our training and discipline" (Neville et al., 2021, p. 1249). Friedline et al. (2023) critique the social work profession's "limited commitments to advancing antiracism and dismantling white supremacy" (p. 89) despite an ethics code that compels social workers to end discrimination and societal injustice. They outline action steps in the domains of Research and Knowledge Development, Education and Teaching, and Service. These action steps are distinguished by their broad reach and structural focus (e.g., "Support future BIPOC scholars by disrupting structural barriers that result in educational disparities starting in elementary school," p. 90), including recommendations for changing the reward system in higher education. In psychiatry, Cénat (2020) outlined guidelines for an antiracist care and treatment plan organized around four main axes: an awareness of racial issues, an assessment adapted to the real needs of Black individuals, a humanistic approach to medication, and a treatment approach that addresses the real needs and issues related to the racism experienced by Black individuals.

In general, these antiracist approaches to training, research, and practice share a number of features including:

- An emphasis on the institutionalized nature of racism and the need for multi-systems approaches to structural transformation;
- A focus on "centering the margins," that is denaturalizing whiteness as the default frame of reference, and honoring the wisdom, experiences, and perspectives of BIPOC, especially those most harmed by structural violence (i.e., epistemic justice);
- An intersectional perspective that recognizes that individuals can be multiply marginalized and shaped by interlocking structures of oppression related to race, ethnicity, gender, sexual orientation, etc.;
- A move away from individual-level factors and outcomes to focus on collective empowerment and healing; and
- Community-based partnerships to develop anti-oppressive programs, interventions, research that reflects the priority concerns of impacted communities.

While these antiracist frameworks provide a blueprint for much-needed structural reform in the mental health field, there are a number of challenges to implementation. For starters, racial trauma and internalized oppression can make it hard for BIPOC in the mental health professions to see the ways in which we may have assimilated to white supremacist ideology, which includes "learning, knowing, and being taught one's social, cultural, political, and racial positioning, or 'place' in dominant White space" (Settles et al., 2019, as cited in Liu et al., 2019, p. 144). Especially for BIPOC situated in predominantly white institutions, exposure to racism at multiple levels – interpersonal, institutional, structural – can feel like being caught in a poisonous web that they cannot escape. And yet there are countless examples of BIPOC who are radically challenging the systems they are in, strategically and persistently carving out alternative career paths that honor their values and collective commitments, and transforming society and institutions for the better. Drawing on Indigenous African and Latine cultural practices that center storytelling as a tool for meaning-making, resilience, and healing (Cervantes, 2020; Chioneso et al., 2020), the current volume narrativizes the courage, costs, and collective efforts behind a transformative career in mental health for BIPOC.

Our Goals and Hopes

In assembling this collection, our goal was to nurture and inspire BIPOC students and professionals in social work, psychology, counseling, and psychiatry (and their white allies) to envision a justice-oriented career path that prioritizes healing and liberation for themselves and their communities. Our hope was that we could create a "counterspace" outside of our mainstream institutions for communion and co-mentoring, a space for healing and restoration for all of us who feel traumatized, invisible, or alone in the struggle (Solorzano et al., 2000).

Toward that end, we gathered a group of leading BIPOC mental health scholars, practitioners, activists, and changemakers to reflect and to share their experiences and wisdom about how to build a meaningful and transformative career. Through their first-person accounts of oppression, awakening, healing, and protest, they show us how we can navigate oppressive institutional practices, reclaim our power, and create pockets of resistance, community, and joy. Because culture and context matters, the authors situate their learnings and advice in relation to their specific positionalities, settings, and roles. They are clinicians and researchers, DEI consultants and activists, media contributors and journal editors, department chairs and university administrators, policymakers and CEOs. Behind their impressive titles and long list of achievements, they recount the messy, relational, and political aspects of the work, the fortitude required to navigate anti-Black racism and other forms of oppression on the job, the inner work of decolonizing the mind, and the cultural strengths and values that sustain them.

How to Read This Book

The book is organized around the choice points and action steps involved in developing a culturally affirming and transformative career in mental health. Part I (Finding and Owning Your Voice) examines the process of shedding internalized narratives of inferiority and non-belonging, and owning your authentic voice. Part II (Taking a Leap) delves into career decision points where we choose or create a path or combination of paths (e.g., academia, clinical practice, training and consulting, organizational leadership), and redefine the boundaries to better reflect our values and commitments. In Part III (Leading for Change and Impact), we explore strategies for transitioning to positions of leadership and influence, and leveraging one's power across diverse institutions including the media, higher education, clinical settings, government, and the non-profit sector. We close with a final summary section (Part IV) reviewing key themes of the book, with final reflections and advice for BIPOC and for white racial justice allies.

Although this book is organized according to a general developmental career sequence with chapters clustered by professional practice arena, we invite you to start wherever you would like. Explore the topics and stories that speak to your heart. Share the lessons and recommendations with your friends, colleagues, and mentors and brainstorm how to implement them at an institutional level. Envision a career path tailored to your unique voice, talents, and values. Dream big and change the world.

References

Associated Press (2020). *The Associated Press Stylebook*. Basic Books.

Buchanan, N. T., Perez, M., Prinstein, M. J., & Thurston, I. B. (2021). Upending racism in psychological science: Strategies to change how science is conducted, reported, reviewed, and disseminated. *The American Psychologist, 76*(7), 1097–1112. doi:10.1037/amp0000905

Cénat, J. M. (2020). How to provide anti-racist mental health care. *The Lancet. Psychiatry, 7*(11), 929–931. https://doi.org/10.1016/S2215-0366(20)30309-6

Cervantes, A. (2020). *Testimonios*. In L. Comas-Díaz & E. Torres Rivera (Eds.), *Liberation psychology: Theory, method, practice, and social justice*. American Psychological Association. https://doi.org/10.1037/0000198-008

Chae, D. H., Yip, T., Martz, C. D., Chung, K., Richeson, J. A., Hajat, A., Curtis, D. S., Rogers, L. O., & LaVeist, T. A. (2021). Vicarious racism and vigilance during the COVID-19 pandemic: Mental health implications among Asian and Black Americans. *Public Health Reports, 136*(4), 508–517. doi:10.1177/00333549211018675

Chaudhary, A. M. D., Naveed, S., Siddiqi, J., Mahmood, A., & Khosa, F. (2020). US Psychiatry faculty: Academic rank, gender and racial profile. *Academic Psychiatry, 44*(3), 260–266.

Chen, C. Y., Kahanamoku, S. S., Tripati, A., Alegado, R. A., Morris, V. R., Andrade, K., & Hosbey, J. (2022). Systemic racial disparities in funding rates at the National Science Foundation. *eLife, 11*. https://doi.org/10.7554/eLife.83071

Chioneso, N. A., Hunter, C. D., Gobin, R. L., McNeil Smith, S., Mendenhall, R., & Neville, H. A. (2020). Community healing and resistance through storytelling: A framework to address racial trauma in Africana communities. *The Journal of Black Psychology, 46*(2–3), 95–121. https://doi.org/10.1177/0095798420929468

Cho, K. S., Banda, R. M., Fernández, É., & Aronson, B. (2022). Testimonios de las atravesadas: A borderland existence of women of color faculty. *Gender, Work, and Organization*. https://doi.org/10.1111/gwao.12894

Dickinson, K. L., Roberts, J. D., Banacos, N., Neuberger, L., Koebele, E., Blanch-Hartigan, D., & Shanahan, E. A. (2021). Structural racism and the COVID-19 experience in the United States. *Health Security, 19*(S1), S14–S26. doi:10.1089/hs.2021.0031

Ferguson, I. (2007). *Reclaiming social work: Challenging neo-liberalism and promoting social justice*. SAGE.

Friedline, T., Cross, F., Doyle, K., Lacombe-Duncan, A., & Schultz, K. (2023). Dismantling white supremacy and promoting antiracism in social work: Tensions, paradoxes, and a collective response. *Journal of the Society for Social Work and Research*, 14(1), 87–99. https://doi.org/10.1086/721800

Goings, T. C., Belgrave, F. Z., Mosavel, M., & Evans, C. B. R. (2023). An antiracist research framework: Principles, challenges, and recommendations for dismantling racism through research. *Journal of the Society for Social Work and Research*, 14(1), 101–128. https://doi.org/10.1086/720983

Hermann, M. A., & Neale-McFall, C. (2020). COVID-19, academic mothers, and opportunities for the academy. *Academe*, 106(4), 37–39.

Hswen, Y., Xu, X., Hing, A., Hawkins, J. B., Brownstein, J. S., & Gee, G. C. (2021). Association of "#covid19" versus "#chinesevirus" with Anti-Asian sentiments on Twitter: March 9–23, 2020. *American Journal of Public Health*, 111(5), 956–964. https://doi.org/10.2105/AJPH.2021.306154

Li, W., & Lartey, J. (2023). *New FBI data shows more hate crimes: These groups saw the sharpest rise*. The Marshall Project, March 25. www.themarshallproject.org/2023/03/25/asian-hate-crime-fbi-black-lgbtq

Lin, P. S., & Kennette, L. N. (2022). Creating an inclusive community for BIPOC faculty: Women of color in academia. *SN Social Sciences*, 2(11), 246. https://doi.org/10.1007/s43545-022-00555-w

Liu, W. M., Liu, R. Z., Garrison, Y. L., Kim, J. Y. C., Chan, L., Ho, Y. C. S., & Yeung, C. W. (2019). Racial trauma, microaggressions, and becoming racially innocuous: The role of acculturation and white supremacist ideology. *The American Psychologist*, 74(1), 143–155. https://doi.org/10.1037/amp0000368

Metzl, J. M., & Hansen, H. (2014). Structural competency: Theorizing a new medical engagement with stigma and inequality. *Social Science & Medicine*, 103, 126–133. doi:10.1016/j.socscimed.2013.06.032

Mitchell, S. M., & Hesli, V. L. (2013). Women don't ask? Women don't say no? Bargaining and service in the political science profession. *PS, Political Science & Politics*, 46(2). doi:10.1017/S1049096513000073355–369.

Mogro-Wilson, C., Negi, N., Acquati, C., Bright, C., Chang, D. F., Goings, T. C., Greenfield, J. C., Gurrola, M., Hicks, T., Loomis, A., Parekh, R., Strolin-Goltzman, J., Valdovinos, M. G., Walton, Q. L., & Windsor, L. (2022). Reflections from academic mothers of young children on social work research and education. *Journal of Social Work Education*, 58(1), 9–33. https://doi.org/10.1080/10437797.2021.2014726

Mude, W., Oguoma, V. M., Nyanhanda, T., Mwanri, L., & Njue, C. (2021). Racial disparities in COVID-19 pandemic cases, hospitalisations, and deaths: A systematic review and meta-analysis. *Journal of Global Health*, 11, 05015. doi:10.7189/jogh.11.05015.

Neville, H. A., Ruedas-Gracia, N., Lee, B. A., Ogunfemi, N., Maghsoodi, A. H., Mosley, D. V., LaFromboise, T. D., & Fine, M. (2021). The public psychology for liberation training model: A call to transform the discipline. *The American Psychologist*, 76(8), 1248–1265. doi:10.1037/amp0000887.

Robertson, C., & Gebeloff, R. (2020). How millions of women became the most essential workers in America. Sec US, *New York Times*, April 18. www.nytimes.com/2020/04/18/us/coronavirus-women-essential-workers.html

Rubin-Miller, L., Alban, C., Artiga, S., & Sullivan, S. (2020). COVID-19 racial disparities in testing, infection, hospitalization, and death: Analysis of epic patient data. *Kaiser Family Foundation*, 2020916. https://madison365.com/wp-content/uploads/2020/09/KFF-Epic-Analysis_COVID19-and-racial-disparities.pdf

Settles, I. H., Buchanan, N. T., & Dotson, K. (2019). Scrutinized but not recognized: (In)visibility and hypervisibility experiences of faculty of color. *Journal of Vocational Behavior, 113*, 62–74. http://dx.doi.org/10.1016/j.jvb.2018.06.003

Shim, R. S. (2021). Dismantling structural racism in psychiatry: A path to mental health equity. *The American Journal of Psychiatry, 178*(7), 592–598. doi:10.1176/appi.ajp.2021.21060558.

Solorzano, D., Ceja, M., & Yosso, T. (2000). Critical race theory, racial microaggressions, and campus racial climate: The experiences of African American college students. *The Journal of Negro Education, 69*(1/2), 60–73.

Staniscuaski, F., Kmetzsch, L., Soletti, R. C., Reichert, F., Zandonà, E., Ludwig, Z. M. C., et al. (2021). Gender, race and parenthood impact academic productivity during the COVID-19 pandemic: From survey to action. *Frontiers in Psychology, 12*, 663252. doi:10.3389/fpsyg.2021.663252.

UCLA School of Law, Critical Race Studies Program. (n.d.). *CRT Forward interactive map.* CRT Forward. https://crtforward.law.ucla.edu/map/

Wood, J. L., Hilton, A. A., & Nevarez, C. (n.d.). *Faculty of color and white faculty: An analysis of service in colleges of education in the Arizona public university system.* http://caarpweb.org/wp-content/uploads/2015/06/8-1_Wood_p85.pdf

Yearby, R., & Mohapatra, S. (2020). Law, structural racism, and the COVID-19 pandemic. *Journal of Law and the Biosciences, 7*(1), lsaa036. https://doi.org/10.1093/jlb/lsaa036

Finding and Owning Your Voice

Part I

The chapters in this section explore the process of identifying and grappling with internalized narratives of inferiority and non-belonging, and reclaiming your authentic voice. These processes often unfold during the early career phase, as BIPOC confront pressures to assimilate to white supremacist and colonial ideologies in educational and training settings.

In **Chapter 1**, Linda P. Juang, a Taiwanese American developmental psychologist living in Germany, discusses how ethnic-racialized identities can support us in navigating academic pathways that may not always affirm and value who we are. She shares how engaging readings and work from minoritized historians, writers, and scientists can further a strengths-based understanding of who we are in relation to the work we do and the careers we are building. In **Chapter 2**, Nari Yoo and Sophia Williams Kapten share advice for international and BIPOC students applying to graduate programs in social work and psychology, including tips for financing your education and coping with the isolation of being the first to study abroad or attend college. In **Chapter 3**, psychologists Iris Yi Miao and Xiang Zhou explore common challenges faced by international trainees in clinical psychology and related fields, including acculturative stress and restrictive immigration policies, and reflect on what they wish they had known as students. Among other lessons, they found that acquiring greater structural awareness of the systemic barriers they faced allowed them to externalize some of their burdens and empowered them to advocate for themselves. In **Chapter 4**, Hector Y. Adames and Nayeli Y. Chavez-Dueñas, a queer, Afro-Dominican

DOI: 10.4324/9781003309796-2

psychologist and a Mexican immigrant psychologist of Indigenous descent, use intersectionality theory to illustrate the connections between identity, systemic oppression, and resistance within the context of graduate school.

The next set of chapters introduces anti-oppressive frameworks for clinical training and research to inoculate trainees against the pain of internalized oppression and racial othering by grounding in cultural and communal strengths. In **Chapter 5**, Eunjung Lee, Ran Hu, and Tolulola Taiwo-Hanna use their own experiences as Asian immigrant and Black Canadian clinicians to discuss how they cope with racial microaggressions and corresponding racial enactments in their interactions with clients, colleagues, and agencies. In **Chapter 6**, E. J. R. David explores how colonial research and education have damaged the Filipino community and offers five tips to decolonize research and heal from the wounds of colonization. In **Chapter 7**, Kevin Cokley reflects on his experiences of the imposter phenomenon at various stages of his career in academia as a Black man and shares advice for the next generation of minoritized scholars. Jeffrey Proulx follows in **Chapter 8** with reflections on his early career journey as a researcher in the field of Indigenous wellness, and the importance of allyship, discipline, strategic planning, and long-term vision in shaping innovative research pathways to affect health equity in marginalized populations.

We close this section with an edited and condensed Community Conversation on the topic of Finding Your Voice with contributors Sophia Williams Kapten, E. J. R. David, Nayeli Y. Chavez-Dueñas, Hector Y. Adames, and Derek Suite (**Chapter 9**).

Ethnic-Racialized Identities as Strengths

1

Navigating Academic Pathways That Affirm and Value Who We Are

Linda P. Juang

Let me introduce myself. I am a second-generation Taiwanese American who grew up in Minnesota and who now lives in Berlin, Germany. I went to the University of Minnesota to study child development and then to Michigan State University in East Lansing to study developmental psychology. For much of my life, I have lived and worked in spaces that were mostly white. In snowy East Lansing I wrote a dissertation titled *Autonomy and Connectedness Among Asian American College Students* because, I admit, I wanted to better understand myself. From there, my work continued to focus on minoritized youth growing up in immigrant families. I wondered how youth made sense of themselves and their ethnic-racialized identities while living in inequitable societies. I started my research in the US and continue here in Germany, a context where there is still little attention to such issues from a psychological perspective. What I learned over the years from these experiences is that the research that helped me figure out who I am as a minoritized scholar could, at the same time, make a contribution to the field because it focused on a population that was often overlooked in studies of adolescence. This fits into the now well-documented phenomena that if you are an underrepresented minoritized scholar, you are more likely

DOI: 10.4324/9781003309796-3

to include underrepresented minoritized people in your scholarly work (Roberts et al., 2020).[1] You should know that if you engage in me-search, you will be expanding scientific knowledge in important ways, not least by contributing to a more representative knowledge base. You will strengthen the field, for the better.

Today, I am a Professor of Inclusive Education at the University of Potsdam. I am one of the few professors in Germany with a non-German citizenship[2] and one of the very few women of color.[3] This severe lack of representation is a problem because who we are contributes to how we engage in our work. Our lived experiences and backgrounds contribute to the research questions we study, populations we are interested in, who we include in our studies, how we interpret data, and theoretical frameworks that we engage with (Nzinga et al., 2018; Roberts et al., 2020; Syed et al., 2018). If only a narrow range of diversities are represented among researchers, our knowledge will be flattened and incomplete. In other words, our identities are central to the science or work that we do.[4] Therefore, in this chapter, I focus on three aspects of ethnic-racialized identity – content, contexts, and configurations – to reflect on how these aspects contribute to navigating an academic career that affirms and values who we are.

The Contours of Identity

Galliher et al.'s (2017) identity framework distinguishes between identity content, contexts, and configurations. Reflecting on these dimensions helps us think about how our ethnic-racialized identities contribute to our strengths

---

1 Roberts et al. (2020) analyzed over 26,000 empirical articles in cognitive, developmental, and social psychology and showed that white researchers are more likely to have white participants in their studies and less likely to have People of Color. Researchers of Color are more likely to have participants of Color in their studies and less likely to have white people. If the field is dominated by people racialized as white, this makes a difference for who is included (or excluded) in our science.

2 7.4% of professors in Germany are international (have a non-German citizenship) and the percent of international professors has increased by only 0.1% since 2011 (German Academic Exchange Service, 2023).

3 Because official data on ethnicity or racialized groupings are not gathered here ("race" is closely tied to its misuse and abuse during the Holocaust, resulting in a strong taboo on collecting such data, Juang et al., 2021), there are no clear numbers on what racialized groups are underrepresented, making it difficult to see where disparities lie.

4 Marsh and Furlong's (2002) aptly titled paper "A skin, not a sweater" argues how our ontological and epistemological positions are always present when doing our research.

and assets as we navigate the pathway to become mental health practitioners and scholars in our various communities.

Ethnic-racialized identity refers to the overlapping ethnic and racialized aspects of how individuals think and feel about being a member of their ethnic-racialized groups (Umaña-Taylor et al., 2014). From developmental and social identity perspectives, a strong ethnic-racialized identity provides a sense of belonging to a valued social community (Erikson, 1968; Tajfel & Turner, 1986). Aspects to consider are identity content (*what* defines our identities), identity contexts (within and through *which contexts* do our identities develop) and configurations (how our multiple identities *go together*). I describe each of these aspects and discuss how they can further our own understanding of who we are in relation to the work we do and the careers we are building.

Identity Content – Who Are You as a Minoritized Scholar?

A method to reveal the *what* in identity are studies taking a narrative approach. If I were to ask you to *think of a time in an academic setting when you were aware of your ethnicity*, what would you say? Who was there, what was happening, and how did you feel?[5] (Please take a few moments to think about how you would respond.) The narratives that we tell (and re-tell) to ourselves and to others reveal how ethnicity and racialized or minoritized experiences are reflected in our lives. Importantly, these narratives also reveal something beyond the self: they shed light on the broader sociocultural context or societal structures that both constrain and afford our identity development (Fish & Counts, 2020; McLean & Syed, 2015). In thinking of a time when you were aware of your ethnicity in academia, for instance, you get a sense of whether your various identities are valued by the broader society. Do some of your identities enjoy privileges? Or are the identities that are important to you marginalized? Which identities are you open about and which identities do you feel like you have to hide? If your story does not fit into the master narrative – a culturally shared script reflecting a norm for the way we are supposed to be – what alternative narratives do you create? And how do we create alternative narratives

---

5 This type of prompt has been used in several field-changing studies of ethnic-racialized identity, e.g., Syed and Azmitia (2010).

beyond what society tells us who we are (or were) and what we can or cannot be? To create alternative narratives, regardless of where we are living in the world, we must learn our histories.

I read Erika Lee's (2015) book *The Making of Asian America: A History* five years ago, when I was 47. It took me this long to have a more solid understanding of my shared history. Asians have been in the US far longer than many think they have (Filipinos have been in the US since the 1500s), they have fought in every major war since the 1800s,[6] and have participated alongside African American, Latinx, and other minoritized communities protesting war and imperialism, fighting for civil rights and fair labor.[7] We were there all along, we just have not been included in the telling and re-telling of our stories.

The longer that I live outside the US, the more I also identify with the Asian diaspora, finding points of connection with Asian-heritage individuals growing up in Germany and Europe. Understanding that Asian American and Asian European identities are also political identities (Maeda, 2009) connects me to those who are collectively racialized not just as "Asian," but also as "other," as "foreign," and as an immigrant. As we learn more and build on the histories that connect us to minoritized people in other times and places,[8] we clarify and strengthen our identities. Not being able to access our histories means denying the important contexts of our identities, limiting the ability to understand ourselves.

---

6 I had never seen photos of veterans of the US American Civil War or WWII who were Asian American until several years ago. This website *Belonging On and Off the Battlefield: Asian Americans in the US Military* has a good overview: www.loc.gov/ghe/cascade/index.html?appid=6301eee806184a9c885374869c325ba4&bookmark=Civil%20War

7 To learn of the ways that minoritized people have been systematically marginalized and excluded can be painful, so finding and connecting with people sharing similar experiences will be important to do.

8 The historian Olivette Otele's book *African Europeans: An Untold History* (2020) is another good example of the importance of history for identity. Otele documents how African people have been a part of Europe since antiquity, through trade and migration and also through colonization, slavery, and empire. Knowing about the presence of African Europeans is not enough. We need to also know their stories and contributions to art, science, music, and European society in general. This is important for who is seen as European. The myth that European = white is not true. Indeed, professional societies such as the American Psychological Association (APA) contribute to this racialized myth by offering guidelines that indicate that it is acceptable to use "European-American" or "white" interchangeably (APA, 2022). This myth erases a rich history of diverse peoples. It is so important to read the work of historians. It makes us rethink and interrogate

Identity Contexts – Are We in Spaces That Affirm or Undermine Our Identities?

We know what kind of contexts affirm identities. For young people, academic spaces and curricula that value and acknowledge diverse identities and emphasize equity, openness, and inclusion, promote a sense of belonging and create a context for youth to not just survive but thrive (Bañales et al., 2021; Celeste et al., 2019; Dee & Penner, 2016; Gay, 2013). As an early career scholar, do you have spaces that affirm your identities rather than undermine them? If you are "the only" in your department (e.g., the only Asian-heritage queer person) and feel isolated and not affirmed, you may need to look beyond your departments or other places of work to find safer spaces and communities. And, you may need to look for ways to try and shift the culture in your organizations to create that community for yourself. We need to find those safer spaces, find allies, and find people we trust.[9]

Relationships are important contexts for developing our identities. It is not new advice to say that establishing relationships with mentors is essential. Most of us have been advised to seek out mentors at different points in our career, to include those who are a few steps ahead of us, and those much further ahead. Both offer different types of support and insights at different stages. No one had told me to find a mentor for my non-academic life, but this is important too. Academia is a big part of my life but so are my family, my friends, and my relationships. Find people who are living the kind of life that you admire. For me, there are two people about a decade older than I am who I see as mentors. They have managed to raise children, have good relationships with their adult children, are doing interesting and important projects as well as living a life that centers, I believe, on relationships. Finding non-academic mentors in addition to academic mentors at different life stages helps.

---

identity labels, such as who is really "American," "German," or "European." If you are a minoritized scholar of color, know this history, it is yours too. One of my favorite short articles is by one of the few classical historians of color: Nandini B. Pandey (2020). The Roman roots of racial capitalism. *The Berlin Journal, 34*, 16–20. www.americanacademy. de/the-roman-roots-of-racial-capitalism/

9 Finding people you trust is important not just for your psychological well-being but academic well-being. Here is a good article by Ijeoma Opara on *How to protect research ideas as a junior scientist* that highlights the importance of creating a "trusted circle" of scholars who you can share ideas with: www.nature.com/articles/d41586-022-03750-0

It is also important to find spaces in academia that you think *deserve* to have you. Instead of feeling like we always need to fit into a particular space, we need to also consider whether spaces acknowledge and truly value what we bring. Do the people around you listen to what you have to say? Do they take the time to provide critical yet constructive feedback on your work? Do you feel like your ideas, inputs, and questions are taken seriously? This space ideally also allows for rest. In our work we are rewarded for doing a lot in a short amount of time even if it means late nights, few breaks, and ultimately harming our health. And for those from traditionally excluded groups, the additional stress of feeling you have to constantly prove that you belong may push you to work even more. A critique of these pressures, as the theoretical physicist Chanda Prescod Weinstein points out so eloquently in her book *The Disordered Cosmos*,[10] is that "Our academic and economic structures are set up with capitalist incentives to keep it to yourself when you realize something is wrong and to favor quick, superficial work over work that requires deep, plodding thought" (p. 159). Do the spaces you inhabit allow for deep, plodding thought? Relatedly, do the spaces you inhabit allow for rest and the refusal to be overworked and undone?

One way I try to create such a space is to protect and prioritize time for writing, which often is slow and plodding (for me anyway). Writing is revision and resistance.[11] In our research group we meet once a month in person to write together in the same space for support and encouragement. We also have mini online-writing days, checking in with each other in the morning, writing for several hours until lunch time, then checking in before getting on with the rest of the day. It is a small thing to do, but sometimes these small things can help along the way. So I would encourage you to find a group to write with, not only for being productive, but to have a protected space to be quiet, for a few hours or a day, to think and write.

---

10 I highly recommend *The Disordered Cosmos: A Journey into Dark Matter, Spacetime, and Dreams Deferred*. If you were ever told that "fill in the blank" program/university/field of study was not meant for someone like you or that you were not good enough, this book shows that gatekeepers and institutions sometimes are full of it.

11 Writing is so important. The short video "While I Write" by artist scholar Grada Kilomba is a powerful reminder of what the act of writing does: "While I write, I am not the 'other,' but the self; not the object, but the subject . . .": www.nytimes.com/2021/10/12/arts/design/amant-kilomba-portuguese-artist.html. I also really like Anthony Ocampo's article urging us to think about *who* we are writing for: https://magazine.catapult.co/dont-write-alone/stories/anthony-ocampo-why-doctoral-students-phds-need-to-study-creative-writing. Finally, I try to read William Zinser's book *On Writing Well* every several years. He reminds us that writing clearly is an act of social justice. If we are not clear in our writing, we are withholding knowledge.

Identity Configurations – How Do We Make Sense of Our Multiple Identities?

Our multiple identities can be configured in different ways. They can be in conflict, be compartmentalized, or cohere (Galliher et al., 2017). How do your identities configure? Do some of our identities seem to be in conflict with one another? Do responsibilities to your family conflict with needs associated with building a successful career, such as moving across the country to take another position? Or do you compartmentalize different aspects of yourself, relying mostly on activating one identity in some situations and contexts, with some individuals and not others? Importantly, how do our central identities cohere? Coherence is described as having a "sense of harmony among identity contents, at various levels" (Galliher et al., 2017, p. 2014). How do we weave together our complex identities to simultaneously hold and embrace identities that society may tell us are incompatible or in conflict? Finding spaces that allow for this complexity is important. Prescod Weinstein's book *The Disordered Cosmos* is a wonderful example of how a scientist who happens to be queer, Black identified, Jewish, and living with a disability, is able to hold all these identities and flourish in the field of physics, dominated by cis-heterosexual white men. It is not easy, and sometimes the fun of physics is outweighed by the racism, sexism, ableism, and patriarchy that she experiences regularly. Yet she is a singular voice in physics not in spite of, but because of, her refusal to leave important parts of herself behind while doing science.

In the same way, your particular social location – that unique configuration of living within overlapping societal structures that informs and reacts to your identities – provides you with a way of looking at things that others may not have. If you are made to feel different, if you feel out of sync with others, if you don't see people who look like you in your department or in the spaces that you work in, this also means that you can offer something unique – not just your perspective but your experiences and expertise in how you view the world and create knowledge. Indeed, there is evidence that traditionally underrepresented early career scholars innovate (i.e., create more novel work) than majority students (Hofstra et al., 2020).[12]

---

12 The study included an analysis of over 1 million US PhD recipients' theses and tracked their academic career. Innovation was defined as introducing novel linkages among scientific concepts. Importantly, the study also documented the unfortunate reality that despite being more likely to innovate, underrepresented PhD students are less likely to benefit (e.g., get an academic position) from this innovation compared to their majority peers.

In thinking of my particular social location and my various identities it is helpful for me to remember that I am, like some of my papers, a work in progress. The writer Kiese Laymon talks about life as a constant revision. This ability to be open to revision, to work on ourselves, our multiple and complex identities, figuring out who we are and trying to understand ourselves and the world around us, is something we will do for the rest of our lives if we want to grow. He says that revising is love, because if you love something, you go back to it, over and over. In an interview he says:

> So for me, it was just the notion that revisitation is part of love. Like, we love songs. Often we go back and listen and listen and listen. And those re-listenings give us different portals of entry into us, into the song-maker, into all kind of stuff. And also, to revise in love, you have to listen to people outside of yourself. *You have to listen to other visions of yourself. You have to mind other people's visions of who you are to them.*[13]

What I take away from this idea of revision as love, revision as revisiting yourself over and over from different angles and perspectives and being reflected back from how other people see you, is that we need to constantly view and work on our kaleidoscope of identities to be able to understand who we are in the work we do. Find someone who can help you see something in you that you may not yet see yourself. Believe in your particular perspective and identities as a contribution in your work. We will always be a work in progress. Our multiple identities and the way they configure will always be a work in progress.[14]

---

13 https://lithub.com/kiese-laymon-on-revision-as-love-and-love-as-revision/, italics are mine to highlight how we need other people to show possibilities of ourselves. Kiese Laymon is a 2022 McArthur Fellow. Here is a thoughtful two-minute video where he talks about why the practice of revision (not being afraid to look back and grapple with what we have done to be able to do our best) is so important for life: www.youtube.com/watch?v=ZcCZwLr9DwA

14 This phrase "A work in progress" sticks in my head because it is the title of a middle school children's book about a boy who struggles with body issues, finally accepting who he is and finding his self-worth. Jarrett Lerner is the author of that book, a very talented children's book author who happens to be the son of my graduate school advisor Jacqueline Lerner.

Final Thoughts

In this chapter I talked about how the content, contexts, and configurations of our identities invite areas for reflection. Here are six things I hope you take away from this chapter:

1. Know that your ethnic-racialized identities reflect unique perspectives and experiences that strengthen your work.
2. Find people you trust. They may be in spaces beyond your department or organization.
3. Find non-academic mentors whose life (and not just work) you admire.
4. Create space for allowing slow, plodding thought.
5. Remember that writing and revision can be acts of resistance and love.
6. Remember that we are always works in progress.

You chose this book because you are on your way to a career in mental health and may be seeking out some inspiration for this path. Know that there are people out there who care about you, who share similar experiences, who know what it is like to question ourselves along this pathway. Find strength in this community. I wish you well.

Acknowledgements

Thank you to the editors Doris Chang and Linda Lausell Bryant for the invitation to contribute a chapter to this important book! Thank you to my dear colleague and friend Lisa Kiang for providing critical and kind feedback on an early messy draft. Finally, thank you to the early career PhD students currently in my research group who also read through and commented on an earlier draft of this chapter: Tuğçe Aral, Sharleen Pevec, Karla Morales, Gyeongah Jang, Jannis Niedick, Oktay Balci, and Zhihao Zhong. Our conversations always leave me feeling inspired by how smart, thoughtful, and truly good-hearted you all are. You were on my mind when I was writing this chapter.

References

Advance, H. E. (2018). *Equality & higher education: Staff statistical report 2018*. www.ecu.ac.uk/publications/equality-highereducation-statistical-report-2018/

American Psychological Association. (2022). *APA style and grammar guidelines.* https://apastyle.apa.org/style-grammar-guidelines/bias-free-language/racial-ethnic-minorities

Bañales, J., Pech, A., Pinetta, B. J., Pinedo, A., Whiteside, M., Diemer, M. A., & Romero, A. J. (2021). Critiquing inequality in society and on campus: Peers and faculty facilitate civic and academic outcomes of college students. *Research in Higher Education.* https://doi.org/10.1007/s11162-021-09663-7

Celeste, L., Baysu, G., Phalet, K., Meeussen, L., & Kende, J. (2019). Can school diversity policies reduce belonging and achievement gaps between minority and majority youth? Multiculturalism, colorblindness, and assimilationism assessed. *Personality and Social Psychology Bulletin, 45*(11), 1603–1618. https://doi.org/10.1177/0146167219838577

Dee, T., & Penner, E. (2016). *The causal effects of cultural relevance: Evidence from an ethnic studies curriculum* (No. w21865; p. w21865). National Bureau of Economic Research. https://doi.org/10.3386/w21865

Erikson, E. H. (1968). *Identity: Youth and crisis.* Norton.

Fish, J., & Counts, P. K. (2020). "Justice for Native people, justice for Native me": Using digital storytelling methodologies to change the master narrative of Native American peoples. In K. C. McLean (Ed.), *Cultural methodologies in psychology: Describing and transforming cultures.* Oxford University Press. https://doi.org/10.31234/osf.io/y2w3v

Galliher, R. V., McLean, K. C., & Syed, M. (2017). An integrated developmental model for studying identity content in context. *Developmental Psychology, 53*(11), 2011–2022. https://doi.org/10.1037/dev0000299

Gay, G. (2013). Teaching to and through cultural diversity. *Curriculum Inquiry, 43*(1), 48–70. https://doi.org/10.1111/curi.12002

German Academic Exchange Service. (2023). *Facts and figures on the international nature of studies and research in Germany and worldwide.* doi: 10.3278/7004002vkew

Hofstra, B., Kulkarni, V. V., Munoz-Najar Galvez, S., He, B., Jurafsky, D., & McFarland, D. A. (2020). The diversity–innovation paradox in science. *Proceedings of the National Academy of Sciences, 117*(17), 9284–9291. https://doi.org/10.1073/pnas.1915378117

Juang, L. P., Moffitt, U., Schachner, M. K., & Pevec, S. (2021). Understanding ethnic-racial identity in a context where "race" is taboo. *Identity, 21*(3), 185–199. https://doi.org/10.1080/15283488.2021.1932901

Lee, E. (2015). *The making of Asian America: A history.* Simon and Schuster.

Maeda, D. J. (2009). *Chains of Babylon: The rise of Asian America.* University of Minnesota Press.

Marsh, D., & Furlong, P. (2002). A skin, not a sweater: Ontology and epistemology in political science. In D. Marsh & G. Stoker (Eds.), *Theory and methods in political science.* Palgrave Macmillan.

McLean, K. C., & Syed, M. (2015). Personal, master, and alternative narratives: An integrative framework for understanding identity development in context. *Human Development, 58*, 318–349. https://doi.org/10.1159/000445817

Nzinga, K., Rapp, D. N., Leatherwood, C., Easterday, M., Rogers, L. O., Gallagher, N., & Medin, D. L. (2018). Should social scientists be distanced from or engaged with the people they study? *Proceedings of the National Academy of Sciences, 115*(45), 11435–11441. https://doi.org/10.1073/pnas.1721167115

Otele, O. (2021). *African Europeans: An untold story.* Basic Books.

Pandey, N. B. (2020). The Roman roots of racial capitalism. *The Berlin Journal, 34*, 16–20.

Roberts, S. O., Bareket-Shavit, C., Dollins, F. A., Goldie, P. D., & Mortenson, E. (2020). Racial inequality in psychological research: Trends of the past and recommendations for the future. *Perspectives on Psychological Science.* https://journals.sagepub.com/doi/10.1177/1745691620927709

Syed, M., & Azmitia, M. (2010). Narrative and ethnic identity exploration: A longitudinal account of emerging adults' ethnicity-related experiences. *Developmental Psychology, 46*(1), 208–219. https://doi.org/10.1037/a0017825

Syed, M., Santos, C., Yoo, H. C., & Juang, L. P. (2018). Invisibility of racial/ethnic minorities in developmental science: Implications for research and institutional practices. *American Psychologist, 73*(6), 812–826. https://doi.org/10.1037/amp0000294

Tajfel, H., & Turner, J. C. (1986). The social identity theory of intergroup behavior. In W. Austin & S. Worchel (Eds.), *Psychology of intergroup relations* (2nd ed.). Nelson-Hall.

Umaña-Taylor, A. J., Quintana, S. M., Lee, R. M., Cross, W. E., Rivas-Drake, D., Schwartz, S. J., Syed, M., Yip, T., Seaton, E., & Ethnic and Racial Identity in the 21st Century Study Group. (2014). Ethnic and racial identity during adolescence and into young adulthood: An integrated conceptualization. *Child Development, 85*(1), 21–39. https://doi.org/10.1111/cdev.1219612

Applying to Graduate School

2

Tips and Strategies for BIPOC and International Students

Nari Yoo and Sophia Williams Kapten

This chapter emphasizes personal experience and testimony as a vehicle for communicating knowledge about graduate school admissions in psychology and social work for Black, Indigenous, and People of Color (BIPOC) and international students. We are writing this chapter because we have taken nontraditional journeys in our respective fields. What do we mean by nontraditional? First consider these statistics. According to the American Psychological Association (2022), 84.4% of psychologists are white, and this statistic has been relatively stable since 2011. Furthermore, 68.8% of social workers are white, according to a 2017 survey by the National Association of Social Workers (Salzburg et al., 2017). From this perspective, we are describing BIPOC and international students entering graduate programs in psychology and social work as nontraditional.

We also are using this descriptor to capture a path into and through graduate school that is a bit more complicated, riddled with barriers that require creative solutions. For example, we found creative solutions to address a compromised undergraduate GPA, contended with the isolation of being the first person in their family to study abroad, navigated graduate studies as the first in their family to attend college, and found ways to exist authentically among people who do not share their mother language. Perhaps you are reading this chapter with similar struggles or other challenges.

DOI: 10.4324/9781003309796-4

We are writing this chapter to encourage you and offer our perspectives about how to pursue your graduate degree.

There are many valuable published resources available that outline the necessary steps in applying to graduate school (Harvard University, 2022; Norcross & Sayette, 2022; Prinstein, 2023; Reyes, 2005). However, our goal is to supplement these resources with information about what you may experience if you too identify as a nontraditional student. In this chapter, we discuss our experiences navigating the application process. You will find a list of tips that you might find helpful as you embark on your journey through graduate school admissions. Although we are writing with a specific population in mind, the tips and strategies may be useful for both BIPOC and international students, given their frequently overlapping identities.

Positionality

We will start by first introducing ourselves.

Sophia. I am a 38-year-old, cis- Black American woman, mother, wife, and clinical psychologist. I was raised by my mother, who gave birth to me as a teenager with no reliable financial or familial support. I am the first in my immediate and extended family to graduate from college and complete a doctorate. As a result, I am also swimming in student loan debt, which is the troubling side of this accomplishment and an unfortunate burden many first-generation BIPOC college students live with (Arnold, 2020; Havens, 2021).

My journey into graduate school was difficult, largely because upon entering college I struggled to keep up with the university's demands. I had been a good student leading up to college, I had been mentored to get into college, but as a college student, I didn't know how to matriculate through university and couldn't imagine my life after graduation. It was not until my final year of college that I understood what was required of me to perform well in school. I graduated from college with a 2.9 GPA, few meaningful relationships with professors, little confidence in myself as a writer or researcher, and a wish to be the kind of scholar I knew I was capable of being.

Three years after graduating from college, when I decided that I wanted to apply to graduate school, I knew I was ill-prepared. I felt deeply insecure about my candidacy yet I was determined to show myself and others that I was capable of more. So, I quit my job, moved in with my very skeptical mother, and poured myself into master's programs applications. After completing a stressful and at times lonely master's program, I took a two-year break from school to reground myself, during which time I worked in marketing. When I knew I was ready to resume my studies, I reconnected with my research lab and faculty advisor from my master's program and began attending lab meetings during my lunch break. By this point, I'd learned the importance of maintaining meaningful relationships in academia and developing my independent voice as a researcher.

I applied to PhD programs twice. The first year that I applied, I only focused on the program from which I earned my master's degree and I received a conditional admissions offer contingent upon passing a comprehensive exam. I studied the best way I knew, failed that exam, and therefore was not admitted into the program. I was devastated and felt like my performance on that exam confirmed what I already feared was true: that I was not smart enough to be a doctoral student. While this fear remained, what I also knew was that the career path that I was on was not satisfying, and the only vision I had for myself included the completion of my doctorate. The following year, I applied to the same institution, among others. This round of applications left me with two offers. One offer in a program housed at one of the most renowned Historically Black Colleges or Universities (HBCU) in the country. Another offer was extended to me by the institution where I received my master's degree. Although I longed for a Black academic community, particularly after my isolative experience in my master's program, I turned down the offer from the HBCU. I accepted the offer from the institution where I received my Master's degree because it offered me the most money and afforded me with the opportunity to study with my graduate faculty advisor of interest. Later, this faculty advisor would become my dissertation chair and truly one of the most amazing mentors I could ever ask for.

Nari. I am a 29-year-old cisgender Korean woman, an international student, and a PhD student in social work. I earned my bachelor's and master's degree in social welfare in South Korea and moved to New York in 2021 for my PhD. As an undergraduate, I researched career paths in my home country without considering the specific requirements for studying abroad since it never seemed affordable. Until I learned that there were fully funded doctoral programs in the United States (US) that don't require proof of bank statements, I never dreamed of studying in the US. When I learned that these were available, I began to explore program and career options. I was fortunate that my family was emotionally supportive, but they knew little about studying abroad and academia, so I had to figure it out on my own.

At first, I didn't know anything about studying abroad and who to ask or how to find information. I started by googling information on how to study abroad for social work programs in the US. I first looked into study-abroad opportunities for a master's degree. For international students, however, obtaining scholarships for a master's program in social work or psychology seems to be especially difficult. I could not afford the tuition fees or living costs, and I was unable to provide proof of financial support. As a result, I decided to pursue a doctoral degree because more fully-funded programs were available. It took me a considerable amount of time to do research on how to apply to doctoral programs at US universities. Throughout the application process, I experienced a high level of anxiety and suffered from hyperventilation due to a sense of uncertainty. My constant question was: Am I competitive enough to be admitted *over* domestic applicants? Now, as a 4th-year doctoral student, I have learned that being an international student is a strength since the social work field and academia always need culturally diverse professionals.

As I managed the entire process of applying and making decisions for a doctoral program in the US from start to finish on my own, I became more equipped with the skills to gather information, secure resources, and pursue my dream without giving up. At first, it was not an easy task for me. I spent about a year organizing what needed to be done, researching how to handle administrative tasks in a foreign language, and other cultural differences in administrative processes. However, besides practical and logistical advice, there are a few things I would like to share that I wish I had known earlier. In what follows, we will share tips and strategies that we have learned along the way and feel are crucial for you to know about applying to graduate programs in psychology and social work.

Financing Your Education

Graduate School Is Expensive and Financial Support Is Critical

Particularly in today's climate, where student debt is discussed more openly, it feels important to be transparent about the expense of graduate school education. Your financial aid options will vary depending on your background. Regardless of the path you take, keep in mind that having a plan for funding your graduate education is critical and it has been shown that students with stable financial aid are more likely to graduate on time (Maher et al., 2004; Maton et al., 2011). To this point, it is not only important to think about the application process but also about how to matriculate through your program.

Some BIPOC students, particularly first-generation students of color, may find securing stable financial aid particularly difficult. For this reason, student loans are often the best if not the only choice, particularly for those entering a master's program. At the doctoral level, more funding streams may be available. You can learn more about these opportunities by attending the program's open house, asking about scholarship opportunities, or contacting professors of interest. Master's students at schools without PhD programs are more likely to receive paid teaching or research assistantships than graduate students at schools with PhD programs. A Fulbright scholarship is also an option for international students seeking a master's degree.

If you are an international student, you can pursue your master's degree in your home country or in a more affordable program abroad and then apply for a PhD program in the US. The Council on Social Work Education (CSWE) offers an *International Degree Review* that recognizes a Master of Social Work or Social Welfare from a foreign country equivalent to an MSW from the US, depending on the curriculum. For a foreign degree to be recognized as equivalent, I (Nari) recommend taking as many social work courses and completing as many practicum hours as possible. Alternatively, advanced standing MSW programs in the US allow you to save about one year of tuition and living expenses once you receive accreditation for a foreign master's degree in social work.

Financial Aid Considerations: From Application Through Matriculation

It is also important to consider the expense associated with applying to graduate school. Keep in mind that application fees are expensive, GRE registration is expensive, and upon acceptance to graduate school, there is a laundry list of expenses to cover. As you consider the various expenses and funding sources that may be available to you as a graduate student, we urge you to also consider that you may have to work in order to apply for and matriculate through your graduate program. While this reality is seemingly obvious, the experience of balancing work and school can be frustrating.

Further, the funding streams listed above may also require some form of labor in addition to your school work.

As you prepare to enter graduate studies, we want you to have a realistic perspective about both the work-related demands that you will need to balance along with your academic requirements. In the absence of a financial safety net, we both had to work multiple part-time jobs before and during the application process, which was difficult, and we also felt guilty that we could not solely focus on the application as other applicants did. However, once you are admitted to graduate school, you may have a greater chance of finding an on-campus job as a teaching/research assistant.

Choosing a University and Faculty Advisor

The Location of the School May Affect Your Experience

As an international PhD student, you will be required to adjust to a new country, a new local community, and an unfamiliar academic system. As a result, we want you to be aware that acculturative stress and related mental health concerns are common (Yakushko et al., 2008). This applies to BIPOC students as well. The racial composition of states in the US is highly diverse, with variations in the state-level percentage of non-Hispanic whites ranging from 35% to 92%, according to the 2021 American Community Survey. As a BIPOC student, you may find yourself in a predominantly white institution (PWI) or a new local community with a racial climate different from what you are used to. This does not necessarily mean that you should avoid the area, but it is worth examining whether the school or program has various support systems in place for BIPOC students.

The following questions may help you assess whether a school's location may exacerbate your challenges as an international or BIPOC student. What are the differences between the community where you live now and the one where your school is located? What is the ethnic makeup of the program and town (Jindal-Snape & Rienties, 2016)? How welcoming is the town for newcomers and immigrants of your race or ethnicity? Can you access the resources you might need (e.g., counseling services in your native language, and ethnic foods and ingredients)? Does the program offer stipends suitable for the cost of living in your area (see www.phdstipends.com)? Does the school/program have student groups, initiatives, or programming that are inclusive of your cultural identity?

Consider How Responsive the Program Is to Their Students' Needs

Consider how many PhD students drop out of the program of interest and how much freedom current students have in changing labs or advisors. This is a particularly important consideration for international students because studying with a student visa requires students to remain enrolled in school. Withdrawal from a program means you will be forced to leave the country. Therefore, it is important that prior to choosing a graduate program that you consider how flexible and responsive this program is to students' needs and concerns, so that dropping out is not the only option. Furthermore, as an international student, if you find yourself in a program that is not meeting your needs, it might be difficult for you to protest if you are not a permanent resident (Fleming, 2022), and you may have to remain silent. For your mental health, look for programs that indicate a concern for students' well-being, happiness, and ability to shift their research specialization if desired.

Seek Out Faculty Mentors Who Honor Your Humanity

Research compatibility is one category to consider when determining which faculty advisor and thus which program to attend. However, we think it is important to clarify what compatibility means in more detail. Ideally, your faculty advisor is guiding and shaping you into who you hope to become; however, keep in mind that this process is symbiotic and the form it takes will be greatly influenced by who they are as well (Freire, 1970). As you are researching faculty advisors, do not simply read their research. Instead, we recommend that you also assess how much their work, their analysis, and the thrust behind their research resonates with your spirit. We also recommend that you review the courses that they teach and the syllabi associated with these courses. While doing so, not only ask yourself if you could envision teaching a similar course but also assess whether you feel in alignment with how they describe the course and the reading materials they have included on the syllabus.

We offer these recommendations because we want you to have some awareness about the "tools" (Lorde, 2003), the scholarship, the epistemology, and the values that your potential advisor will implicitly or perhaps explicitly use to inform the mentorship process. Particularly for students of color and international students at PWIs, your relationship with your faculty advisor can transform your experience in your program and can serve as a space of refuge. We want you to have as much knowledge as possible about the intellectual structures that keep your potential space of refuge in place so that you have some sense of the dependability of this space throughout your journey.

Centering Your Background and Your Voice

Bring Your Cultural Perspective to Your Personal Statement

One of the concerns that we find with the admissions process is the emphasis on program fit and the impression that this language may leave on candidates of color and international students. Let us be clear, fit is important; however, from whose perspective is fit being considered? Are you considering whether you fit into the program or whether the program fits with who you are and hope to become? As you begin the personal statement writing process, we advise you to center the richness of your experience and consider ways in which the program of interest will be nourishing for you.

Consider weaving into your statement your multicultural and/or multilingual experiences. You may be uniquely positioned to write critically about the differences between how mental health and wellness is discussed in your native language/country compared to English/the US. Perhaps, you are seeking a program with a global perspective on training and practice. Regardless of how you decide to present yourself in your personal statement, we recommend that you embrace and speak from the parts of you that are full of cultural knowledge, even if those are the parts of you that you think are incongruent with academia. Keep in mind that your voice deserves and needs to be heard!

Research Starts in Your Heart: Explore Your Convictions

Your growth as a researcher is not about how smart you are but rather about asserting your voice into the proverbial conversation. Asserting your voice is no small act. In fact, it is an expression of resistance or a way to talk back to "the logic of domination" (Rosales & Langhout, 2020). Do not let the sometimes esoteric process of graduate study frighten you from speaking and participating. If you wish to pursue a PhD, be intentional and explore your heart prior to applying. If you are in a master's program, this is an excellent time to do this exploration. Pursuit of a PhD is not only about getting a diploma but also about finding your voice as a researcher. Rather than centering gaps in published research, center longings in your heart. What do you wish to know more about? How much does available theory and research fulfill your interest? Allow yourself to be guided by your convictions, your dreams, your aches, and your joys, especially when self-doubt and symptoms of imposter syndrome creep up.

Creating Community to Manage Isolation

Community Can Be the Antidote: Make It, Build It, Create It

Graduate school requires support. The more support, the better. As you evaluate different programs, consider how you can find the support, resources, community, financial aid, and mentorship that you need to thrive in graduate school. If there is a limited community in your target program or department, you may need to cultivate connections with students and faculty at other universities. You can develop networking skills, attend conferences, join electronic mailing lists, and make individual contacts (Vasquez et al., 2006). If there is a gap in the academic community available to you, you can turn to your friends and loved ones for nourishment. Keep in mind that your personal life does not have to stop while you are in graduate school. In fact, your personal life might provide you with the ongoing nourishment you need to get through the more challenging aspects of graduate school.

I (Sophia), offer this recommendation from a position of experience. I found my first year of graduate school particularly isolating. I felt fortunate to have the support of my partner and friends to lean on. With time, I developed meaningful bonds with others in my program. As a graduate student, I was very intentional about maintaining a rich personal life. I did not want my life to be governed by academic requirements and demands. Nor did I want to neglect my relationships outside of school. I had to keep a strict schedule to ensure that there was adequate time for both my personal and academic interests. For example, while my partner slept, I often stayed up working. If I made weekend plans with friends, I made sure to wake up early and study before I went out. As you evaluate graduate school options, keep your personal life and social needs in mind. Consider how close you would like to be to your friends and family. While balancing work and your personal life requires a great deal of effort, maintaining such a balance is a never ending challenge and school is no reason to deprive yourself of the warmth of friends and family.

Some of you may be wondering about the best time to apply to graduate school, especially if you want to start a family in the near future. I decided to have a child while pursuing my doctoral degree, timing the pregnancy to coincide with my internship year. Although this was a decision made with intention, I wrestled with a lot of doubt and fear throughout my pregnancy. I have no clear answers or advice for those interested in expanding your family while also working toward your graduate degree. Such a decision could turn into a serious distraction; however, as in my case, it could also provide you with a sense of community that is so very important while completing graduate school.

If you want to start a family while you are in school, you may want to consider the program's proximity to family and friends. My mom occasionally flew into town to offer support, but it was challenging to juggle childcare, work, and school without family close by. There were many days when my partner had to take over childcare duties so that I could write my dissertation.

Although starting a family while in graduate school was difficult at times, I also found that as a mother I felt better equipped to practice psychotherapy. I knew maternal transference and countertransference more intimately. I knew the depths of pain and love, the demands of parenting, the exhaustion of caregiving, and the faith required to move through seasons of darkness. As you live your life more fully you may find that you can enter into your work as a therapist or researcher more fully. Balancing the personal and the professional is no small task. However, moving toward the fullness of the human experience will not only make your journey throughout graduate school richer but also will provide you with a much needed social-emotional safety net. As you plan your journey through graduate school, I urge you to consider how you can maintain or even grow not only in your scholarship but also in your humanness and your connectedness to others.

Organize or Join a Support Group for International PhD Applicants in Your Home Country

For me (Nari), support groups played a vital role in sustaining and completing the graduate school application process. If you can, join an existing group; if one doesn't exist, create a small support group of other international applicants in your home country. A group of three to four people is sufficient, and it is okay if everyone has different disciplines of interest. Along with motivating each other, a support group can provide constructive feedback on your application package. You could organize study groups for standardized tests (GRE or TOEFL), academic English writing, or book clubs. The graduate school application process is arduous and challenging, particularly for international applicants, and some give up during this process. A support group of individuals with similar goals will assist you in moving forward. They also become another *family* in the US, as they experience similar or different challenges from different positions during your study abroad journey. When you travel to different areas or relocate, they can also be a great source of support. Beginning with the application stage, try to create such a support group (or friends) and cherish each other.

Navigate Academia by Using Social Media to Network

Networking in the US could be characterized as the strength of weak ties (Granovetter, 1973). In order to benefit from networking, even a weak connection can be valuable in and of itself. If networking in person seems difficult, consider leveraging social media (Hamid & Bukhari, 2015). We recommend that you join online academic communities such as NextGen Psych Scholars Program, Project Short, academic Twitter, now known as X. "Academic Twitter" used to refer to a loose community of scholars who use Twitter as part of their academic identity (Gregory & Singh, 2018). There is no need to post anything; by simply following professors, clinicians, and PhD students you can learn about the projects they are working on, application tips, and funding opportunities.

Familial Isolation or Rejection May Make Your Admissions Journey Challenging

You may encounter familial doubt or disapproval; you are not alone. Before applying to graduate school, I (Sophia) muscled my way back into my mother's home because I knew I needed her help. She was very alarmed by what appeared to be a regression in my development, from being entirely independent to fully dependent on her help. You may find your family similarly confused by your interest to pursue graduate education. Research has found that first-generation college students are less likely to receive encouragement from their families and may experience more disapproval or criticism from loved ones for pursuing graduate school (Redford & Mulvaney Hoyer, 2017; Richardson & Skinner, 1992). We note this research not to be alarmist but rather to provide some insight into the pushback that first-generation BIPOC students have reported in the past. If you find yourself in this place, let this be a reminder that you are not alone. Today, my mother (Sophia) is one of my biggest cheerleaders. She doubted my judgment but I now understand this doubt was rooted in fear of a path that she knew very little about and that she could not fully advise me on. You too might encounter fear-based disapproval. However, keep in mind that fear is not a great place from which to make decisions. Instead, follow the light of your convictions.

Conclusion

Let this chapter be a reminder that graduate school is possible even if it feels out of reach. We hope that our words help you feel less alone when facing similar issues. There are certainly additional challenges in regards to graduate school applications as a BIPOC or international student. However, we would like to reiterate the unique strengths that you possess. Your presence is critical to the field, particularly to the BIPOC clients searching for clinicians who identify with their ethnic-racial identity. You have strengths that the field needs. Consider that the dimensions of your background that you feel insecure about may also be points of connection that will help you better understand your clients. Elevating equity and inclusion in mental health research and practice calls for unique voices like yours.

References

American Psychological Association. (2022). *Demographics of US psychology workforce [interactive data tool]*. American Psychological Association. www.apa.org/workforce/data-tools/demographics

Arnold, C. (2020). Graduates of historically Black colleges may be paying more for loans: Watchdog group. *NPR*, February 5. www.npr.org/2020/02/05/802904167/watchdog-group-minority-college-graduates-may-pay-higher-interest-rates

Fleming, N. (2022). *Underpaid and overworked: researchers abroad fall prey to bullying*. Nature Publishing Group. https://doi.org/10.1038/d41586-022-02142-8

Freire, P. (1970). *Pedagogy of the oppressed*. Seabury Press.

Granovetter, M. S. (1973). The strength of weak ties. *American Journal of Sociology*, 78(6), 1360–1380. https://doi.org/10.1086/225469

Gregory, K., & Singh, S. S. (2018). Anger in academic Twitter: Sharing, caring, and getting mad online. *tripleC: Communication, Capitalism & Critique. Open Access Journal for a*

Global Sustainable Information Society, 16(1), 176–193. https://doi.org/10.31269/triplec.v16i1.890

Hamid, S., & Bukhari, S. (2015). *Information seeking behaviour and international students: The role of social media in addressing challenges while abroad.* https://repo.uum.edu.my/id/eprint/15627/

Harvard University. (2022). *Harvard Psychology's PhD resources and online tips page (PRO-TiP).* Harvard University Department of Psychology, September 30. https://psychology.fas.harvard.edu/pro-tip

Havens, T. (2021). Educational redlining: The disproportionate effects of the student loan crisis on Black and Latinx graduates. *The Vermont Connection*, 42(1), 11. https://scholarworks.uvm.edu/tvc/vol42/iss1/11/

Jindal-Snape, D., & Rienties, B. (2016). *Multi-dimensional transitions of international students to higher education.* Routledge.

Lorde, A. (2003). The master's tools will never dismantle the master's house. *Feminist Postcolonial Theory: A Reader*, 25, 27.

Maher, M. A., Ford, M. E., & Thompson, C. M. (2004). Degree progress of women doctoral students: Factors that constrain, facilitate, and differentiate. *The Review of Higher Education*, 27(3), 385–408. https://doi.org/10.1353/rhe.2004.0003

Maton, K. I., Wimms, H. E., Grant, S. K., Wittig, M. A., Rogers, M. R., & Vasquez, M. J. T. (2011). Experiences and perspectives of African American, Latina/o, Asian American, and European American psychology graduate students: A national study. *Cultural Diversity & Ethnic Minority Psychology*, 17(1), 68–78. https://doi.org/10.1037/a0021668

Norcross, J. C., & Sayette, M. A. (2022). *Insider's guide to graduate programs in clinical and counseling psychology: 2022/2023 edition.* Guilford Publications.

Prinstein, M. (2023). *Mitch's uncensored advice for applying to graduate school in clinical psychology.* https://mitch.web.unc.edu/wp-content/uploads/sites/4922/2017/02/MitchGradSchoolAdvice.pdf

Redford, J., & Mulvaney Hoyer, K. (2017). *First generation and continuing-generation college students: A comparison of high school and postsecondary experiences.* https://vtechworks.lib.vt.edu/handle/10919/83686

Reyes, J. (2005). *The social work graduate school applicant's handbook: The complete guide to selecting and applying to MSW programs.* White Hat Communications.

Richardson, R. C., Jr., & Skinner, E. F. (1992). Helping first-generation minority students achieve degrees. *New Directions for Community Colleges.* https://doi.org/10.1002/cc.36819928005

Rosales, C., & Langhout, R. D. (2020). Just because we don't see it, doesn't mean it's not there: Everyday resistance in psychology. *Social and Personality Psychology Compass*, 14(1). https://doi.org/10.1111/spc3.12508

Salzburg, E., Quigley, L., Mehfoud, N., Acquaviva, K., Wyche, K., & Sliva, S. (2017). *Profile of the social work workforce.* www.socialworkers.org/LinkClick.aspx?fileticket=wCttjrHq0gE%3D&portalid=0

Vasquez, M. J. T., Lott, B., García-Vázquez, E., Grant, S. K., & Vestal-Dowdy, E. (2006). Personal reflections: Barriers and strategies in increasing diversity in psychology. *The American Psychologist*, 61(2), 157–172. https://doi.org/10.1037/0003-066X.61.2.157

Yakushko, O., Davidson, M. M., & Sanford-Martens, T. C. (2008). Seeking help in a foreign land: International students' use patterns for a US university counseling center. *Journal of College Counseling*, 11(1), 6–18. https://doi.org/10.1002/j.2161-1882.2008.tb00020.x

Experiences of International Graduate Students in Training in Health Service Psychology and Related Mental Health Disciplines

Challenges and Reflections

Iris Yi Miao and Xiang Zhou

> During the first week of graduate school, I followed a group of domestic BIPOC students from orientation to a social mixer for graduate students of color. I was surprised to discover that I was the only international student there, only to find out later that no international students received the email invitation to the social mixer. The department's administrative assistant informed me, "Because of how our university system documents students' demographics, international students are not included on the students of color listserv. In fact, the enrollment data on the university website has all international students as a separate category alongside other races . . ."
>
> (Author: Xiang Zhou)

Many international students who are Black, Indigenous, and other People of Color (BIPOC) encounter similar career development challenges as

DOI: 10.4324/9781003309796-5

their domestic counterparts, such as those related to ethnocultural identity development, mentorship, or racial microaggressions. However, as illustrated by the vignette above, international and domestic BIPOC students are often classified as mutually exclusive entities within the university, with implications for how resources are allocated. While the presence of international students diversifies the US education system and provides a useful global perspective, they are not always included in campus conversations on diversity, equity, and inclusion, thus rendering their experiences invisible and leaving their professional development concerns unaddressed (Xu & Flores, 2022). For example, in 2013, 4.29% (N=845) and 8.34% (N=218) of doctoral students identified as foreign nationals in APA-accredited Clinical Psychology and Counseling Psychology programs, respectively (American Psychological Association, 2013).

In this chapter, we, two former international trainees in the mental health field, provide a brief review of the pertinent literature, share an example from our lived experience, and conclude with reflections on our own journeys and practical takeaways for other international trainees pursuing mental health training in the United States. To contextualize the experiences and practical lessons offered in this chapter, we begin by sharing our positionalities. Both of us are early-career psychologists who are originally from small cities (in the Chinese context) in the southern and central parts of China. Thus, in addition to common experiences shared by all international trainees, the two of us also share somewhat similar challenges with respect to institutionalized Sinophobia as well as opportunities and support offered within our diasporic community (Gulamhussein et al., 2023). However, we also have considerable differences in our perspectives situated in our positionalities – Iris identifies as a cisgender woman. She obtained an undergraduate degree then a PhD in Clinical Psychology in US institutions, and is currently a postdoctoral fellow specializing in clinical neuropsychology in an academic medical center. Xiang identifies as a cisgender queer man, who graduated from a counseling psychology PhD program and is currently at a tenure-track position in an R1 US institution.

Before we unpack the struggles and challenges of international trainees, it is critical to acknowledge their unique assets and contributions. Apart from their substantial contributions to the US economy, international students are active participants in cultivating a more inclusive and interconnected global environment. Within the field of mental health, international students can often bring first-hand experiences and non-US-centric perspectives to enhance the multicultural competence training of all students (Lee, 2013). Some subfields in mental health such as counseling psychology have championed the internationalization movement (Forrest, 2010; Xu & Flores, 2022). That is, US-based research, theories, and practices, by ignoring advancements made outside the US cultural context, are vulnerable to cultural encapsulation. The voices of international students can contribute to the critical examination and decolonization of the status quo of mental health training. Last but not least, the United States, as one of the most popular destinations for studying abroad, hosts more than 1 million international students (Open Doors Report, 2020). Former international trainees who become faculty provide further mentorship, advocacy, and intellectual contribution to diversify the field of mental health (Consoli et al., 2022). Clinicians who have personal experiences as international students are often hired by university counseling centers to meet the mental health crises across US campuses as international student specialists.

Common Stressors Faced by International Students in Mental Health Training Programs

In spite of the heterogeneity within international students with respect to countries of origin and languages spoken, the literature has identified several stressors commonly experienced by international trainees in psychology and related fields of mental health in the United States. In the next section, we will outline some common challenges faced by international trainees. While we would like to acknowledge that this may not be an exhaustive list, these are common concerns that empirical research has identified and that the authors have personally experienced during their graduate school years.

Academic and Acculturation-Related Challenges

International students across all fields of study often face academic challenges when adjusting to US educational and mentorship practices. Mental health training programs can bring additional barriers to this academic adjustment. Clinical work inherently requires international trainees to have a more advanced and nuanced understanding of the English language and US culture, which may take years to acquire. Similar to domestic BIPOC students, international students report challenges in finding culturally competent supervisors. It is even rarer for multilingual trainees to find linguistically competent supervisors if they intend to gain experiences to practice in languages other than English. Furthermore, international students' development in clinical competence often intersects with their personal growth and acculturation/enculturation to the US, thus necessitating supervisors to be able to initiate culturally informed supervision conversations around their personal development (Zhou et al., 2019).

Financial Struggles

In addition to academic and acculturation challenges, many international students also experience substantial financial struggles. Aside from the higher tuition compared to their domestic counterparts, international students are required to maintain full-time status throughout their course of study by immigration policies. Federal laws impose restrictions on international students' employment opportunities: they are generally not permitted to work off-campus unless the position is related to their area of study, and there is a 20-hour per week time limit for on-campus employment (Lee, 2013; McFadden & Seedorff, 2017). Therefore, despite the majority of international students being self-funded, they have limited access to financial resources. Additional factors play a role in limiting international graduate students' income sources. For example, they are ineligible for federally based financial aid, such as work-study programs. Many prestigious fellowships and scholarships (e.g., the National Science Foundation graduate student fellowship) also exclude foreign nationals, even when their funding mission is to advance ethnic and racial diversity (e.g., Ford fellowship). Further, these exclusionary policies disadvantage international students seeking to demonstrate their ability to secure research grants, an important criterion in evaluating candidates on the academic job market.

Stressors Related to Immigration-Related Policies

Immigration-related policies deeply impact the clinical training experiences of international psychology trainees at both pre-doctoral and postdoctoral levels. While clinical practicum is an integral part of training for accredited doctoral programs in applied psychology, the majority of clinical placements are off-campus, such as community outpatient clinics and academic medical centers. Even for the predoctoral internship, a mandatory requirement for doctoral programs in psychology, international trainees have to submit requests for employment authorization (Curricular Practical Training CPT or Optional Practical Training OPT) to the US Citizenship and Immigration

Services (USCIS). While CPT allows them to work off-campus during their academic training, it typically requires the position to be part time. Students can also apply for full-time CPT but they may be ineligible for post-graduation employment (i.e., postgraduate OPT) if they maintain more than one year of full time CPT. OPT authorization permits international trainees to gain work experience in the United States for up to 12 months (e.g., a post-doc training position). In order to complete the predoctoral internship, international psychology trainees often opt to use either pre-completion OPT (in which case, they may not be able to apply for postgraduate OPT and will have to leave the US after graduation), or full-time CPT (in which case, they may negotiate with their internship sites to shorten the internship length to less than 12 months) (Illfelder-Kaye, 2006; Lee, 2013).

For the trainee who has successfully navigated these constraints at the predoctoral level and wishes to pursue licensure in the US, fulfilling licensing requirements within the one-year limit of OPT is challenging. Most states' licensure boards in professional psychology require formal postdoctoral training that typically lasts more than one year (Raney et al., 2008). These challenges require the international trainees to be well informed of specific regulations and keep abreast of recent updates, while serving as a liaison between their international student office and graduate department. They may take on the responsibility to increase awareness and provide education surrounding these concerns to their clinical training directors at school and/or at the off-campus placements.

These immigration-related policies are complicated and often carried out differently across universities. For example, one university may mandate all trainees to submit CPT documentation for a part-time unpaid clinical practicum, while another university may not require any documentation at all. We illustrate this complexity with a personal anecdote from Iris.

Untangling the Threads: A Personal Journey in Navigating Immigration Policies in Graduate Training

Stumbling across the field of neuropsychology was a serendipitous discovery during my first year in a clinical psychology program. As one of the few students who pursued this subspecialty in my program, I was the only one who identified as an international student. My initial excitement about being able to bridge my passion for the brain and human behavior was quickly quelled when I learned about the two-year fellowship requirement in order to become a board-certified clinical neuropsychologist. With several years of experience living as an international student under my belt, I was mindful that the ever-evolving visa regulations could potentially pose a significant barrier to my professional pursuit. Such restrictions became especially pronounced during the application process for predoctoral internship and postdoctoral fellowship. As one of the fastest-growing subspecialities in psychology, the demand for internships offering training in neuropsychology continues to soar. My status as an international trainee imposed further constraints: I was precluded from applying to medical centers that require citizenship or permanent residency as well as VA hospitals. After successfully matching at a site that offered rigorous training in both neuropsychology and rehabilitation for internship, I was soon confronted with another similar but more formidable challenge. With OPT, I am permitted to work up to 12 months following the completion of my doctoral degree, however, the board-eligible fellowship positions usually have a minimum two-year requirement.

Through friends and my internship director, I connected with other international trainees who were on a similar path and who graciously shared their experiences with me. While juggling a full-time internship, I spent many nights and weekends contacting training directors to inquire about their institutional policies regarding international trainees. This information is not readily available in application guidelines and is often subject to change. Training directors generally had to clarify further details with their colleagues in Human Resources. While some offered hope, many correspondences led to disappointment.

Meanwhile, I learned about other trainees who pursued different pathways in order to complete their training, including getting a second graduate degree in a STEM-related field (which would qualify them for an OPT extension), or advocating for Classification of Instructional Programs (CIP) code conversion in their home institutions. Currently, the federal government does not classify Clinical, Counseling Psychology, and Applied Psychology as a STEM (science, technology, engineering, and mathematics) field, despite the fact that the study of the scientific basis of psychology is an integral component of these programs alongside robust training in statistics and research. Such regulations preclude many international students from pursuing a postdoctoral fellowship that requires more than a one-year commitment or from obtaining licensure in states that have specific requirements for postgraduate supervised hours. However, students in programs with a designated CIP code that is one of the STEM fields may be eligible for an additional 24-month period of temporary training in their field of study. Thus, some programs have re-identified themselves with STEM-qualified CIP codes such as experimental psychology or developmental psychology (American Psychological Association, 2022) to make it easier for international students to complete their training.

One important lesson learned was the importance of advocating for myself as an international trainee – especially in light of the increasingly hostile environment, exclusionary policies, and anti-immigration sentiment in the current socio-political climate (Anandavalli et al., 2020). Because international students are viewed by many as holding educational and economic privileges, the systematic challenges we face are often rendered invisible or trivialized. Thus, bringing these conversations to the forefront promotes social change. I also had to "unlearn" the inclination to view myself as the cause of my challenges, and instead advocate for myself in a system that was unaware of the needs of international trainees.

Lessons Learned and Recommendations for International Trainees

Lastly, although we have personally encountered many of the aforementioned obstacles, we also benefited from the wisdom of predecessors and allies throughout this journey. We would like to offer a list of ten things "I wish I had known . . ." to our younger selves who navigated this process. As each international trainee carves out their unique career roadmap, there is no one-size-fits-all set of instructions. Therefore, we share our individual insights gleaned from our own experiences in hope that they may be helpful for individuals who are currently on this path, or contemplating studying psychology or a related field in the United States:

I wish that I had known . . .

1. **. . . that the US higher education system needs to be changed and can be changed by me.** Because the United States is the largest host nation for international students, I used to think that the US higher education had been perfectly set up for international students' success. This is far from the truth. There are many systematic barriers that do not take into consideration our academic needs in mental health training. This shift in perspective allowed me to externalize some of the burdens and guilt I have carried.
2. **. . . that racism can permeate classrooms and therapy spaces.** Whether overt or subtle, discrimination seems to seep into our lives. My training

as a psychologist heightened my awareness of social inequities and discrimination. However, the training curriculum, usually focused on raising white students' awareness of how these issues affect their patients, rarely addresses how these issues affect minority students on a personal and professional level. Unlike domestic students of color, my upbringing outside the US also leaves me less equipped to navigate these situations. Cultivating critical consciousness, accurately labeling these experiences for what they are, and reflecting on our own internalized racism constitute initial steps toward addressing structural racism and its impact on mental health.

3. **. . . that I could seek out a network of mentors, instead of relying on one mentor for all my needs.** My mentor is great, but they are as busy as most professors, and they are limited in their expertise in certain areas. For the longest time, I was afraid of offending them by seeking out additional mentorship under the assumption that we should only be working with the mentor we applied to work with. In cultivating a wider network of mentors, it is also important to seek out peer mentorship. Make connections with other international trainees and colleagues to draw on their wisdom and support to survive and thrive.

4. **. . . more about how to prepare myself for teaching.** Teaching undergraduates without prior experience was daunting. Grasping US classroom dynamics, creating rapport with students without being able to draw on shared cultural references, and teaching in my second language felt overwhelming. In addition to proactively engaging in pedagogical training, I discovered the immense importance of granting myself grace, seeking support, and, notably, establishing clear boundaries for my class preparation time (two hours max per week).

5. **. . . that some American students struggle with writing, too.** Okay, writing in English is hard. Writing in my second or third language, I wrongly believed I was a poor writer. Learning that native English speakers also grapple with academic writing provided some solace. Academic writing demands specific skills that are often not intuitive even for native speakers accustomed to essay writing. This shift in perspective motivated me to work on my writing rather than seeing it as a personal flaw.

6. **. . . the extent to which my visa status would impact me.** As discussed above, there is so much hidden or obscure information about visa-related issues for international students that is not readily available on institutional websites. Once, I accepted a practicum site when I was struggling financially and this site offered a small stipend. It was only

after I began that I learned that if I accepted this small stipend, I would no longer be able to use my CPT for my predoctoral internship.

7. **. . . that I would need to mourn many transnational losses.** For the longest time, I didn't talk about how two grandparents passed away during graduate school. Not only because they are important to me, but also because it felt surreal that I was not able to be there due to travel and financial restrictions. Thus, I was not able to experience the grief of this loss together with my family. Only later on did I realize that so many international students have gone through similar transnational losses – parents' major illness, missing a best friends' wedding, or a young nephew who no longer recognizes them after a long period of graduate study. These transnational losses are hard to speak about with our domestic counterparts. Acknowledge your feelings, build a support system, create rituals for special occasions even while abroad, and consider seeking help from another mental health professional.

8. **. . . that sometimes just participating is not enough.** Growing up in an environment where advocating for oneself may be mistaken as a sign of hubris, I always thought that my work would be acknowledged if I kept my head down and worked hard enough. However, self-actualization in a professional environment in the US often requires self-advocacy and leadership skills. I started to understand that many concerns related to minoritized students reflect larger systemic issues and institutionalized cultural norms. I now feel empowered to engage in advocacy for myself and other international trainees within the systems we occupy.

9. **. . . that being born outside of the US and having been raised in an environment with different worldviews and belief systems does not make me an outsider.** Instead, these experiences offer me the gift of viewing things from various lenses and allow me to connect with people in unique and creative ways.

10. **Lastly, I wish my younger self had known that there are many routes leading to success.** There is no singular definition for success. In times of stress or adversity, I will strive to cultivate flexibility, take on the challenges with resilience and relish the lessons I have learned from them.

In closing, this chapter has delved into the multifaceted experiences of international students pursuing higher education and clinical training within a US context. Through an exploration of the existing literature, and sharing of personal narratives and insights, we offered a glimpse of the complexities of this journey. Our hope is that this chapter serves as a resource for you, providing practical suggestions to better prepare you, and fostering a greater understanding of the unique experiences of international trainees in mental health disciplines. By acknowledging these challenges and striving to address them, our goal is to collectively work toward creating a more equitable and nurturing environment for individuals like you who aspire to contribute to the field of mental health.

References

American Psychological Association. (2013). *Total number and percentage of students who are foreign nationals in APA-accredited doctoral programs by area, 2008–2013* [data set]. www.apa.org/ed/accreditation/about/research/doctoral-foreign-nationals.pdf?_ga=2.81362583.1451343986.1664239658-1113347154.1662781742

American Psychological Association. (2022). *Welcoming changes to international student visas.* January 26. www.apaservices.org/advocacy/news/international-student-visas

Anandavalli, S., Harrichand, J. J., & Litam, S. D. A. (2020). Counseling international students in times of uncertainty: A critical feminist and bioecological approach. *Professional Counselor, 10*(3), 365–375. https://doi:10.15241/sa.10.3.365

Consoli, A. J., Çiftçi, A., Poyrazlı, Ş., Iwasaki, M., Canetto, S. S., Ovrebo, E., Wang, C. D., & Forrest, L. (2022). International students who became US Counseling Psychology faculty members: A collaborative autoethnography. *The Counseling Psychologist, 50*(6), 874–910. https://doi.org/10.1177/00110000221098377

Forrest, L. (2010). Linking international psychology, professional competence, and leadership: Counseling psychologists as learning partners. *The Counseling Psychologist, 38*(1), 96–120. https://doi.org/10.1177/0011000009350585

Gulamhussein, Q., Zhou, X., Kim, A. Y., & Lee, R. M. (2023). Incorporating diaspora into the developmental science of immigrant communities. In D. P. Witherspoon & G. L. Stein (Eds.), *Diversity and developmental science.* Springer International Publishing. https://doi.org/10.1007/978-3-031-23163-6_12

Illfelder-Kaye, J. (2006). Tips for trainers: International students on F-1 visas. *APPIC Newsletter, XXXI*(1), 12. www.appic.org/Portals/0/Newsletters/2006/May_2006.pdf

Lee, K. C. (2013). Training and educating international students in professional psychology: What graduate programs should know. *Training and Education in Professional Psychology, 7*(1), 61–69. https://doi.org/10.1037/a0031186

McFadden, A., & Seedorff, L. (2017). International student employment: Navigating immigration regulations, career services, and employer considerations. *New Directions for Student Services, 158*(2017), 37–48. https://doi.org/10.1002/ss.20218

Open Doors Report. (2020). *The 2020 open doors report on international educational exchange.* November 16. www.iie.org/Why-IIE/Announcements/2020/11/2020-Open-Doors-Report

Raney, S. C., Hwang, B. J., & Douce, L. A. (2008). Finding postdoctoral training and employment in the United States. In N. T. Hasan, N. A. Fouad, & C. Williams-Nickelson (Eds.), *Studying psychology in the United States: Expert guidance for international students.* American Psychological Association.

Xu, H., & Flores, L. Y. (2022). Facilitating the professional development of international counseling psychology students: Introduction to special issue. *The Counseling Psychologist, 50*(6), 746–750. https://doi.org/10.1177/00110000221092684

Zhou, X., Zhu, P., & Miao, I. Y. (2019). Incorporating an acculturation perspective into the Integrative Developmental Model (IDM) in supervising international trainees. *Training and Education in Professional Psychology.* http://dx.doi.org/10.1037/tep0000278

Intersectionality and Graduate Students of Color

4

Addressing the Interplay Between Identity, Systemic Oppression, and Resistance

Hector Y. Adames and
Nayeli Y. Chavez-Dueñas

Education is powerful. When grounded in the values and praxis of human rights, education has the potential to be a source of liberation. This assertion is echoed by many of our ancestors. The whispers of Nelson Mandela remind us that "education is the most powerful weapon you can use to change the world" (Nelson Mandela Centre of Memory, 2012, para. 13). Poetic words from bell hooks proclaim that "the classroom remains the most radical space of possibility in the academy" (1994). And Cesar Chavez's resounding chants declare that "you cannot uneducate the person who has learned to read. You cannot humiliate the person who feels pride. You cannot oppress the people who are not afraid anymore" (1984, para. 13). From this stance, education is expansive; it is more than the curriculum – it is also a source of resistance, liberation, and possibility.

The central purpose of this chapter is to underscore the critical need to honor the intersectional experiences of all Students of Color pursuing

DOI: 10.4324/9781003309796-6

careers in mental health. To meet this goal, we introduce and use the theory of intersectionality and its three domains (i.e., weak, strong, and transformative) to describe the interplay between identity, systemic oppression, and resistance. Within each domain of intersectionality, strategies for Students of Color to survive and thrive while in graduate school are offered. We believe in the power of working together to build educational environments anchored in respect and dignity for the rights of Students of Color, as etched in the writings of Mandela, hooks, and Chavez. Let's begin!

A Brief Overview of Intersectionality

Creating learning environments where Students of Color can flourish requires us to understand how oppression operates in the day-to-day lives of students. At its core, oppression is a power imbalance between social groups driven by ideologies that some groups are superior to others (Nelson & Prilleltensky, 2010).

The theory of intersectionality, an analytical framework used to study, understand, and challenge systems of oppression and inequities, can stimulate and expand our thinking on how multiple forms of oppression (e.g., racism, sexism, heterosexism) impact students' experiences and access to opportunities. Created by Black feminist activists, intersectionality describes and illustrates how systems of oppression (e.g., racism, sexism, cissexism, heterosexism, ableism, ethnocentrism) overlap and interact to uniquely impact the lives of minoritized groups (Crenshaw, 1989, 1991).

Over the past decade, intersectionality has increased in popularity across the social sciences (Moradi & Grzanka, 2017), including psychology (Cole, 2009). For instance, intersectionality has been used to create psychometric scales (Lewis & Neville, 2015) and psychotherapeutic treatment approaches (Adames et al., 2018), and has been applied to ethics (Pope et al., 2021). Additionally, scholars have introduced and described a classification system to organize three domains of intersectionality, including (a) *weak intersectionality*, which centers on multiple identities, (b) *strong intersectionality* underscoring systems of inequities and oppression, and (c) *transformative intersectionality* focusing on ways to challenge and dismantle systems of oppression (Dill & Kohlman, 2011; see also Adames et al., 2018).

Honoring All of Me: Graduate Students Deepening Self-Knowledge

> Our humanity is defined and distinguished by the development of knowledge and in particular self-knowledge, therefore it is critical for each generation to learn who and what they are.
>
> (Akbar, 1998, p. 1)

Who are we? How do we begin to know ourselves and define who we are? The process of answering these questions are the goals of identity studies in the social sciences. In psychology, theorists have explained how people navigate and answer these defining questions. For instance, Eric Erickson's idea of identity describes how biological, psychological, and societal demands, including oppression, influence people's notion of the self (Adames & Chavez-Dueñas, 2021; Erikson, 1980; Syed & Fish, 2018). Our siblings in sociology have also tackled similar questions albeit with a different focus. Their theories underscore the importance of individuals connecting with a group of people with similar values, ideologies, and practices (e.g., social identity theory) as another source to answer the question of "who I am" (Adames & Chavez-Dueñas, 2021). Part of coming to know who we are (self-definition) takes shape in the context of being known by others (Blatt, 2008). To illustrate, Adames and Chavez-Dueñas state

> that identity is shaped by how individuals connect, disconnect, identify, or not identify with various social group categories (e.g., race, ethnicity, gender, sexual/affectional orientation) in which society structurally places them (e.g., Asian, African American, Indigenous, lesbian, gay, bisexual, transgender). In other words, a person's ideologies, feelings, and behaviors are also shaped by their social group membership and the structural power that these groups have within a given society.
>
> (Adames & Chavez-Dueñas, 2021, p. 60)

Understanding, taking pride, and honoring all parts of our identity and the unique experiences that arise from their interconnection is critical for surviving and thriving in various spaces, including graduate school. Concurrently, we must remember how our identities are weaponized against us in a culture grounded in white supremacist capitalist heterosexual cisgender patriarchal values – resisting internalizing such narratives becomes equally vital. In the following two sections we briefly share glimpses of our narratives to help illustrate the role that identity plays in our process as mental health professionals as a prelude to suggestions for you to reflect on your identity and its role in your graduate school journey.

Hector Y. Adames[1]

I am a cisgender, queer AfroLatino immigrant from Quisqueya, the island divided by superimposed borders now called Haiti and the Dominican Republic. I was born on the island of Quisqueya, the first space in the Americas where Black, white, and Indigenous People met. I come from a land and people who are intimately wrapped by a history of destruction and survival. As a queer man of African descent living in the 21st century of US American imperialism, my experiences of oppression, survival, and resistance reverberate in and outside the academy. These historical and contemporary realities influence all of who I am.

I am the first in my family to attend college and earn a graduate degree in Clinical Psychology. Echoes of my experiences of being in a foreign land and developing as an AfroLatinx Queer immigrant reverberate in my role as a psychologist, professor, and scholar-activist. These experiences also guide my ethics – valuing curiosity, embracing questions, honoring differences anchored in social and racial justice, and the unwavering belief in the transformative power of supporting others. I've devoted my career and talents to speaking the unspoken by naming and studying systemic forces that brutalize people through words, policies, and practices while developing methods that humanize and celebrate the strengths of those who coloniality aims to vanish. To echo Junot Diaz, also from Quisqueya, "all of us must be free, all of us must be free, all of us must be free or none" (2016, 4:22).

Nayeli Y. Chavez-Dueñas[1]

I am a cisgender, heterosexual, genderqueer Mexican Immigrant of Indigenous descent living in the land of the Sauk, Mesquakie, Potawatomi, Kickapoo,

---

1 Portions of the brief narratives were first published in Adames, H. Y., Chavez-Dueñas, N. Y., Vasquez, M. J. T., & Pope, K. S. (2023). *Succeeding as a therapist: How to create a thriving practice in a changing world*. American Psychological Association.

and Winnebago People. My upbringing in Michoacan, Mexico, and my immigration to the United States as a teenager have shaped my professional and personal life. Remnants of colonization remain alive on both sides of the US-Mexican border. Many of the laws, policies, and practices across the globe are anchored in the pillars of coloniality. These pillars are designed to control, dehumanize, and criminalize people for simply being Black, Brown, Indigenous, and existing outside the gender binary, to name a few. Simply put, we pay a heavy price for nurturing and exercising the audacity to cross the imaginary borders established by imperialism to maintain power. It is these experiences and realities that my work in psychology seeks to name, describe, and address.

I am one of nine children raised by a strong, determined woman who struggled to make ends meet. My mom was my living book, my constant source of wisdom, support, and love. She would often say, *"A dios rogando y con el mazo dando,"* which translates to "Begging god while working hard with a hammer," connotes that god helps those who help themselves. This proverb serves as a reminder to me and my siblings that hope is not just about dreaming and having faith that something will happen; instead, it is about working to make our dreams a reality. She taught me to imagine and work for dreams that may seem impossible to others. She embodied hope in action – a kind of hope that defies logic, a hope that propelled her to leave Michoacán and immigrate to the United States. Thanks to the lessons I learned from my mother, the strengths I carry from my ancestors, and my family's sacrifices, I became the first person to graduate from high school, attend college, and earn a doctoral degree. These achievements fueled my determination to learn, write, work, and use my skills to help dismantle the systems that oppress, dehumanize, and criminalize the hopes of Communities of Color.

We both often talk about our graduate school experiences and how we attended a predominantly white institution (PWI), in rural America, with no faculty that looked like us and very few Peers of Color. We often wonder, "How did we make it through" which ignites an anxious giggle that kind that transports us back to defending our comprehensive exams and dissertations in buildings with names and portraits of only white men, reading required literature void of the rich histories of People of Color and research that pathologized our communities, and being denied the same opportunities offered to our white peers (e.g., authorship on papers and presentations, leadership opportunities). Along the way, we had to find ways to survive and even thrive despite our challenges. The following guiding principles about identity helped us navigate graduate school, and we hope they can also be valuable to you.

Know and Be Proud of Who You Are

You cannot depend on the system to teach you who you are. Instead, we invite you to seek opportunities to build and expand your knowledge about who you are and where you come from. Read literature, poetry, and stories created by and for people in your community. Watch documentaries, listen to music, and talk to elders who often hold rich narratives. Connect with the many ways your people have contributed to society and the world at large.

Learn and Internalize the Psychological Strengths of Your People

Oppression is not new. Unfortunately, People of Color have endured injustice and dehumanization for centuries. We've had no choice but to create and learn strategies to survive. These methods are what people in our communities have used to cope, resist, persist, and even thrive in the face of relentless oppression. Collectively, our psychological strengths are the things that help us to keep on keeping on. Learning and internalizing our people's psychological strengths can be an antidote to moments of helplessness and hopelessness.

Remember That You May Feel Lonely, but You Are Not Alone

Being a graduate Student of Color in a PWI is not easy. You may be the only racial-ethnic minoritized person in most of your classes. Perhaps you are one of the few Women of Color or the only Queer Person of Color in your program. Onlyness is desolate, making us feel like there are few people with whom we can connect. During these instances, remember that the work, sacrifice, and advocacy of countless People of Color and allies helped create opportunities for you to be in a graduate program. You may feel lonely, but you are not alone. You represent the dreams of all those who came before you and those who sacrificed and are supporting you (e.g., family, chosen family, friends, partners, and mentors).

Graduate Students Understanding and Navigating Systems of Oppression

> If you don't understand racism, what it is and how it functions, everything else you think you know will only confuse you.
>
> (Fuller, n.d., para. 1)

Malcolm X described education as the passport to the future. Building on this stance, education helps us understand who we are, where we come from, and where we want to go. However, this goal is challenging for Students of Color who often must navigate and learn in an educational system built on the pillars of white supremacist capitalist heterosexual cisgender patriarchal values. For instance, higher education often reflects the expectations, values, and traditions of the people it was created to educate (i.e., white, cisgender, able bodied, heterosexual men). From Galton's classist, racist, and sexist theory of intelligence (see Helms, 2012) to the current backlash on Critical Race Theory (e.g., Oklahoma House Bill 2988 banning using the 1619 Project and prohibiting teachers from discussing white privilege in the classroom) and beyond, there are no shortage of examples to support the assertion that the educational system in the US continues to erase the history and experiences of Communities of Color and other minoritized groups.

Mental health graduate programs are not immune from perpetuating the erasure of People of Color and other oppressed communities. For many Students of Color, Queer Students of Color, Women of Color, and the like, the information they are expected to learn in educational settings often fails to reflect their lived experiences and their communities' rich histories. To illustrate, when the experiences of oppressed communities are included in the curriculum, stigmatizing and deficit-based frameworks are typically used. This practice leads to myopic and pathologizing descriptions of minoritized groups that uphold negative stereotypes and strengthen biases grounded in white supremacist capitalist heterosexual cisgender patriarchal values. In the current higher education system, minoritized students often struggle to find faculty who understand their experiences and can help them navigate the unique challenges of graduate school. In 2021, the American

Psychological Association (APA) recognized how it has failed Students of Color. The apology states how

> a general lack of faculty and Advisors of Color to assist with navigating and completing graduate programs has placed great burdens on current Faculty of Color to support Students of Color and champion all university-related issues pertaining to race and diversity, all of which is a consequence of racial disparities in the field and discipline of psychology which may be rooted in negative training-related and other experiences of Faculty and Students of Color.
>
> (APA, 2021, para. 20)

It is not surprising that Students of Color often report feeling unwelcome and that their experiences of racism and other forms of oppression are invalidated in psychology and related graduate programs (Curtis-Boles et al., 2020). The impact of these experiences contributes to the underrepresentation of Students of Color in the mental health field. To illustrate, in 2020, APA reported that 84.5% of the psychology workforce self-identified as white (APA, 2022), and 69% of doctoral degrees in psychology awarded in 2018 were earned by white students (APA, 2020).

Given their underrepresentation, students who experience multiple forms of oppression need resources and tools to succeed and navigate epistemic violence and toxic academic environments. Below we offer guidance to help students navigate the negative experiences they are likely to encounter while in graduate school.

Resist Internalizing the Imposter Syndrome Narrative

While it is true that systems are not built with minoritized groups in mind, this does not mean that we do not belong or deserve to be in these spaces. The countless hurdles we are required to jump through to make it to the same place as our counterparts more than prove that we deserve to take up space. We are not imposters. Instead, we are the opposite. We have more than earned the right to be in the halls of academia. If and when you sense or notice yourself beginning to internalize the imposter syndrome narrative, remind yourself of the following:

- Stop and reflect on what an imposter is – someone who does not belong or deserve to be where they are. It's a person who has not earned their place due to unearned advantages (i.e., privileges). As someone who has had to overcome the barriers that prevent people like you from entering academic spaces, you have had to work twice, sometimes three times as hard as your peers, to be where you are today. So, who is the imposter? Are you really an imposter?

- Despite the countless ways multiple forms of oppression (e.g., racism, sexism, cissexism, heterosexism, ableism) try to destroy or defer our academic dreams, you still made it to the same place as your peers. You have more than earned your place in your program! Don't minimize this accomplishment.
- Contemplate on who benefits from having you feel like you don't deserve to be or belong in graduate school? What can you do to resist buying into this narrative?

Build and Nurture Connections

Surviving and thriving in systems not built by us and for us is difficult, and we cannot do it alone. As a graduate student, you will need a community to support you as you navigate systems anchored in white supremacist capitalist heterosexual cisgender patriarchal values. This group can validate and affirm all of who you are – a community that is there during moments when the system injures you. People that will remind you that the problem is not inside of you. Having a squad that understands what it is like to be you, supports you, and helps you navigate challenging times is the fuel to get you through when you feel like giving up.

Resist Seeking Validation from the Oppressor and the Systems They Created

Experiencing compassion and being treated with respect and dignity not only feels good but is a healthy need. It is vital to pause and reflect on where, and to whom we go to meet these human needs. Suppose we seek compassion, respect, and dignity from the wrong places (e.g., white supremacy culture, ethnocentric spaces, heterosexist, and transnegative people). In that case, we will not only be left feeling depleted but also empty or perhaps confused. The outcome may be disorienting and painful, and we may blame ourselves for our human reactions. We invite you to resist the temptation to seek and expect approval from such sources. Instead, connect with people who genuinely understand and can validate your experiences. People who will support you and help you find or create ways to meet your goals. People who will not require you to change the essence of who you are for a degree.

Graduate Students Engaging in Acts of Resistance

> I am no longer accepting the things I cannot change, I am changing the things I cannot accept.
>
> (Davis, n.d., para. 1)

Being a graduate Student of Color who is also a member of multiple oppressed communities may contribute to feelings of helplessness, a common theme throughout this chapter. You may feel like you are swimming against the current and that there is very little you can do to change the system. However, this is a fallacy. History is filled with examples of oppressed people creating ways to resist and persist, even in spaces and places designed to cause them harm. Similarly, graduate students have engaged in actions to honor their dignity and right to a life of self-determination. You don't have to be the exception. Consider the following acts of resistance to use as you complete your graduate degree.

Protect Your Mind, Body, and Spirit

- There is no better act of resistance than caring for ourselves in a world that seeks to destroy our dreams and harm our existence. Our graduate school years allow us to engage in many activities and projects. It is a great time to be thoughtful about what you commit to doing. Remember that it is okay to say no to things; we can't do it all at the same time. It is vital to take time to rest, recharge, and replenish your energy. Your wellness matters!
- Think about your relationship with your spirit and create ways to develop or strengthen your connection. Some people do this through their faith or by spending time in nature or with animals. Others use art to connect to themselves.
- Experiencing joy and laughter is vital for physical and mental health. Engage with people and activities that bring joy into your life. Stop and allow yourself to experience these moments. Joy is a form of resistance. You deserve it!

Planning and Taking Strategic Actions of Resistance

Political engagement and student activism at postsecondary institutions in the United States have a long history. Students and faculty have organized, led, and joined several political movements throughout the decades, from the Civil Rights Movement to the more contemporary movements such as the DREAMers and Black Lives Matter movements. These forms of engagements are filled with wisdom we can adopt and tools we can use to build community, organize, and collectively resist legalized oppression in and outside academia. One of the tools you can use is the power of the pen. We encourage you to expand the definition of activism to include scholarship as a form of resistance. Reflect on the following:

- How can you use your own scholarship to resist perpetuating paradigms in mental health that stigmatize and pathologize minoritized groups and communities?
- How is your current research helping to change the narrative about oppressed communities?
- What can you do to make your scholarship accessible to the public instead of falling prey to the status quo of academics talking only to each other. Giving science and knowledge away is an act of resistance.

Learn but Do Not Internalize the Curriculum

As a graduate student in mental health, you will be expected to become familiar with the field's major theories, frameworks, and interventions. Whether or not you agree with the content, you need to learn the information to do well in courses, obtain the degree, and pass licensure exams. However, you can still question and recognize the shortcomings of dominant theories and practices. When we have a solid grasp of existing theories and frameworks we are better equipped to understand and address its epistemic violence. From this stance, resistance is twofold: (a) needing to meet the curriculum's learning objectives to complete degree requirements in a system that often expects people like us to fail WHILE (b) being creative in not internalizing how mainstream psychology invisibilizes oppressed communities and pathologizes our cultural values and traditions.

Conclusion

The premise of this chapter centers on the importance of honoring all of who we are. We accomplish this by building and nurturing a community that supports and celebrates our existence. In the words of Subcomandante Marcos, "We are nothing if we walk alone, but we are everything if we walk together in step with other dignified feet" (Marcos, 1994, para. 6). In closing, we invite you to never forget that the field of mental health does not define your worth as a person and the value of your community. Period!

References

Adames, H. Y., & Chavez-Dueñas, N. Y. (2021). Reclaiming all of me: The Racial Queer Identity framework. In K. L. Nadal & M. Scharron del Rio (Eds.), *Queer psychology: Intersectional perspectives*. Springer. https://doi.org/10.1007/978-3-030-74146-4_4

Adames, H. Y., Chavez-Dueñas, N. Y., Sharma, S., & La Roche, M. J. (2018). Intersectionality in psychotherapy: The experiences of an AfroLatinx queer immigrant. *Psychotherapy, 55*(1), 73–79. https://doi.org/10.1037/pst0000152

Akbar, N. (1998). *Know thy self*. Mind Productions & Associates, Inc.

American Psychological Association. (2020). *Psychology's workforce is becoming more diverse: News on psychologists' education and employment from APA's center for workforce studies.* www.apa.org/monitor/2020/11/datapoint-diverse

American Psychological Association. (2021). *Apology to People of Color for APA's role in promoting, perpetuating, and failing to challenge racism, racial discrimination, and human hierarchy in US resolution adopted by the APA council of representatives.* www.apa.org/about/policy/racism-apology

American Psychological Association. (2022). *Demographics of US psychology workforce.* www.apa.org/workforce/data-tools/demographics

Blatt, S. J. (2008). *Polarities of experience: Relatedness and self-definition in personality development, psychopathology, and the therapeutic process.* American Psychological Association. https://doi.org/10.1037/11749-000

Chavez, C. (1984). *Cesar Chavez address to the Commonwealth of California Club.* www.awb.com/dailydose/?p=1660

Cole, E. R. (2009). Intersectionality and research in psychology. *American Psychologist, 64*(3), 170–180. https://doi.org/10.1037/a0014564

Crenshaw, K. W. (1989). Demarginalizing the intersection of race and sex: A Black feminist critique of antidiscrimination doctrine, feminist theory and antiracist politics. *University of Chicago Legal Forum, 1989*(1), 139–167. http://chicagounbound.uchicago.edu/uclf/vol1989/iss1/8

Crenshaw, K. W. (1991). Mapping the margins: Intersectionality, identity politics, and violence against women of color. *Stanford Law Review, 43*(6), 1241–1299. https://doi.org/10.2307/1229039

Curtis-Boles, H., Chupina, A. G., & Okubo, Y. (2020). Social justice challenges: Students of color and critical incidents in the graduate classroom. *Training and Education in Professional Psychology, 14*(2), 100–108. https://doi.org/10.1037/tep0000293

Davis, A. Y. (n.d.). *Angela Y. Davis quotes.* Goodreads. www.goodreads.com/quotes/7767240-i-am-no-longer-accepting-the-things-i-cannot-change

Diaz, J. (2016). Acceptance speech, Hispanic Heritage Awards, Washington, DC, September 22. www.pbs.org/video/hispanic-heritage-awards-29th-hispanic-heritage-awards-junot-diaz-full-speech/

Dill, B. T., & Kohlman, M. H. (2011). Intersectionality: A transformative paradigm in feminist theory and social justice. In S. N. Hesse-Biber (Ed.), *Handbook of feminist research: Theory and praxis* (2nd ed.). SAGE.

Erikson, E. H. (1980). *Identity and the life cycle.* W. W. Norton & Co.

Fuller, N., Jr. (n.d.). *Neely Fuller, Jr. quotes.* Goodreads. www.goodreads.com/quotes/2586703-if-you-don-t-understand-white-supremacy-racism-everything-that-you-do

H. B. 2988, 2022 Reg. Sess. (Okla. 2022). http://webserver1.lsb.state.ok.us/cf_pdf/2021-22%20INT/hB/HB2988%20INT.PDF

Helms, J. E. (2012). A legacy of eugenics underlies racial-group comparisons in intelligence testing. *Industrial and Organizational Psychology, 5*(2), 176–179. https://doi.org/10.1111/j.1754-9434.2012.01426.x

hooks, b. (1994). *Teaching to transgress: Education as the practice of freedom.* Routledge.

Lewis, J. A., & Neville, H. A. (2015). Construction and initial validation of the Gendered Racial Microaggressions Scale for Black women. *Journal of Counseling Psychology, 62*(2), 289–302. https://doi.org/10.1037/cou0000062

Marcos, S. (1994). *Utne reader visionary: Subcomandante Marcos.* www.utne.com/politics/utne-reader-visionary-subcomandante-marcos-zapatista-communicator/

Moradi, B., & Grzanka, P. R. (2017). Using intersectionality responsibly: Toward critical epistemology, structural analysis, and social justice activism. *Journal of Counseling Psychology, 64*(5), 500–513. https://doi.org/10.1037/cou0000203

Nelson, G., & Prilleltensky, I. (2010). *Community psychology: In pursuit of liberation and well-being* (2nd ed.). Palgrave Macmillan.

Nelson Mandela Centre of Memory. (2012). Lighting your way to a better future: Speech delivered by Nelson R. Mandela at launch of Mindset Network. http://db.nelsonmandela.org/speeches/pub_view.asp?pg=item&ItemID=NMS909&txts

Pope, K. S., Vasquez, M. J. T., Chavez-Dueñas, N. Y., & Adames, H. Y. (2021). *Ethics in psychotherapy and counseling: A practical guide* (6th ed.). Wiley.

Syed, M., & Fish, J. (2018). Revisiting Erik Erikson's legacy on culture, race, and ethnicity. *Identity: An International Journal of Theory and Research, 18*(4), 274–283. https://doi.org/10.1080/15283488.2018.1523729

Addressing Racial Microaggressions and Racial Enactments in Therapy for BIPOC and Immigrant Clinicians

5

Eunjung Lee, Ran Hu and Tolulola Taiwo-Hanna

When a client and a mental health clinician converse in a session, all intrapsychic and interpersonal psychotherapy components mirror and represent marked and unmarked social norms, expectations, and power. Psychotherapy is a microcosm of society. It is thus inevitable that racist structures and governing race-related dominant values seep into therapy encounters. Since the 1970s, most of the multicultural therapy literature has focused on training white therapists to work with culturally diverse clients (Lee et al., 2018). Meanwhile, this very focus on white clinicians' experiences and learning needs in multicultural scholarship has worked to erase the presence, experiences, and learning needs of Black, Indigenous, and People of Color (BIPOC) clinicians.

This chapter examines the experiences of BIPOC clinicians with racial microaggressions and corresponding racial enactments in their interactions with clients, colleagues, and agencies. The term microaggression was originally described by Black psychiatrist Chester Pierce as "subtle, stunning, often automatic, and non-verbal exchanges, which are 'put downs'" (Pierce et al., 1978, p. 66). More recently, racial microaggressions have been defined as "brief and commonplace daily verbal, behavioral, or environmental indignities, whether intentional or unintentional, that communicate hostile, derogatory, or negative racial slights and insults toward people of color"

DOI: 10.4324/9781003309796-7

(Sue et al., 2007, p. 271). Sue et al. (2007) presented different types of racial microaggressions such as alien in their own land, ascription of intelligence, color blindness, myth of meritocracy, pathologizing cultural values, second-class citizen, and environmental microaggressions. While several studies illustrate how therapists enact racial microaggressions toward BIPOC clients (Lee et al., 2018), few have addressed how racial microaggressions and racial enactments may be directed toward and experienced vicariously by BIPOC clinicians. Therefore, this chapter contributes to addressing this gap and, more importantly, invites BIPOC clinicians to critically reflect on their own therapeutic encounters and how these encounters have impacted the very *person* of who we are as BIPOC clinicians (Aponte et al., 2009).

We are three BIPOC clinicians with years of clinical practice experience and currently in varying stages of academic social work in Canada as a doctoral student (TTH), an early career researcher (RH), and a tenured full professor (EL). While TTH was born and raised in Canada, the other two authors are im/migrants to North America initially as international students and then employed as clinicians. While we all are very much privileged with access to education, employment, and socioeconomic status that many BIPOC do not have, we have experienced ongoing racism and racial microaggressions in our respective clinical practice work. In this chapter, we take turns sharing our own practice experiences of racial microaggressions, while locating ourselves as culturally fluid subjects and contextualizing our practice settings. In particular, we explore three themes: racial enactments in cross-cultural therapy, vicarious exposure to microaggressions in our work with racially or ethnically similar clients, and the complexities of decision-making regarding how to respond to microaggressions in the moment. We use first-person voice when sharing these examples to allow not only the context but also the internal processing of the clinician to be visible to the readers.

Racial Enactments in Cross-Cultural Psychotherapy Encounters

The first author (EL) has over 25 years of clinical practice experience working in outpatient mental health settings in South Korea and North America with culturally diverse clients. One client, Paul (pseudonym), was a white male of British descent working as a medical technician at the same hospital where I worked. Due to his ongoing anxiety and depression, his family physician recommended individual psychotherapy, and he was referred to the outpatient clinic. Paul presented himself as a polite, engaging, and thoughtful person in sessions, accepting the clinician's guidance in reflecting on his earlier and present relationships and their meanings and impacts on him. He often brought a cup of coffee, a plastic water bottle, and/or some snacks to sessions, which he did not necessarily consume during the sessions, but consistently left behind as garbage. At first, I did not notice and without much thought, would quickly clean up before inviting in the next client. Over time, I began to notice my resentment of repeatedly cleaning up after him. One day, as he was preparing to leave at the end of the session, I slipped into an enactment when I asked him, without much reflection, "Are you going to leave your garbage behind today as well?" He apologized, picked up after himself, and left.

Since my own comment was not premeditated, I later reflected on what was going on between me and the client. Freud (1915) pointed out that what is unbearable in one's psyche is repressed deeply, yet seeps out in slips of tongue, jokes, bodily symptoms, and affective residues. An enactment in therapy broadly refers to a therapist's inadvertent actualization of a client's transference as their countertransference experience (Ivey, 2008). Also, as I could not ignore how the labor of cleaning up messes and garbage is represented in society – as the work of someone of a lower social class – I interpreted his actions toward me, a racial other, as a racial microaggression. Racism not only governs our daily life and structural levels of organizations and policies, but also governs our internalized worlds in a racialized society. Thus, racial microaggressions may be one such psychic derivative that Freud noted – a manifestation of one's disavowed psychic reality – that softly otherizes and deeply wounds BIPOC people.

Once I was able to identify his actions as a racial microaggression, it opened space for me to clinically reflect on this racial enactment through the lenses of my own internal experience, the therapeutic relationship, and the clinical issues the client initially brought to therapy. First, I asked myself why I kept cleaning up after him so naturally, only to feel resentful later? Were my actions unconsciously being shaped by my early years of immigration when my credentials from South Korea were not recognized and I had to exert extra effort to prove that I deserved to be valued the same as white social workers? At the same time, had I internalized the expectation that as an Asian woman, I would remain invisible and not make any fuss about the extra workload, an enactment of the well-known model minority stereotype? Was I feeling uneasy and insecure about the fact that I was the only non-doctorate (at that time) racially minoritized social worker in the outpatient psychiatry psychotherapy institute (the other therapists were white male psychiatrists and one white female doctoral-level psychologist)? I was frequently questioned directly and indirectly by many white and BIPOC clients who wondered why they were assigned to me – meaning a racialized clinician with a social work degree who spoke English as a second language.

Once I reflected on what I had contributed to the racial enactment, I was able to see what was happening in the therapeutic relationship more clearly. When a client leaves something tangible or intangible to a clinician, it is a genuine offer of their sufferings or illnesses – derivatives of their psychic pains (Marcus, 2012). What was Paul leaving behind for me? Did he want me to feel what he was feeling in life? The feelings I had included resentment, insecurity, distaste, non-belonging, and feeling small, dismissed, and disrespected. I wondered if this array of feelings was the unconscious communication that he might be displacing as transference projected onto me. This series of critical clinical reflections in the personal and interpersonal realms required meaningful examination in relation to the client's presenting conflicts and issues.

Paul was a single white heterosexual male, the youngest of three children of British parents. He described his father as a physician and stern, and his mother as suffering from long-standing depression. His brothers were both physicians and while growing up, Paul always felt that he was not meeting the expectations of his father, making him feel like that he did not belong, a second-class citizen of the family. In sessions, he often described experiences of being mistreated during interactions with his parents and brothers over family gatherings. At the same time, he also projected his feelings of inadequacy and insecurity onto minoritized others in his job and communities. Although I felt like I was understanding his experiences, it was not until I made the link between his sufferings and the racial microaggression that I really felt it on a visceral level. He was not only using this transferential enactment in the form of a racial microaggression to communicate his experience to me, but he also showed how this racial idea was deeply entrenched in his psyche and enacted in various parts of his life.

With these three levels of critical clinical reflection, I was able to bring up this observation when the next opportunity presented itself. In that session, Paul described his weekend grocery shopping where he witnessed a Black mother shopping with a toddler fussing to such an extent that the mother could not finish the shopping. He made a comment about "how inconsiderate she was that she did not bother putting things back in their original place before she left the store." When I inquired as to why he was so upset, he noted that "she was not supposed to do that." When I inquired further about how he would have felt if she was a white mother, he paused and reflected. Given the strength of our alliance, he did not feel that I was accusing him of being racist but acknowledged that he might have not had the same reaction to a white mother, and may have assumed that both the child and mother had had a long tiring day. He then noted that he had different standards for different people, which was not fair. At that point, I asked if he noticed that he left things behind after sessions for me to clean up. He apologized, yet admitted that he started to notice this pattern once I mentioned it. He acknowledged that given his own hierarchical family dynamic, he could see that he had a tendency to rank others as "first- or second-class citizens" as well. After this critical point of conversation, Paul began to resist any dismissive treatment by members of his family, in hierarchical work relationships between medical doctors and technicians, and in his interactions with BIPOC individuals, including me. One day, as he was picking up his coffee cup after the session, he appreciated me noticing the subtle and non-verbal micro-exchanges in our therapeutic interactions that signified both clinical and racial issues in our lives.

Vicarious Exposure to Racial Microaggressions in Our Work with Racially Similar Clients

The second author (RH) identifies as a migrant woman, born and raised in China. She has lived in North America for 14 years. Her migration experience as a constant temporary visitor in both the United States and Canada has been critical to the shaping of her own exploration into her (assigned) identity as a woman of color across personal, professional, and academic settings. This case example, drawn from her counseling work with im/migrant women survivors of trafficking, illustrates how in racially or ethnically matched clinician–client dyads, BIPOC clinicians may experience vicarious exposure to racial stress through their clients' direct experiences of racial microaggressions.

Mei (pseudonym) is a Chinese migrant woman living in an anti-trafficking transitional housing facility serving a culturally diverse client population. In one of our counseling sessions, Mei shared an incident where she felt judged by one of the housing managers (woman-identified, American-born) when she had accidentally put a piece of foil wrap in the microwave while heating up her lunch. Mei described that the housing manager appeared to be "very upset" and said to her, "This is dangerous! Everybody here knows how to use a microwave. You don't have microwaves in China?" Listening to my client describe this incident with the housing manager made me feel unsettled. The three of us quickly convened to clarify that Mei was aware of how to use a microwave safely but was just emotionally overwhelmed as the "incident" happened. Even though the conversation concluded on a pleasant note, I continued to feel unsettled and confused about what the "incident" was that needed to be addressed. Was it only about resident safety in the kitchen? Was it necessary for me to clarify that microwaves do exist in China? Why did I feel unsettled? To some extent, I almost felt I was being subtly attacked. It was not until almost a year later, at a social work continuing education workshop, that I recalled Mei's experience of this racial microaggression and its vicarious impact on me, neither of which, unfortunately, was explicitly named and addressed during my conversation with Mei and the housing manager.

As shown in this clinical encounter, clinicians' vicarious exposure to clients' experiences of racial microaggressions can provoke a wide range of emotions and introduce a number of clinical challenges. First, the clinician might struggle with identifying and naming the incident as a form of racial microaggression. Second, clinicians who have internalized a particular racial microaggression may attempt to normalize the incident, especially given the "micro" nature of these types of incidents (e.g., justifying the housing manager's concerns about residents' safety). Further, clinical decisions, for example about whether to "address the incident with the manager," might be complicated by structurally and organizationally constructed power differentials that exist between BIPOC im/migrant clinicians and their non-immigrant colleagues and supervisors. Clinical supervision that lacks racial and cultural consciousness may further compound how BIPOC clinicians experience and address these incidents. For example, the supervisor might not recognize the racial microaggression, or shift the burden of addressing the microaggression back to the racialized clinician by "reaffirming" that the clinician is the "cultural expert."

Finally, challenging and avoiding the normalization of racial microaggressions requires that the BIPOC clinician recognize and reflect on their possible internalization of microaggressions experienced vicariously. Supervision and consultation with trusted colleagues can be useful. Supervisors and clinicians must practice critical reflexivity on an ongoing basis, including recognizing the prevalence of racial microaggressions in the workplace and proactively reflecting on how their own experiences of racialization and power held in the organization may shape their assumptions and ways of communicating and relating to others.

Navigating Racial Microaggressions as "the Angry Black Woman"

The third author (TTH) is a Black, dark-skinned second-generation immigrant with Nigerian-born parents and also a first-generation, cis-gender Canadian woman. Two years after getting my MSW degree, I was working in an interdisciplinary organization that supports individuals experiencing acute psychiatric symptoms. Of note, the team I worked with here was quite ethno-racially diverse. At that time, I worked with a client named Betty (pseudonym), a middle-aged white woman, who presented with clinical depression. While conducting my initial psychosocial assessment, she accused me of yelling at her, and demanded to know why I was so angry. I recall being quite puzzled as I had not raised my voice or altered my tone in our brief time together. I inquired as to what I had said or asked that elicited that judgment, but she would not tell me. Instead, she requested that we meet at another time when I had "calmed down."

After this interaction, I reflected on my tone, the questions I had asked, and my use of self (particularly body language) during the psychosocial assessment. When I could not identify any specific issues, I wondered if the client perceived me as being angry because of something I had actually said, or if it was due to my Blackness. I remember dismissing the thought of racism immediately as I was mentally exhausted just thinking about how I would need to judge the validity of the evidence to determine if the situation was a racial microaggression. Instead, I set my attention to writing an action plan for how I might approach her in session the following day.

During our daily staff meeting the next morning, the client's nurse for the day, a Black male, shared that Betty did not wish to work with him because in her words, he was "angry and aggressive," and she "did not feel safe" working with him. Further, she provided no specific examples of what he did to make her feel this way. The silence in the room after he gave this report was deafening; even I did not speak up about my own experience with Betty. I did eventually check-in with the nurse later and told him about my encounters with Betty even though I did not feel emotionally prepared to share my experience with the whole team that morning.

Black people are often stereotyped as angry, aggressive, and dangerous (Walley-Jean, 2009). In the early days of my practice, I attempted to pre-emptively mitigate this stereotype by speaking softly, carefully crafting my every word, hiding my hair under a straight weave, and dressing in more neutral tones to avoid standing out too much. What I wish I had known then is that regardless of how quiet I am, my presence, to some, would always be loud. At that time, I stuck with my "softer" Black girl approach, and to some extent it was effective. I was able to establish a rapport with Betty by asking her if moving forward, we could use immediacy to identify when she felt unsafe with me so that I could adjust my mannerisms or tone in the moment. This "solution" worked, but at what cost? One of the questions I have had to discern throughout my practice is when to address racism directly with my clients. In hindsight, it may have been appropriate for me to ask her in our later sessions, after an alliance had been established, if she had initially felt unsafe or threatened because of my racial identity. Had she denied this, the question would have still brought her unconscious bias to her conscious awareness, even if she ultimately chose not to address this. Had she accepted, it might have provided us with an opportunity to work together and address this racial bias as a target in our therapeutic work.

Further, I would advise BIPOC practitioners to seek support, and to identify who they can debrief these kinds of situations with, even before they arise. It likely would have bolstered me, and perhaps prevented me from feeling so isolated in my experience. It also may have freed me from the moral distress I experienced by not speaking up regarding the racist incident (Campbell et al., 2016). Though I checked in with the nurse privately, this was a missed opportunity to facilitate a discussion with our team about the barriers that Black clinicians face in the context of anti-Black racism. Notwithstanding, it is not our job alone to identify these teachable moments. Any team member could have initiated a discussion about racial microaggressions toward BIPOC individuals in practice, yet no one did.

Conclusion

In this chapter, we illustrated different ways that racial microaggressions have surfaced in three BIPOC clinicians' therapeutic encounters with clients. Racial microaggressions can be racially enacted within therapeutic interactions, vicariously experienced by clinicians, and provoke feelings of isolation in the absence of others who validate their experiences. While the examples we provide are specific to the authors' positionalities and lived experiences as BIPOC clinicians, we hope that they invite other BIPOC clinicians to reflect on and share their own experiences and lessons learned from their own race-related clinical encounters. Fricker (2007) notes that when one's experiences are acknowledged as valid sources of information, one's dignity and humanity are truly valued. It is critical that we remind ourselves not to dismiss racial undercurrents and messages that are subtle, non-verbal, and marked as normative in practice and society.

In lieu of a list of practical strategies for managing racial microaggressions in therapeutic contexts, we invite the reader to engage in a process of self-reflection: When have you experienced racial microaggressions in practice? What did you do? Upon reflection, what do you wish you could have done? Where might you need to have grace for yourself, and how can you practice this even now? What might you do in the future if a similar situation arises? Most importantly, to whom can you turn for support?

Addressing the challenges of racial microaggressions requires a multilevel approach with attention to structural and organizational (in)equities. We must, first of all, recognize that racial microaggressions can be experienced, both directly and vicariously, at intrapsychic and interpersonal levels; they can also be legitimized by structurally and organizationally produced power differentials. Supervision is imperative to processing microaggressions and planning next steps. Beyond ensuring ongoing check-in with supervisees, supervisors, especially when supervising a clinician with different cultural and racial experiences, should not assume their knowledge of microaggression but humbly collaborate with the supervisee in co-learning, processing, and addressing micro-aggressive incidents and the impacts on the supervisee. Ongoing workshops on racial microaggressions, such as intergroup dialogues, may be useful when thoughtfully planned, including consideration of organizational hierarchies and power differentials rooted in societal racial injustice. It is also necessary for supervisors or teams with BIPOC clinicians to check-in with them regularly to ensure that they are working in an inclusive and affirming professional environment. While having open dialogue about experiences of microaggressions with colleagues and supervisors is an important step, it is imperative for BIPOC clinicians to reflect on their safety and readiness for such conversations and to give themselves permission to prioritize their own well-being in deciding how best to proceed.

At the organizational level, the leadership team must proactively promote a type of organizational culture that is conducive to staff's learning and growth in recognizing and addressing microaggressions, whether directly or vicariously experienced. Due to power differentials and employees' diverse experiences of and exposure to cultures and racialization processes, encountering and addressing incidents of microaggression can evoke anxiety and fear. Therefore, developing organizational policies that are not based on individual blame and punishment, but instead facilitate cross-cultural, relationship-focused, and open dialogue, is crucial not only for strengthening the organization's capacity to respond effectively, but also for reducing moral distress among BIPOC clinicians when racial microaggressions are dismissed.

References

Aponte, H. J., Powell, F. D., Brooks, S., Watson, M. F., Litzke, C., Lawless, J., & Johnson, E. (2009). Training the person of the therapist in an academic setting. *Journal of Marital and Family Therapy, 35*(4), 381–394. https://doi.org/10.1111/j.1752-0606.2009.00123.x

Campbell, S. M., Ulrich, C. M., & Grady, C. (2016). A broader understanding of moral distress. *The American Journal of Bioethics, 16*(12), 2–9. https://doi.org/10.1080/15265 161.2016.1239782

Freud, S. (1915). *The unconscious.* In J. Strachey (Ed. & Trans.), *Standard edition* (Vol. 14). Hogarth.

Fricker, M. (2007). *Epistemic injustice: Power and the ethics of knowing.* Oxford University Press. https://doi.org/10.1093/acprof:oso/9780198237907.001.0001

Ivey, G. (2008). Enactment controversies: A critical review of current debates. *International Journal of Psychoanalysis, 89*(1), 19–38. doi:10.1111/j.1745–8315.2007.00003.x

Lee, E., Tsang, A. K. T., Bogo, M., Johnstone, M., & Herschman, J. (2018). Enactments of racial microaggression in everyday therapeutic encounters. *Smith College Studies in Social Work, 88*(3), 211–236. https://doi.org/10.1080/00377317.2018.1476646

Marcus, E. (2012). *Psychosis and near psychosis: Ego functions, symbol structure, and treatment.* Springer. https://doi.org/10.1007/978-1-4613-9197-5_1

Pierce, C. M., Carew, J. V., Pierce-Gonzales, D., & Wills, D. (1978). An experiment in racism: TV commercials. In C. Pierce (Ed.), *Television and education.* SAGE. https://doi.org/10.1177/001312457701000105

Sue, D. W., Capodilupo, C. M., Torino, G. C., Bucceri, J. M., Holder, A. M. B., Nadal, K. L., & Esquilin, M. (2007). Racial microaggressions in everyday life: Implications for clinical practice. *American Psychologist, 62*(4), 271–286. https://doi.org/10.1037/0003-066X.62.4.271

Walley-Jean, J. C. (2009). Debunking the myth of the "Angry Black Woman": An exploration of anger in young African American women. *Black Women, Gender + Families, 3*(2), 68–86. https://doi.org/10.1353/bwg.0.0011

Decolonizing Research   **6**

Some Tips to Heal the Damages of a Sick World

E. J. R. David

Colonial research and education have been the tools that erased my peoples, our ways, and our worldviews (Constantino, 1970). Colonial research and education were the tools through which my peoples' bodies and cultures were inferiorized, the tools through which my peoples' minds were colonized. My peoples and I have struggled – and continue to struggle – to unlearn generations of colonial programming and heal from its deep and insidious, but at the same time pervasive and wide-ranging, damages. I share a bit of my journey here.

I grew up in the Philippines where light skin was admired, English was valued, and Indigenous peoples were regarded as uncivilized savages. The research that guided what was taught in our schools reinforced and perpetuated these dehumanizing messages. I grew up in a context wherein everything that was "Made in the USA" is valued and associated with better quality, while anything "Local" or "Made in the Philippines" is regarded as cheap, of poor quality, and only for the poor. I grew up surrounded by relatives, friends, teachers, elders, and authority figures who talked about ways to make their skin color lighter, or at least, ways to prevent their skin from getting too dark. I was schooled in an Americanized educational system where English was used for teaching, where I was taught that Spain discovered and civilized my peoples – then the US liberated us – and where I was inculcated with American values and ideals. My teachers taught me that America was the land of milk and honey.

DOI: 10.4324/9781003309796-8

The reward systems in colonial and even postcolonial Philippines were designed to be pro-white. Thus, for Filipinos, our success and even our survival depended on how much we understood and adopted whiteness. So before I – and many other Filipino immigrants like me – even got to the US, we have already been socialized for generations to be pro-white (David & Nadal, 2013) and to believe that being pro-white is necessary to succeed.

The education I received in the US when I moved here as a 14-year-old, unsurprisingly, did not challenge the miseducation I received in the Philippines. The US was founded on stolen Indigenous lands, and was built on the backs of enslaved Black people. This country was founded on the myth of white supremacy. So it's not surprising that the institutions in this country – especially the educational institutions where research mostly resides – also reflect white supremacy. White supremacy is the air that this country breathes. It is not surprising, then, that the people who are trying to be a part of this country – like me and other immigrants – end up breathing this air of white supremacy. It's inevitable. The reward system in this country is designed to reward people for being pro-white. In this country, pro-whiteness is required to succeed, and many of us have come to believe that pro-whiteness is required to survive.

Pro-whiteness is part of the Americanization process.

Damages of a Sick World

The research on how oppression affects People of Color and other oppressed groups is clear: oppression can lead to poor mental health, trauma, poor self-esteem, lower life satisfaction, substance use, suicidal ideation (for a review, see David & Derthick, 2018). But oppressed peoples don't just deal with the oppression we directly experience. We also are forced to deal with the oppressive experiences that our friends and family face. But not only that, we also feel the oppressive experiences faced by other people who we don't even know but who look like us or who we have a shared identity with. When we see maltreatments of our people, when we see on TV how our people are dehumanized and othered and inferiorized or terrorized or murdered, we feel that. It makes us anxious, stressed out, scared, and maybe even depressed too. Vicarious oppression affects us too (Chae et al., 2021).

To take this concept of vicarious oppression even further, the oppressive experiences of our ancestors also affect us today. Historical trauma can be passed down to later generations (Brave Heart et al., 2011). There is emerging epigenetic research that supports this (Kellerman, 2013; Yehuda et al., 2016). All of those historical experiences of racism, of colonialism, of imperialism that regarded our communities as savages, as uncivilized, as inferior – those messages that damaged and messed up our ancestors – they can still inflict damage on us today.

Even further, many of us have internalized these oppressive messages and have succumbed to them, coming to accept and believe that our peoples are indeed inferior (David, 2014). Today many of us feel ashamed or embarrassed of our roots. Many of us might use skin-whitening products, or straighten our hair. Many of us might look down on other people in our communities, and even be hostile to and inflict violence on those who we think are not "Americanized enough." We make fun of their accents, and regard them as backward or less intelligent. Many of us even get to the point where we minimize the oppressive experiences we've faced, thinking that such oppression is OK because at least we're here, and that we should just work harder on our accents, work harder on our jobs, work harder on being American – work harder on becoming white – so that we can avoid racism. Many of us have become convinced that the closer we are to whiteness, then the better off we will be.

So sure, the damages of living in a sick, oppressive world include well-known mental health consequences: distress, trauma, low self-esteem, anxiety, depression, substance use, suicide. But the effects of living in an oppressive world also include loss of culture, loss of pride, loss of connection to our ancestors, loss of identity, and loss of connection with our peoples, therefore putting us in a vulnerable position to replace what was our own with what this sick, oppressive world tells us is better. Putting us in a vulnerable position to accept white supremacy.

It was not until I was lucky enough to attend college and graduate school, and was given the opportunity to learn about the history of my people and critique the systems – including colonial educational and epistemological systems – that perpetuated our oppression, that I began to unlearn white supremacy as the standard. But this learning and unlearning should not be just left up to luck, or only be available to the privileged few. It has to be more accessible so we can cease conducting oppressive research and move toward more healing ways of knowing.

Five Tips Toward Decolonizing Research

So what kind of research can help us heal the damages of an oppressive world? Decolonizing research is research that heals and corrects for the injustices and harms done by a sick world – including the harms done by research and education itself – by centering and valuing the experiences, worldviews, and ways of knowing and doing of historically oppressed peoples (Smith, 1999). And the research must not just heal, liberate, and empower individuals and communities, it must also be research that heals and improves a broken, sick society.

For research to be healing, I have five general tips.

Tip #1: Look Beyond the Individual

We as a field have prioritized and overly valued intra-individual factors (i.e., genes, biology, thoughts, feelings, behaviors), with the assumption that these are universal across all peoples. This is a direct result of Western dominance in psychology, in that the way we've approached psychological science is a reflection of Western values and emphasis on individuality, reductionism, elemental thinking, and breaking things down to separate parts. The way that we do psychology has evolved toward a strong focus on identifying and modifying factors that are inside individuals (Jessor, 1958; Rose, 1998).

But we've learned that even the most basic intra-individual factors and processes are influenced by our environment (Henrich et al., 2010). For historically oppressed groups, this is especially important because many of our concerns don't exist because of us, or because of something within us. Our problems are not because of something inherent about us, or because of internal processes – like our cognitions or perceptions. What's wrong is not inside us, and our suffering isn't because of something inherent about us or our community. This tendency to problematize our peoples is very colonial. This tendency to make our bodies, our worldviews, our cultures, and our ways of life the problem is very colonial.

Our problems and struggles exist because of oppressive environments. So we must look at extra-individual factors: Colonialism, neocolonialism, racism, all forms of oppression. We must go beyond our focus on individual thoughts, feelings, and behaviors, and also be influenced by other works in critical race theory, postcolonial studies, ethnic studies – works that encourage divergent thinking and shift our focus to oppressive systems (Rappaport, 1981).

Tip #2: Make Social Change

Because we tend to focus on intra-individual factors to explain phenomena, we then also tend to intervene on the individual level. We try to change the way a person thinks, the way they feel, and how they behave and react. Our interventions have focused on helping people and communities cope and tolerate an oppressive environment. This tendency to look for individual-level factors to explain phenomena, and consequently our tendency to focus on making intra-individual changes, ultimately just keeps the status quo. Individual-focused work keeps an oppressive system in place.

We must challenge our focus on individual-level factors that lead to our tendency to blame victims of oppression for their own oppression. One way to make social change is to move beyond simply being scholars to being "Scholactivists." Researchers, academics, and scholars historically influence society indirectly through "third parties" or – using academic terms – through mediating variables. Some examples of these mediating variables include activists, reporters or journalists, policymakers, or administrators. Not only was our influence indirect, it was also passive in that we tend to just completely depend on third parties; an almost complete or full mediation to influence society. We simply hope that somehow our work will get noticed, that it will be read, inspire, spark action, and be shared with and applied to society.

Over the past few years, however, there has been a growing movement among scholars to no longer be so passive. Many scholars no longer just hope that their message will be conveyed through mediators. They now want a direct effect, or at least a more active, significant role in influencing society. Scholars are becoming more like activists (Nadal, 2017).

To do this, we need to develop and engage in new skills like advocacy, community organizing, consulting, and writing op-eds, magazine articles, blog posts, or other publications for "general audiences" to make psychology more accessible. We need to go beyond our conventional roles and be more useful to society. We need to give psychology away (Miller, 1969). We must remember that most people also aren't privileged enough to go to college or attend conferences and hear presentations. Therefore, we need to go beyond hotel ballrooms, classrooms, and lecture halls and present our work to the community. We need to go to community halls, churches, and recreation centers to share and apply our work with the people who we are supposed to be serving in the first place.

Tip #3: Regard Values as Strengths

From the beginning of this chapter and through the discussions I've shared so far, I have revealed a little bit of myself, my struggles, and my values – I have revealed my heart. And although I now believe this is OK, this hasn't always been the case. There was a time when I felt bad for being so passionate in my work, for being so involved and emotional and connected. I felt like I was less of a researcher and scholar for not being separate, distant, and objective enough. I used to believe that my intimate connections with my work somehow make it less rigorous and less valid. But I don't believe this anymore.

In the field of psychology, in our effort to become a legitimate science, we've come to subscribe to notions of objectivity. We were taught to see values – including our own – as confounding variables, as noise, as mess, as limitations in our research. We began to believe that we must be separate and distant from our "subjects" (Bornstein, 1999; Mascolo, 2016). We have been brainwashed to believe that to be true scholars we must become uninvolved robots. But this is the farthest thing from reality, especially for members of historically oppressed groups.

For many of us, we do the work we do because it is personal to us, it is close to our hearts, and because we care. We do this work for our communities, our ancestors, our elders, and our youth. This is our heart's work. So to pretend that this is noise and a limitation is not only untrue and not a reflection of reality, it is also wrong. It is wrong because the fact that we care, the fact that our work is our passion, the fact that it is close to our hearts is not a limitation – it's a strength (e.g., Brayda & Boyce, 2014; Ghaffari, 2019; Hill, 2000; Watts et al., 1999). Colonial science has convinced us that our involvement and enmeshment are weaknesses, when in reality they are strengths. We must resist this.

Tip #4: Have a Strengths Orientation

A strong reflection of how colonial our typical scientific approach has been is our tendency to focus on what's wrong with people and communities;

their deficits, illnesses, and diseases (Seligman & Csikszentmihalyi, 2000). This is reflective of one of the more critical features of colonization. Based on Frantz Fanon's works, Becky Tatum (2000) proposed a four-phase model of colonialism. According to Tatum, the first phase is the forced entry of a foreign group into a new territory with the intention of exploiting its natural resources. To facilitate this, the second phase is when everything of the colonizer is associated with superiority and everything of the colonized is associated with inferiority. This is done to create a clear contrast between the supposedly more civilized, more advanced, more enlightened ways of the colonizer and the supposedly primitive and savage ways of the colonized. Once this is accomplished, then a justification is established to put domination and oppression into practice, which is the third phase. The fourth phase is when systems are put in place to train, educate, civilize, tame, or save the "savages."

Mirroring what typically happens during colonialism, we as scholars, scientists, or researchers have been trained to identify issues, deficits, and other things we must fix and correct in the communities we are "interested" in. We tend to focus on finding things we must educate people about, or train them how to do; things we must do to bring them up to our level, enlighten them, civilize them. Again, this is very colonial. We must fight this tendency, and we must balance it out by also looking at people's and communities' strengths. We must also learn from communities and see how different ways of conceptualizing phenomena and solutions can be applied to addressing many of the most pressing issues facing our world today.

Tip #5: Reverse the Expert–Subject Dynamic

Another strong reflection of how colonial our typical scientific approach has been is the typical distinction and power differential between the researcher and subject, between the "expert" and the "naïve layperson." This is very colonial. Once again, this contrast between the supposedly more educated, more aware, more knowledgeable, more enlightened "researcher" and the naïve other clearly mirrors the dynamic between the supposedly superior, more civilized colonizer and the inferior, savage, primitive, barbaric, backward colonized. This power differential between the researcher and subject must be challenged, and changed (Andress et al., 2020). In fact, we must reverse it. We must yield the power. The communities must lead. Instead of being the expert researcher, or teacher, or leader, or doctor from so and so university, when we go out to the community we are simply collaborators (Wallerstein & Duran, 2003). We are allies. We are accomplices.

So we need to stop our standard operating procedures, evaluate them, critique them, and constantly gauge how (in)appropriate, (in)compatible, and (dis)empowering or colonial they are. Then we must collaborate. We should not conduct research on communities; instead we must do research *with* them. Communities must lead and have control over every phase of the research from developing the topics and questions and methods of inquiry, to who owns the data, all the way to how and to whom the findings are disseminated. Most importantly, we must listen. We must regard the experiences, the voices, and the lived realities of oppressed peoples as equally valid and legitimate as the dominant "theories" and the "scientific knowledge" we are trained in. We must center the voices of the people who we are purporting to serve.

Conclusion

I want to close with a quote from James Baldwin (1962), who said: "Many of them indeed know better, but as you will discover, people find it very difficult to act on what they know. To act is to be committed and to be committed is to be in danger."

I think many of us – especially those of us in academia – do know better, and now it's a matter of acting on what we know. I understand that many of us feel powerless and vulnerable, and so acting on what we know might be difficult. Many of us might feel like we don't have a choice but to play the game right now, and just survive it and hopefully get to a point in our lives where we have enough power to then act on what we know. I understand that. But please remember that if you commit to act on what you know – if you take a risk and put yourself in danger to do what you know is right – there are many of us with you. You are not alone.

References

Andress, L., Hall, T., Davis, S., Levine, J., Cripps, K., & Guinn, D. (2020). Addressing power dynamics in community-engaged research partnerships. *Journal of Patient-Reported Outcomes, 4*(1), 24. https://doi.org/10.1186/s41687-020-00191-z

Baldwin, J. (1962). A letter to my nephew. *The Progressive.* https://progressive.org/magazine/letter-nephew/

Bornstein, R. F. (1999). Objectivity and subjectivity in psychological science: Embracing and transcending psychology's positivist tradition. *The Journal of Mind and Behavior, 20*(1), 1–16. www.jstor.org/stable/43853874

Brave Heart, M. Y., Chase, J., Elkins, J., & Altschul, D. B. (2011). Historical trauma among Indigenous Peoples of the Americas: Concepts, research, and clinical considerations. *Journal of Psychoactive Drugs, 43*(4), 282–290. doi:10.1080/02791072.2011.628913.

Brayda, W. C., & Boyce, T. D. (2014). So you really want to interview me? Navigating "sensitive" qualitative research interviewing. *International Journal of Qualitative Methods, 13*(1), 318–334.

Chae, D. H., Yip, T., Martz, C. D., et al. (2021). Vicarious racism and vigilance during the COVID-19 pandemic: Mental health implications among Asian and Black Americans. *Public Health Reports, 136*(4), 508–517. doi:10.1177/00333549211018675.

Constantino, R. (1970). The mis-education of the Filipino. *Journal of Contemporary Asia, 1*(1), 20–36.

David, E. J. R. (2014). *Internalized oppression: The psychology of marginalized groups.* Springer.

David, E. J. R., & Derthick, A. O. (2018). *The psychology of oppression.* Springer Publishing.

David, E. J. R., & Nadal, K. L. (2013). The colonial context of Filipino American immigrants' psychological experiences. *Cultural Diversity and Ethnic Minority Psychology, 19*(3), 298–309. https://doi.org/10.1037/a0032903

Ghaffari, R. (2019). Doing gender research as a "gendered subject": Challenges and sparks of being a dual-citizen woman researcher in Iran. *Anthropology of the Middle East, 14*(2), 130–142.

Henrich, J., Heine, S. J., & Norenzayan, A. (2010). The weirdest people in the world? *Behavioral and Brain Sciences, 33*(2–3), 61–83.

Hill, J. (2000). A rationale for the integration of spirituality into community psychology. *Journal of Community Psychology, 28*, 139–149.

Jessor, R. (1958). The problem of reductionism in psychology. *Psychological Review, 65*(3), 170–178. https://doi.org/10.1037/h0045385

Kellerman, N. P. F. (2013). Epigenetic transmission of holocaust trauma: Can nightmares be inherited? *The Israel Journal of Psychiatry and Related Sciences, 50*(1), 30–39.

Mascolo, M. F. (2016). Beyond subjectivity and objectivity: The intersubjective foundations of psychological science. *Integrative Psychological & Behavioral Science, 50*, 185–195.

Miller, G. A. (1969). Psychology as a means of promoting human welfare. *American Psychologist, 24*(12), 1063–1075. https://doi.org/10.1037/h0028988

Nadal, K. L. (2017). "Let's get in formation": On becoming a psychologist–activist in the 21st century. *American Psychologist, 72*(9), 935–946. https://doi.org/10.1037/amp0000212

Rappaport, J. (1981). In praise of paradox: A social policy of empowerment over prevention. *American Journal of Community Psychology, 9*(1), 1–25. https://doi.org/10.1007/BF00896357

Rose, S. (1998). What is wrong with reductionist explanations of behaviour? *Novartis Found Symposium, 213*, 176–186. doi:10.1002/9780470515488.ch13.

Seligman, M. E. P., & Csikszentmihalyi, M. (2000). Positive psychology: An introduction. *American Psychologist, 55*(1), 5–14.

Smith, L. T. (1999). *Decolonizing methodologies: Research and Indigenous peoples.* Zed Books.

Tatum, B. L. (2000). Toward a neocolonial model of adolescent crime and violence. *Journal of Contemporary Criminal Justice, 16*(2), 157–170. https://doi.org/10.1177/1043986200016002003

Wallerstein, N., & Duran, B. (2003). The conceptual, historical and practical roots of community based participatory research and related participatory traditions. In M. Minkler & N. Wallerstein (Eds.), *Community based participatory research for health.* Jossey Bass.

Watts, R. J., Griffith, D. M., & Adbul-Adil, J. (1999). Sociopolitical development as an antidote for oppression – theory and action. *American Journal of Community Psychology, 27*, 255–271.

Yehuda, R., Daskalakis, N. P., Bierer, L. M., et al. (2016). Holocaust exposure induced intergenerational effects on FKBP5 methylation. *Biological Psychiatry, 1*(80), 372–380.

Coping with Racism and Oppression in Higher Education

Overcoming the Impostor Phenomenon

Kevin Cokley

As I enter into my 25th year as a professor, I still wonder how a little Black boy from the small rural town of Pilot Mountain, NC was able to obtain a doctoral degree in counseling psychology. It was a dream come true to be hired by Southern Illinois University Carbondale (SIUC) for my first academic position. When the University of Missouri – Columbia recruited and hired me from SIUC, I was so excited to be working at a public flagship school. I was a faculty member in arguably the top counseling psychology program in the country and thought I would end my career there, but life had other plans. After three years I was recruited and hired by the University of Texas at Austin (UT Austin). I'll never forget the level of pride I felt to be working at what has been called a "public Ivy." I distinctly remember looking at the pedigrees of my new colleagues, which included many of the most prestigious universities in the country, and feeling both pride to be associated with them as well as feeling self-conscious about my doctoral pedigree. I wondered whether I truly belonged, even though I had already proven myself as a scholar. I continued "grinding" and proving myself as a scholar and eventually as a leader. While there were challenges during my tenure at UT Austin, I thought of UT Austin as being the pinnacle of my career and my final career destination. I had already far surpassed my own career expectations as I never imagined that I would

DOI: 10.4324/9781003309796-9

ever work at an institution like UT Austin. However, once again life threw me a curve ball. During my 15 years working at UT Austin, I often fantasized about working at my dream institution, the University of Michigan (UM).

In the Fall of 2021, everything changed when I received an email from the Chair of the Psychology Department at UM indicating that both my spouse and I were being targeted for hire. To make a long story short, we were hired and are now full professors at UM! I have been on an improbable academic and professional journey where I have experienced both the lowest of academic and professional lows (e.g., losing my academic scholarship and being put on academic probation in my freshman year, having a promotion and tenure committee give me a negative vote for promotion to full professor) and the highest of professional highs (e.g., receiving an endowed professorship, being inducted as a Fellow in the University of Texas System Academy of Distinguished Teachers). As I reflect on my career it is perhaps serendipitous that a few years ago I came across research on the impostor phenomenon. Throughout my academic and professional career I have constantly battled feelings of impostorism (long before I was familiar with the term). It has often been said among professors that research is "me-search," the idea that a researcher uses their personal experiences when pursuing scientific questions. My positionality as an African American man who has navigated predominantly white and often elite educational spaces as a student and professor has made me particularly susceptible to impostor feelings. In this chapter I will share some personal reflections about the challenges I've faced, issues I continue to grapple with, strengths and supports that have sustained me, and lessons I've learned along the way.

Discovery of the Impostor Phenomenon

Sometime around 2010 as I was conducting a literature search I came across an article by Clance and Imes (1978) that would change the course of my program of research and, in many ways, change the course of my professional life. In that article, Clance and Imes coined the term impostor phenomenon (IP) to describe an internal sense of being an intellectual phony. They believed that IP was particularly prevalent among a group of high-achieving women they had worked with in individual psychotherapy, interactional groups, and college classes. Yet, in spite of their demonstrated excellence, the women believed they had fooled others into believing they were intelligent.

While Clance and Imes were focused on high achieving women, the article resonated very deeply with me for reasons not necessarily related to gender or sex. I began to reflect on my experiences as a Black undergraduate student, and how gratified I was to know that there was an actual term to describe my feelings and experience in college. I started to look for how race and culture were being addressed in the IP literature. As I began to think more deeply about the article, and other early articles about IP, I wondered how IP impacted African American and other minoritized students. However, I was struck by the fact that race and culture were not typically part of the discussions about IP.

I knew that the IP construct would fit well in my program of research, which focuses on the psychosocial experiences of African American and other minoritized students in predominantly white colleges and universities. Intuitively it seemed to me that minoritized students would have to contend with impostor feelings in predominantly white colleges and universities. This led to my first published empirical study involving IP (Cokley et al., 2013). In that study we found that impostor feelings were stronger predictors of mental health than minority status stress. This finding was significant because it confirmed the idea that IP is an important construct to examine among minoritized students.

Since the publication of that article, there have been additional empirical studies published on IP among African American and other minoritized students (e.g., Bernard et al., 2017; Peteet et al., 2015). Several of these studies have been published by my research lab (e.g., Cokley et al., 2017; Stone et al., 2018). These articles focus on the IP construct, as currently conceptualized, with a minoritized group. One of the articles suggests that IP should be understood using a culturally informed framework (Stone et al., 2018). This perspective was a result of several discussions in my lab where we discussed the idea that IP is experienced differently among minoritized students. We later characterized this as a **racialized impostor phenomenon**. This perspective is largely absent from the traditional IP literature, and I believe has contributed to the current interest in examining IP among minoritized students.

Professional Reflections

I have dealt with impostor feelings at various points throughout my career. My earliest recollections are when I was an assistant professor at Southern

Illinois University Carbondale (SIUC). At the time that I applied I only had one publication. The article was not empirical, and it was published in a relatively new and unknown niche journal, *The Journal of African American Men*. I told the chair of the search committee that I did not have a published empirical study to present, but I did have some data from a research study that I had collected. I was advised that for the purposes of a job talk, I should present some empirical data. (Side note: I was young, naïve, and did not have good professional mentoring to help me navigate this process.) I presented data on a study entitled "An exploratory study of spirituality and racial identity among African American women." I gave the job talk and competently answered the questions during Q&A. Much to my surprise I received a job offer! Later I found out from one of my new colleagues that the position had initially been offered to another individual (a current academic "star" in the field) who turned it down. My colleague disclosed to me that while I was viewed as needing growth in the area of research, my presentation skills suggested that I would be a strong teacher. However, I held onto the comments about me as a researcher. This no doubt fueled my impostor feelings. I was also very aware of the fact that I was the only African American professor in the department, so naturally I wondered about how much my race was a factor in being hired. My impostor feelings were further fueled by walking the hallways of the Psychology Department and seeing the publications of my colleagues prominently displayed on the walls. I did not have any empirical publications to display, so I knew that I had a lot of work to do to prove that I truly belonged there.

As a pre-tenured assistant professor I worked tirelessly to get published. I was single with no family and spent much of my evenings and weekends writing. I was the classic workaholic! I was incredibly happy when I published my first two empirical papers in the *Journal of College Student Development* and the *Journal of Black Psychology*. My publishing strategy was essentially to get published in any journal that was appropriate for the kind of research I was doing. I was not driven by publishing in "mainstream," prestigious psychology journals. It was important for my research self-efficacy to see my name in print.

While the idea of impact factors was just starting to emerge, the prestige of journals was still important in my department. I remember talking to the chair of the Psychology Department about publication outlets. I wanted to know if it was important for me to publish in what was considered to be prestigious journals. His response was that it would be good if I could publish in some top tier journals. Once again, my impostor feelings flared up. Did I really have the ability to publish in a top tier journal? Was I smart enough?

Even though I already had ten empirical publications in rank by my third year (nine first authored), I wondered if I had the ability to publish in my discipline's top empirical journal, the *Journal of Counseling Psychology* (JCP). I decided to submit a manuscript to JCP. After several "revise and resubmits" it was finally accepted! During this time I also had another paper accepted in the *Cultural Diversity and Ethnic Minority Psychology* (CDEMP) journal. I'll never forget how proud I was when the director of the counseling psychology program announced during a program faculty meeting that she had just opened up new issues of the JCP and the CDEMP journals and saw my two sole authored articles published! In spite of the impostor feelings I had during my early years as an untenured assistant professor, I fought through them by working tirelessly on becoming a better researcher.

Immediately after getting promoted and tenured at SIUC, I was recruited away by the University of Missouri – Columbia (a.k.a. Mizzou). This was a significant milestone in my professional journey because Mizzou was the flagship school of Missouri and boasted arguably the top counseling psychology program in the country. I had established myself nationally in the field of counseling psychology. I found myself among some of counseling psychology's biggest names. I was excited to be there and wanted to prove that I belonged. I closely examined my colleagues' publication records, and I saw that they frequently published in the top tier counseling psychology outlets. Once again I received the message that it would be good if I published in the JCP, so that is what I set out to do. It was at Mizzou where I published my most cited article in the JCP.

After three years at Mizzou, I was contacted by a colleague at the University of Texas at Austin (UT) about my interest in applying for a position. While I was happy at Mizzou, I needed to be at an institution where my partner and I could both have tenure-track positions. We applied and were both made offers. I went to UT as a tenured associate professor. Like Mizzou, UT was the flagship school of Texas. Additionally, UT was considered one of the best public schools in the country, a so-called "public Ivy" school. Many of the UT faculty had pedigrees from some of the most prestigious universities in the country. Even though I had proven myself as a scholar and was already a tenured associate professor, I was very self-conscious about my doctoral pedigree. Interestingly, I was most self-conscious around my African American colleagues who would eventually form the African and African Diaspora Studies Department. The pedigrees of many of these colleagues included schools such as Harvard, Stanford, Princeton, Cornel, and NYU among other prestigious universities. I struggled to fit in, partially because I was the only psychologist and partially because I felt that I did not have a prestigious doctoral pedigree. I struggled with what felt like an air and culture of elitism that was at odds with what I understood Black Studies to be about. How much of this was my own insecurity versus the actual climate is difficult to know. What I do know is that I often felt like an impostor whenever I interacted with these colleagues. During faculty meetings they would sometimes use jargon that I was unfamiliar with. To be clear, no one ever explicitly said anything to me about my pedigree. It was just the way that I felt whenever I was around them.

There were times that I did not want to affiliate with these African American colleagues and the quest to departmentalize Black Studies because I did not feel that I fit in. However, with the encouragement of a senior and well-respected African American professor, I persisted and we eventually were able to achieve departmentalization. Sometime around 2012 this senior African American professor told me that I was ready to go up for full professor. In the nascent African and African Diaspora Studies (AADS) department there were no full professors, and politically it was important for us to have full professors. In the Department of Educational Psychology (EDP), the Chair thought I had a good publication record, but was less encouraging because I did not have a record of grant funding. The increased emphasis on obtaining grants was yet another factor that contributed to me feeling like an impostor because I had never been socialized into the grant culture. I had managed to achieve a pretty good publication record without grant funding, and quite frankly the thought of pursuing grants was anxiety-provoking. Nevertheless, we agreed that I had the publication record to go up for promotion to full professor. Because I had a joint appointment in EDP and AADS, I had to go through two promotion processes and two votes in two departments and two colleges (College of Education and College of Liberal Arts).

In EDP, I received a unanimous vote for promotion. In the College of Education promotion and tenure committee, I also received a unanimous vote for promotion. In AADS, I also received a unanimous vote for promotion. However, this was not the case for the promotion and tenure committee in the College of Liberal Arts. This 20-person committee voted 8 in favor of promotion, and 12 against promotion. When the AADS department chair delivered the news to me, it was like someone had punched me in the gut. It was the first time I felt like I was being told that I was not good enough to be a full professor. For a couple of days I sat with knowledge that my colleagues had scrutinized my record and deemed me to not be worthy of becoming a full professor. I experienced an existential crisis as I began questioning whether I was good enough to be a full professor. I also second guessed my decision to have a joint appointment.

As it turned out, the Dean of the College of Liberal Arts disagreed with the vote, and in his letter to the Presidential promotion and tenure committee he recommended that I be promoted. The President of UT ultimately agreed, and I was promoted to full professor! Later I had a debriefing meeting with the Dean of the College of Liberal Arts. He informed me that it was a psychology professor on the promotion and tenure committee who raised concerns about my publication record. There were concerns that I had published too frequently in the *Journal of Black Psychology* and other "minority" journals, and not enough in top tier "mainstream" journals. I found this to be an ill-informed criticism for a couple of reasons. First, when counting the number of publications I had in so-called "minority" journals compared to so-called "mainstream" journals, the numbers were very comparable. Second, this criticism failed to take into account that a content analysis had recognized me as being one of the top contributors to the prestigious *Journal of Counseling Psychology* between 1999 and 2009. The Dean disagreed with the committee's assessment of my scholarship and attributed it to methodological biases (e.g., the psychologist was also critical of my non-experimental, mostly correlational research). This experience was the most emotionally draining and difficult one I've had in the academy. For so many years I had worked hard to publish good research and to prove myself as a scholar, and for a moment all of that was taken from me. I could not help but feel that I had just experienced the racism that causes many minoritized faculty to leave academia (Dolezal, 2022). When I suggested to the Dean that racism may have been a factor in the negative evaluation of my promotion materials, he struggled to acknowledge that racism may have been a possibility.

Recommendations and Strategies

As a scholar on the impostor phenomenon, I often provide recommendations about how to cope with impostor feelings. One recommendation I discuss is being intentional about documenting your academic and professional successes, because individuals experiencing impostor feelings often minimize their successes. I do this by regularly reviewing my publication record and publication metrics. To be honest I'm hesitant to even put this in print for fear that it might be considered to be a form of professional vanity, but honestly I need to do this as a reminder of my professional accomplishments and that

I am worthy of the accolades I have received. A second recommendation is to not suffer in silence, and to discuss your impostor feelings with trusted friends and colleagues. I am transparent about my impostor feelings, and I have found that it is helpful to share these feelings with people. When I do openly share my feelings I receive validation that I am not an impostor. My spouse is my biggest supporter and when I start having doubts she often reminds me about what I have accomplished. A third recommendation is to not be afraid to discuss your failures. No one is perfect. I am transparent about the times that I have failed because it helps other people (and me) feel more comfortable talking about their failures.

Lessons Learned

As I have gotten older and am now seen as a more senior scholar, my priorities have changed. I am no longer consumed with proving myself as I was when I was younger. Don't get me wrong, I still want to be a high achiever. The difference now is I want to achieve to advance the field and leave a scholarly legacy to be proud of rather than achieve to prove myself worthy. In spite of the struggles I have had with impostor feelings throughout my career, the fact of the matter is that my professional achievements have exceeded my greatest expectations. As a more senior scholar now, I wish my younger self would have taken more time to relax and enjoy my family. I say this because for years when I would go home to visit my family, I would spend hours working on manuscripts because I was consumed with getting published. I know that my family saw me (and to a certain extent still sees me) as a workaholic. I wish that my younger self could have been more relaxed. The thing about impostorism is that it makes people work incredibly hard in the constant pursuit of proving themselves as smart enough, as good enough, and as truly belonging.

As a Black man, I have always felt compelled to prove myself in the predominantly white educational spaces where I've been. I am keenly aware of and hypersensitive about the stereotypes regarding the intelligence of Black people and how we could not achieve without the benefit of affirmative action. I think this awareness especially plagues many Black scholars, but likely plagues other minoritized scholars too. My words of wisdom to junior scholars of color are to embrace the fact that you truly belong in academia. You are smart enough, you are good enough, and you do belong. You have earned your right to be in academia, not because of the color of your skin, but because you offer something that is valuable and needed in higher education. Your content expertise combined with your lived experience is an invaluable commodity in academia.

When I think about my 25 years as a professor at four different universities, my legacy will be defined in large part by the Black and other minoritized students I have positively impacted by my mere presence as well as by my teaching, scholarship, and mentorship. I know that I have made a difference in their lives. My presence in the academy has been a source of motivation for many minoritized students. The fact that I was not a perfect student and experienced some academic challenges and professional setbacks yet still became a distinguished full professor is an important example for junior minoritized scholars who are experiencing impostor feelings. Remember this: Just because you feel like an impostor doesn't mean that you are an impostor. When I give talks and workshops on the impostor phenomenon, I frequently share a PowerPoint slide with my picture, professional accomplishments, and the caption: From Impostor to Professor. Given where I've come from, I know that if I can make it, you can make it too!

References

Bernard, D. L., Lige, Q. M., Willis, H. A., Sosoo, E. E., & Neblett, E. W. (2017). Impostor phenomenon and mental health: The influence of racial discrimination and gender. *Journal of Counseling Psychology*, 64(2), 155–166. https://doi-org.proxy.lib.umich.edu/10.1037/cou0000197

Clance, P. R., & Imes, S. A. (1978). The imposter phenomenon in high achieving women: Dynamics and therapeutic intervention. *Psychotherapy: Theory, Research & Practice*, 15(3), 241–247. https://doi-org.proxy.lib.umich.edu/10.1037/h0086006

Cokley, K., McClain, S., Enciso, A., & Martinez, M. (2013). An examination of the impact of minority status stress and impostor feelings on the mental health of diverse ethnic minority college students. *Journal of Multicultural Counseling and Development*, 41(2), 82–95. https://doi-org.proxy.lib.umich.edu/10.1002/j.2161-1912.2013.00029.x

Cokley, K., Smith, L., Bernard, D., Hurst, A., Jackson, S., Stone, S., Awosogba, O., Saucer, C., Bailey, M., & Roberts, D. (2017). Impostor feelings as a moderator and mediator of the relationship between perceived discrimination and mental health among racial/ethnic minority college students. *Journal of Counseling Psychology*, 64(2), 141–154. https://doi-org.proxy.lib.umich.edu/10.1037/cou0000198

Dolezal, J. (2022). Why faculty of color are leaving academe: Too many find themselves disenfranchised, exhausted, and isolated. *The Chronicle of Higher Education*, September 20. www.chronicle.com/article/why-faculty-of-color-are-leaving-academe?cid2=gen_login_refresh&cid=gen_sign_in

Peteet, B. J., Brown, C. M., Lige, Q. M., & Lanaway, D. A. (2015). Impostorism is associated with greater psychological distress and lower self-esteem for African American students. *Current Psychology: A Journal for Diverse Perspectives on Diverse Psychological Issues, 34*(1), 154–163. https://doi-org.proxy.lib.umich.edu/10.1007/s12144-014-9248-z

Stone, S., Saucer, C., Bailey, M., Garba, R., Hurst, A., Jackson, S. M., Krueger, N., & Cokley, K. (2018). Learning while Black: A culturally informed model of the impostor phenomenon for Black graduate students. *Journal of Black Psychology, 44*(6), 491–531. https://doi-org.proxy.lib.umich.edu/10.1177/0095798418786648

Allyship as a Vehicle for Health Equity

8

Reflections on a Career in Community-Based Research with Indigenous and Black Populations

Jeffrey Proulx

I was conducting a literature review on Indigenous mental and physical health in the United States, and I found myself in a state of shock. The statistics outlining the impact of addiction, violence, and intergenerational trauma were jarring, and the anecdotes in the literature resonated eerily with my own family. However, that was not how I remembered family members and this moment forced me to face the discrepancy between my idea of Indigenous families and how science presented these same families. Family for me was a source of humor and wisdom, teaching me valuable skills like shooting a rifle and playing lacrosse. Life on the reservation was characterized by tranquility and simplicity, offering a contrasting world to the busy world of white-dominated spaces. These memories were intertwined with a profound love my family had for their culture, despite the lack of emphasis on Indigenous culture in America in general. And I remembered a lot of laughter in my community.

Initially, I was surprised by the extent of my shock from the readings on Indigenous mental health, realizing that this was akin to a fish recognizing that it is wet. Given the breadth of health disparities such as diabetes, alcoholism, and heart disease in Indigenous communities, the literature

DOI: 10.4324/9781003309796-10

presented pathology as inherent to the landscape of Indigenous health. However, I couldn't ignore the fondness and inspiration I felt when images of uncles or aunties arose while I was conducting my review and I knew that my research models would show how effective that love could be if I could capture that construct. It seemed that the answer to health equity (and ending intergenerational trauma in Indigenous communities) lay in the wisdom and experiences of the people I was interested in.

Path to Graduate School

The literature review I was conducting was part of a summer research project I was conducting as part of the Ronald E. McNair Program at the small liberal arts college I attended as an undergraduate. I am a mixed-race Indigenous scholar, a heterosexual male, who was raised by a single mother until the arrival of an urban Black male figure in our family. Higher education wasn't a common path for individuals in my family due to financial constraints and people I relied on tended to avoid any discussion of college. Although we eventually moved to a town blending lower-income and relatively well-off families when I was younger, I encountered a stark contrast in opportunities. Other kids spoke of attending prestigious institutions like Cornell, Colgate, Columbia, and Wesleyan, which made me acutely aware of the privilege divide because no one in my family life was talking about Wesleyan. The one-and-a-half year McNair program sought to bridge some of those divides at the college level by providing additional hours in the classroom being trained on everything from GRE preparation to formal dinner etiquette as well as paid summer research funding to match some of the same advantages students at Columbia had in the grad school market.

A view of the wider population of underserved students shows that the discrepancies between wealthy and non-wealthy families have varying impacts on people from these non-wealthy communities. Some have internalized societal messages of a racial caste system in America that often turns into lack of confidence in academic achievement. A not-insignificant percentage of underserved students let these messages seep into their subconscious due to the pervasive nature of these messages throughout society, such as the type of person who goes to college and "succeeds" in life. However, I was raised by strong women on both sides of my family, and much of my worldview was informed by the Mohawk tradition of matriarchy. Within the Haudenosaunee Confederacy, clan mothers held authority, a practice that resonated with my upbringing. My bond with the natural world was deepened by the interconnectedness between humans and nature in Indigenous culture, where every day held significance when caring for Turtle Island. It seemed to me that these were strengths that society did not promote or investigate as strengths and my goal was to leverage those strengths toward a better planet.

Lesson #1: Value and Protect the Cultural and Community Strengths You Bring

I downplayed my Indigeneity when interacting with my peers, because not many others were talking about Indigenous well-being/health or intergenerational trauma. This was a time when underserved communities grappled with ubiquitous white-centric values in most areas of society and often traumatizing examples of violence and restrictive policy to maintain white supremacy. In that environment, People of Color found innovative ways to flourish despite systemic barriers. I was delighted to imagine having a bachelor's degree, but McNair solidified my resolve to pursue graduate education, driven in part by the realization that a BS *in psychology* held limited prospects for me. More importantly, my McNair summer research underscored the significant gap in our understanding of Indigenous traditional healing and its potential as a pathway to healing within Indigenous communities.

While existing literature heavily emphasized the pathologies and alcoholism prevalent in Indigenous communities, there was a notable absence of focus on psychological approaches to healing in these communities, specifically healing that involved Indigenous traditional healing. While scholars like Michael Yellow Bird (2013), Edgar and Bonnie Duran (1995), and Maria Yellow Horse Brave Heart et al. (2016) advocated for the incorporation of Indigenous healing methods in Indigenous communities, there remained substantial voids in our knowledge regarding the practical application of traditional healing as a therapeutic modality. Moreover, the field of psychology struggled to fully encompass dimensions integral to Indigenous healing in the research models, despite the growing call for culturally specific healing within non-white communities. Enrolling in graduate school held the promise of equipping me with the requisite tools to conduct research within Indigenous communities, while also enabling me to infuse my work with the inherent strengths deeply rooted in Indigenous heritage. Moreover, much of my interest had become focused on mindfulness and I was interested how mindfulness could be used with Indigenous communities. I understood mindfulness not to be a specifically Indigenous healing method, but over time I came to realize that many Indigenous practices were already "mindful." Notably, I understood that my role as a spokesperson or leader in all of this was not to be the primary focus of my research, but to center the communities I was working with and to develop relationships that would lead to allyship in order to have the most impact.

Most of the "mental health" centers for Indigenous people I visited were addictions treatment centers that catered to all Indigenous people, meaning that there would be several different nations represented in the patient lists. This was a key point to overcome: Indigenous healing was practiced from a pan-Indian approach in many of these centers. That meant that treatments could not be culturally tailored to every patient given the wide variation in histories and cultural activities across Indigenous communities. Further, I asked every person I interviewed if there were Indigenous healing practices that were included in the treatment options at their respective centers and almost all the centers I approached said "no," they did not provide such treatment due to insurance and best-practice models restrictions. To a limited extent, these centers offered some Indigenous practices for healing, such as the model developed from the Red Road to Recovery (White, 2002) that emphasized traditional healing and healers or gestures to Indigenous ceremonies (e.g., smudging before sessions). But there was little from the scientific world that explored the efficacy of these types of endeavors, and I took it upon myself to gather the necessary data and experiences to show whether Indigenous healing practices are more effective than so-called mainstream treatments for Indigenous people. And although it seemed like I was entering a large unknown landscape that did not get a lot of attention in the research-funding world, my travels around California and Oregon and the people that I met made me think very hard about how to make a career out of that kind of work and more importantly provide evidence that Indigenous ways of healing were the "best practices" for Indigenous people if that relationship existed.

Lesson #2: Rely Hard on Your Mentors and Follow Their Advice

I highlighted my McNair training and research in grad school applications, and I got some interviews from the PhD programs I was interested in. Receiving interview offers was an exciting moment for me, especially as these universities emphasized their commitment to diversity and inclusivity in their communications. Not to mention the sense that my entire life course was going to change. I anticipated meeting fellow interviewees from underserved communities hailing from various and culturally diverse backgrounds. However, the reality of those interviews was not what I had envisioned. The notion of diversity seemed to revolve around the assortment of prestigious colleges the candidates came from, rather than their unique personal experiences. When I raised this concern with department representatives, they argued that while their student body might lack diversity, their research subjects were diverse, and they believed their work could positively impact these communities. I couldn't help but wonder why the department didn't actively recruit individuals from these communities, support them in pursuing doctoral degrees, and empower them to contribute to community healing. This situation reminded me of the Mars Rover project discussions in the media at that time, where locating water on Mars was a central topic. I imagined a scenario of a Martian applying to work on the Mars Rover, but the Martian's insight on Mars' water sources took a back seat to a non-Martian candidate's technical skills (and their impressive American college degree), despite the latter having no better understanding of the water's location. My life experiences had taught me the value of local knowledge (and how valuable it would be to have a Martian participate in a project to find water on Mars) and fueled my determination not only to chart my own path but also to create avenues for more individuals from marginalized backgrounds to receive advanced education and to give voice to those communities so we could know where the equivalent of the water was for them.

At about the same time as I was applying to PhD school, I received a National Academies of Science Ford Fellowship. This community of students (fellows) and professors (past fellows) that were primarily from underserved communities quickly felt like family, offering a safe space where I could openly discuss both my personal and professional struggles without fearing repercussions on my career. Their advice encouraged me to remain true to myself, reminding me not to sacrifice my individuality on the altar of academia. They guided me in infusing my work with my identity, passion, and love, showing me how to authentically represent my community and advocate for Indigenous healing practices. They also emphasized the reality that my path might often be in the shadows, underscoring the importance of drawing attention to the burdens Indigenous communities bear and employing persuasive statistical models to demonstrate the efficacy of Indigenous healing. Perhaps most important, these people convinced me that I too was excellent in science and my sense of self-efficacy was quickly boosted. Having a fellowship gave me a lot more say over my graduate school process and opened doors to other institutions where I found that a lot of the work I was preparing to do had already been mastered by other academics; all I needed to do was learn from them.

Lesson #3: Plan Ahead

Right away I recognized that external support was a key to carving my own path and I had a strong feeling that continued external funding (e.g., National Institutes of Health (NIH) funding) would have to carry over into my career if I wanted to have more control over my vocation. Almost immediately I heard about K-awards at NIH and decided I was going to apply for one of those after I had completed my first postdoctoral placement (keep in mind I had only been in graduate school about a week before deciding on my postdoctoral placement plans. Notably, I attribute that foresight to being able to develop the skill sets and pick the opportunities over a five-year span that I needed to toward my K-award goal. It became apparent that looking ahead five years and hitting benchmarks were the keys for building a foundation for a K-award (or any large goal) to simply unfold when the time came). I knew that if I wanted to highlight Indigenous traditions in health-related research, that I would have to expand my abilities to medical research and biomarker testing as well as qualitative methodologies that seemed necessary to draw out the narratives from people that described their resilience and strengths. Eventually, I received that K award, which I crafted as a dream proposal, because I figured that I might as well have written a dream scenario due to the high unlikelihood I would actually get the award: *always pursue your dream idea because someone might be inspired enough to fund it.*

While these insights were a lot to absorb as a first-year PhD student, they illuminated a direction for my future. Though I wasn't entirely clear how to publish manuscripts, secure grants, or navigate the intricacies of academia, I was certain that these would be the foundational elements of my career and that I would have to do a lot of those things to be successful. *All my success is due to the relationships I received both in and out of the academy and my ability to listen to and follow the advice I was given.* I have consistently advocated for students from underserved communities to become part of organizations like the Ford Fellowship or cultural groups on campus, especially those in the sciences (e.g., Society for the Advancement of Chicanos/Hispanics and Native Americans in Science (SACNAS); American Psychological Association's Committee for the Advancement of Racial and Ethnic Diversity, etc.). These organizations provide *community* where like-minded scholars can come together to provide mutual support. I recognized the value of scheduling regular opportunities to engage with fellow scholars from underrepresented backgrounds, both for my own well-being and as a catalyst for my research endeavors. Most importantly the conversations and experiences in these spaces showed me how to engage with the communities I was interested in so that I could be an ally and contributor to those communities. Combined with the excellence I had in my dissertation committee, I felt confident that I had the mentorship I needed to succeed.

Lesson #4: Question Normative Assumptions in Research

A seminal paper by Jackson and colleagues (2010) shed light on the relationship between Black men, depression, health behaviors, and the hypothalamic-pituitary-adrenal (HPA) axis. I heard academics discuss this paper as further proof of how poor health behaviors shielded Black men from stress and buffered HPA axis function, consequently reducing depressive symptoms compared to white men. Yet, the authors noted that these behaviors were also linked to long-term health problems from unhealthy eating, smoking, and alcohol use. Personally, I felt that academia misunderstood this dynamic. I recall accompanying my Black stepfather to visit his wounded Vietnam War veteran brother, and despite societal challenges, they found solace in playing chess and partying. These nights represented moments of strength and camaraderie that were acts of resistance in a time (has much changed?) when systems were put in place to disenfranchise non-Christian-whites from access to the mechanisms of wealth and power. The commitment to freedom and happiness despite the darkness of racism was altogether inspiring for me. It was the togetherness that my stepfather and family enjoyed and their refusal to bow to the racist dictate that non-whites be miserable that stuck out to me as a more fruitful direction for research.

Lesson #5: Dream Big, Aim High

My path eventually led me to an Ivy League campus as a professor. Yet, I was resolute in ensuring that the strengths ingrained in me by my community also found a place within these hallowed halls. There were two driving forces behind this commitment. Firstly, I aimed to equip underrepresented students with perspectives and skills that would empower them to thrive in their college experience. Secondly, I firmly believed that the wisdom of Indigenous cultures and the resilience of Black communities held transformative potential for healing our world.

We have forged allyship with our communities as all the people in our lab are drawn to community-based research that is reflective of those communities' goals and dreams. We also emphasize the importance of using our resources and research goals to provide those communities with opportunities to be true partners in our proposals and learn substantive skill sets that will move people forward. Those skills include advanced research proposal writing and intervention design as our allies engage fully in the process from the beginning to end of our projects. Many of our community partners have been trained to become mindfulness teachers so we can set up people from those communities to become the proponents of mindfulness practice in their own communities, thus ensuring sustained efforts for health and wellness in those communities. More importantly, we trust that the self-efficacy and identity development that arises for communities as a result of engaging in our projects will lead to sustainable health equity in these communities.

Takeaways

Allyship, both with my communities and other scholars, has been the motivation for the work that I do. Along the way, I have learned some important lessons that may be helpful to you as you pursue your own paths: 1) *Value and protect the cultural and community strengths you bring*, 2) *Rely hard on your mentors and follow their advice*, 3) *Plan ahead*, 4) *Question the normative assumptions of research*, and finally, 5) *Dream big, aim high*. Believing in myself and building trust with community members have been foundational in my work. I have been fortunate to be in a situation where I could refine myself as a researcher and person and bring those skills to benefit the people that I love.

References

Brave Heart, M. Y. H., Chase, J., Elkins, J., Martin, J., Nanez, J. S., & Mootz, J. J. (2016). Women finding the way: American Indian women leading intervention research in Native communities. *American Indian and Alaska Native Mental Health Research, 23*(3), 24–47. https://doi.org/10.5820/aian.2303.2016.24

Duran, E., & Duran, B. (1995). *Native American postcolonial psychology.* State University of New York Press.

Jackson, J. S., Knight, K. M., & Rafferty, J. A. (2010). Race and unhealthy behaviors: Chronic stress, the HPA axis, and physical and mental health disparities over the life course. *American Journal of Public Health, 100*(5), 933–939. https://doi.org/10.2105/AJPH.2008.143446

White, W. (2002). Introduction. In *The red road to wellbriety: In the Native American way.* White Bison.

Yellow Bird, M. (2013). Neurodecolonization: Applying mindfulness research to decolonizing social work. In M. Gray, J. Coates, M. Yellow Bird, & T. Hetherington (Eds.). *Decolonizing social work.* Ashgate Publishing.

Finding Your Voice

A Community Conversation

9

*Sophia Williams Kapten[1], E. J. R. David,
Nayeli Y. Chavez-Dueñas, Hector Y.
Adames, Derek H. Suite, Linda Lausell
Bryant and Doris F. Chang*

In this conversation, Linda Lausell Bryant and Doris F. Chang speak with Sophia Williams Kapten, E. J. R. David, Nayeli Y. Chavez-Dueñas, Hector Y. Adames, and Derek Suite about the pivotal moments, turning points, processes, and supports that fostered their ability to develop a voice that is authentic, affirming, and original. Our goal in this conversation, and for this book, is to foster a communal space of sharing and exploration, one that allows for honesty and vulnerability.

Participants

Hector Y. Adames, PsyD is a neuropsychologist and full professor at The Chicago School of Professional Psychology Chicago Campus. He co-founded and co-directs the IC-RACE Lab (Immigration, Critical Race, and Cultural Equity Lab).

---

1 The first five authors are listed in random order, reflecting their equal contributions to this chapter.

DOI: 10.4324/9781003309796-11

Nayeli Y. Chavez-Duenas, PhD is a full professor at The Chicago School of Professional Psychology where she serves as the faculty coordinator for the concentration in Latinx Mental Health in the Counseling Psychology Department. She is the co-founder and co-director of the IC-RACE Lab (Immigration, Critical Race, and Cultural Equity Lab).

E. J. R. David, PhD is a full professor in the Clinical-Community Psychology PhD Program at University of Alaska, Anchorage. He also directs the Alaska Native Community Advancement in Psychology (ANCAP) Program, and co-chairs the Division on Filipino Americans (DoFA) of the Asian American Psychological Association.

Sophia Williams Kapten, PhD is in private practice at Therapists of New York, a team of doctoral level psychotherapists located in Midtown Manhattan. She has held clinical training positions at Mount Sinai, Beth Israel, New York Presbyterian, Columbia University Irving Medical Center, Montefiore Medical Center, The New School's Counseling Center, and Kings County Hospital.

Derek Suite, MD, MS is a board-certified psychiatrist and founder of Full Circle Health. He is the consulting team psychiatrist to the New York Knicks, New York Rangers, and New York Jets and consults for Major League Soccer on restorative practices and cultural sensitivity. He is an Associate Adjunct Professor of Clinical Psychopharmacology at Teachers College, Columbia University in New York.

Finding Your Voice: "The System Wants Us to Think That We're Lost, but We're Not"

The conversation begins with the participants introducing themselves with a story about a key moment of *discovery*, when they realized that the world was not what they thought it was.

Linda: When I was six years old, my mother would make me clean
          the linoleum steps in the hallway that led up to our Brooklyn
          apartment. Like Cinderella, with a bucket and a brush in hand,
          I scrubbed every step. Our landlords were Italian immigrants who
          lived in the ground floor apartment. My mother explained to me

that as Puerto Ricans, we needed to show the landlords that we were clean people, even though it wasn't our job to maintain the hallway. The discovery for me, at this young age, was that there was something about us, as Puerto Ricans, that people assumed was negative, specifically *dirty*, and lazy, unless we could prove otherwise. This connects to my lifelong sense that I always have something to prove, regardless of my accomplishments, and that requires me to go above and beyond.

Doris: The "aha" moment that comes up for me has to do with my waking up to the reality that no matter my efforts to conform to whiteness – culturally, linguistically, behaviorally – I was never going to be perceived as white. My parents immigrated to Texas for educational opportunities, and I grew up seeing very few Asian faces like ours. I was fortunate to have a close-knit group of friends, but everywhere I looked – white people were in charge, the most popular, the *norm*. I remember feeling embarrassed by my Chinese parents, their accents, how they didn't understand certain things about American culture. Like any teenager, I tried really hard to fit in and I thought I was doing a decent job, excelling academically and feeling for the most part that I belonged. It felt like I was leaving my parents' culture behind and that was honestly OK by me. I felt like I was becoming *white*. It wasn't until I got to college that I had my racial awakening. For the first time, I encountered lots of other Asian American kids like me, and I felt really *seen* in a way that I didn't even realize I hadn't been. It started a whole process of learning more about my culture and history, learning Mandarin, and figuring out for myself what it meant to be Chinese American.

Derek: I want to thank you both for sharing. I found myself synergizing with everything you shared, like being marginalized and dealing with opposition. There's just something about when others share their journey, because we never get to talk about it that much. While I can pick a million stories, I'm going with the theme of evolution. I don't think I ever fully understood how powerful this whole process of evolving really is. I started out wanting to be nothing more than an emergency room (ER) physician and geared my entire life toward that, only to find that when I got there, that wasn't who I was. I found that I was more interested in talking to people and having a connection with them. I hadn't evolved yet into understanding that this is who I was. So I stayed in the ER for quite some time as a miserable, unhappy, depressed doctor. I'd go to the park before work and look at the pigeons, envying these lucky birds for having no pressure on them. I guess that's when I knew something was wrong (laughing). At work, doing medical procedures gave me a sense of competence but still, there was no fulfillment for me.

And then I started getting into trouble in the ER, because I was talking to patients and connecting with them. My superiors thought I was just a socializer and not doing my work. When I decided I was going to leave the ER, that's where discovery came in for me. I expressed interest in psychiatry and everyone reacted as if it was a ridiculous choice. In fact, when I tried to resign from the ER, my department chair refused to accept my resignation. Even my family questioned my desire to leave ER medicine, the pinnacle within the hierarchical medical world. I actually considered staying in the ER and pleasing everyone even though I'd be miserable. I think when we are evolving, there's a lot of discomfort until you fight. Evolution is an uncomfortable process of progression. When I went into psychiatry, I felt so fulfilled, though I found all kinds of problems within the mental health system. What Linda shared about having to always prove yourself on every level, that was my experience as a Black male inside of a very Eurocentric system. I started my own practice and decided to go in a more holistic direction, including prayer, stress management, aromatherapy, and mindfulness.

Sophia: I, too, feel a lot of gratitude for this timely discussion. I'm going to ask for grace, here. I am an emotional person, and I'm pregnant with my second child. So I am crying with solidarity and lots of feelings. I did find myself thinking about an ongoing feeling throughout my life. At a really young age, my world was rocked. When I was nine I learned that the person I thought was my father was not. I felt like the world could not be trusted. Where do I belong? This has been a lingering question throughout my life. So the word *discovery* makes me think about my experience throughout life discovering the places where I feel most alive and where it feels as though I belong. So the story that I'm thinking of is one in which I felt something different, like *I belong, like I'm actually connected here.*

When I was pregnant with my first child, I felt super alive in my body and I found myself walking down the street looking at every single person, thinking, *someone birthed you, you were in somebody's body, and they labored you into the world.* Every person's existence amazed me and I felt some solidarity with the person who birthed them. It was both magical and mundane at the same time. I felt connected to all of these people through this experience, and even felt deeply connected to mammals. Feels complicated, but also really nice, too.

Hector: I'm just gonna go with where the Spirit takes me to share. I was born in Quisqueya, the island that is now divided into what we know as the Dominican Republic and Haiti. The question about discovery took me back to my first arrival at JFK Airport when I immigrated to the United States at the age of five. I vividly remember landing in New York City on a windy February night with my mother after a bumpy Eastern Airlines flight. My face being touched by the coldness of winter for the first time. My lanky body gently being zipped up in a navy-blue one-piece hooded snowsuit by two men – my *papi* and *tio*. People around talked in English. The new language and faces were disorienting to me and my developing brain. Meeting my paternal grandmother, cousins, and tias for the first time. All strangers to me. New smells, tall pointy buildings, buzzing cars flooded my senses. No trees in sight, no greenery, no rhythmic dancing blue ocean waves. Over the Throgs Neck Bridge, through the South Bronx, and into Manhattan we drove. Sowing new seeds in a Dominican enclave, our new home away from Quisqueya; my emerging role as a cultural broker.

I am a living testament to the hard work of my working-class parents. My mother worked three jobs to afford to send me to what was considered a "good school." Unfortunately, a "good Catholic school" didn't offer English as a Second Language (ESL) support, and I found it challenging to communicate and understand what was happening in class. I have always been a talker and naturally inclined to dialogue. I remember consistently finding a way to ask, "What's happening?" This trait uniquely served me – I became my own advocate within those foreign white spaces, a responsibility that no child should bear. As a result, I was frequently disciplined for talking and questioning. Reflecting on old class pictures today, I can now contextualize and better understand the challenges I faced back then. I was among the few Students of Color and sported a big, beautiful afro. Furthermore, my gender non-conforming expression was just as pronounced then as it is today. Those were undoubtedly tough years in my educational journey in this country. Looking back is quite painful, and more so because I know many other children of color today are navigating similar spaces. I was thrust into self-discovery without much choice, and this experience has been echoed in various spaces and times throughout my personal and professional life.

As I enter my early 40s, I find solace in the wisdom of Nina Simone, who reminds us of the importance of leaving the table when love is no longer served.[2] Her words have become the guiding compass of my life today. I've realized the power of walking away, forging new paths, and rejecting the scripts imposed upon us as individuals of African descent, immigrants, and queer folx – scripts often forced upon us by society. Instead, I deeply believe we can author counter-scripts and stand in solidarity with those who share our vision of creating new ways of living, loving, and simply existing. Today, I am a clinical psychologist and professor in a graduate program where I support and train the next generation of psychotherapists. I honor my African ancestors, queer siblings of color, and my family through my professional commitment to serving communities of color through my research, writing, and activism. This professional journey has been liberating, allowing me to do work that truly matters to me and my communities. It's a freedom that fills me with hope and inspires a dance within my soul, like my beloved Caribbean's rhythmic dancing blue ocean waves.

E.J.:   There are a lot of stories of discovery, but it was hard for me to think of one because in many ways, I am still in the process of discovering things. I will just share a couple of things that significantly sparked that journey of discovery. I remember when I was 12 years old and I developed my first crush ever on this neighborhood girl. I told my older sister about this exciting feeling, asking for her advice on how I could impress this girl. Her advice was to go into our medicine cabinet and use this bleach to start whitening my skin. She meant well and I didn't question it. By that point, I was used to seeing TV and magazine ads for skin whitening products. I started using skin whitening products, and staying away from the sun so that I would

2 From her 1965 song, "You've Got to Learn" on the album, *I Put a Spell on You.*

not get too dark. Nevermind that this was the Philippines, right by the equator. I grew up with that belief that the lighter skinned or whiter you are, the better off you will be in this world.

I also got other consistent messages that the United States of America was the land of milk and honey, the promised land, which I also believed. I guess my dream came true because I was able to move to the United States when I was 14 years old. That solidified my belief that the closer I am to whiteness, the better off I will be and when I got here, I felt like I was close to achieving it. I wanted to be your typical American boy and separate myself from anything related to my roots. One of my passions is basketball and I remember it was game day in my junior year of high school. During game days, the spirit team and cheer squad would decorate the lockers of the athletes with posters but on this game day, my locker was decorated with a message that stood out from all the other typical good luck messages. It said, "You're Filipino, act like it." That moment made me question myself. How have I been acting? How have I not been acting Filipino, whatever that might mean? That was the beginning of me asking questions about myself and the world. I started thinking about my family. Why did they leave everything that they love, to go to a country that they'd never been to? That set me on this journey of why I do what I do now. I really just wanted to understand myself, my loved ones, and my community better.

Nayeli: I want to share a story of immigration and discovery that has shaped my life. I grew up in Michoacan, Mexico, the ancestral homeland of the Purepecha people. Throughout my childhood, I was surrounded by stories of my aunts and uncles, who had taken a brave step by migrating to the United States in the early 1960s to seek opportunities in the factories of Chicago.

In the early 1970s, one of my uncles achieved a significant milestone by becoming a US naturalized citizen. His accomplishment opened the doors for our family's immigration journey. I recall the hushed conversations among my parents and siblings, speculating about the arrival of a life-changing letter that would grant us access to the so-called American dream. It was a concept I could only grasp as I grew older. My mother's daily prayers were a testament to her unwavering hope that our application would be approved one day and we would embark on a journey to reunite with our extended family in Chicago. This included my brother, whom I had never met because he had migrated the year I was born. Curiosity consumed me about life in a new country. I couldn't comprehend why our Chicago-based aunts and uncles seemed so joyful during their visits to Mexico, adorned in fine clothing and bearing gifts beyond our reach in Mexico. Through their stories, I painted a picture of the US as a land of boundless opportunities and prosperity. The wait was arduous, spanning many years, but one momentous day, we finally received the long-awaited letter from immigration informing us that our application had been approved. At the time, I was 17 years old. However, I was unaware of a crucial detail – only my siblings under 21 could accompany my mother. This unforeseen circumstance separated our family once again. My older brother had turned 21 while we awaited the letter, forcing him to remain in Mexico.

I traveled to Ciudad Juarez with my mom and two sisters, a US-Mexican border town where we went through the visa application process to enter the United States. The experience was challenging; we encountered minimal respect and dignity. We had to undergo a physical exam, background checks, fingerprinting, and an interview. I remember feeling incredibly anxious because I knew that if we didn't pass the entire process, we would be denied entry into the United States and forced to return to Michoacan, where we faced economic hardships. As challenging and frightening as the process was, I believed it would be worth it for the chance to live in a place where everyone had access to food and where poverty did not exist. At last, we were granted a visa and could enter the country. My first revelation occurred when we finally arrived in Chicago. Contrary to the clean, picturesque streets depicted in movies, we found ourselves in a neighborhood where walls were marked with graffiti, houses appeared dilapidated, and a strong smell of garbage permeated the air.

It was hard to believe that this place was the United States. Those first few months in Chicago were a time of many discoveries. My preconceived notions of the United States contrasted starkly with the harsh reality I was living in. Rats, roaches, violence, and poverty surrounded me. I also discovered that some members of my family, who seemed so content during their visits to Mexico, were not as joyful here. They had backbreaking, dangerous, and poorly paid jobs. I began to understand that they were happy when I saw them in Mexico because they were home. I realized they had saved all their money to visit and briefly escape their challenging reality. It was a profound discovery for me to realize that how the United States portrays itself to the world is often disconnected from reality. As a result, many immigrants, like myself, arrive in this country with expectations based on an illusion.

Linda: **Thank you so much for sharing these powerful stories. While the discoveries that each of you shared were tinged with pain, they also opened your eyes to a realization that set you on a new path. In the professional realm, I wonder if others of you have faced similar moments to what Hector shared, that realization that something was not right about the way you were being trained, "that love was not being served there." And you decided to make a different choice that was more authentic to who you are.**

Doris: **For example, E.J., in your chapter, which was about decolonizing research, you wrote, "From the beginning of this chapter, and through the discussions I've shared so far, I have revealed a little bit of myself, my struggles and my values. I have revealed my heart. And although I now believe this is okay, this hasn't always been the case. There was a time when I felt bad for being so passionate about my work. I felt I was less of a researcher and scholar for not being separate, distant, and objective enough. I used to believe that my intimate connections with my work somehow make my work less rigorous and less valid, but I don't believe this anymore." (p. 76) And so to Linda's point, we'd love to know how you went from believing that to believing this.**

E. J.: To be honest with you, it's not just one singular moment. It's many things. Using Derek's evolution theme, with this particular evolution of mine, one of the more important things that helped me get to that realization was understanding that I embarked on this journey initially to try to understand myself better and try to understand my loved ones and community better. I got to the realization that my people were not born feeling less of themselves. We don't have an "I want to move to the United States" gene. It's not individual level factors that pushed us to come to this country; it's not that we were born wanting to be lighter skinned. It's not like we were born wanting to get rid of our brown skin, it's not like we were born trying to get rid of our language, our accents. We were not born in this world with an instinct to value whiteness.

So when did I start questioning my training? Being trained in clinical psychology, a lot of what I was getting was about just needing to help people change the way that they think, feel, behave, and react to the world. All of the interventions were focused on making individual-level changes. And, I began to think, there's got to be something more than just helping people change the way they think about their own oppression, or change the way they feel about injustice. There's got to be something more. When I started getting away from conventional psychology, I started feeling okay about that. I started reading beyond psychology, and listening to people who are not psychologists, focusing on my experiences, and what me and my communities have gone through. It's been a huge mess, with hundreds of years of colonialism. We cannot address such a mess by pretending that we can simplify it and just use a broom to clean it up. We can't just use a broom, we need to use scrubs, we need to use vacuums, we need to use all the different tools to clean up this huge mess, because that's the reality.

What was psychology teaching me with objectivity and a focus on individual level factors? To me, it was just too simplistic and it was not enough. Even though I was trained in psychology, my allegiance is not to psychology. My allegiance is to my community. And I must open myself up to using whatever tools, whatever framework, whatever theories I must use to be responsive to my community.

Sophia: I recently graduated and while in graduate school I really struggled to find a home – a place where I felt comfortable being myself and connected with others who held similar worldviews and values. During one of my practicums, I found myself in a contentious dynamic with my supervisor who was quite esteemed at my site. Despite how well respected she was, I found her theoretical positions offensive and we argued. Her theoretical orientation influenced how she showed up in her clinical work and I did not agree with what she was trying to teach me as it felt counter to the patient-centered and multicultural stance that I wished to practice. The arguing grew much too painful and I had the impression that the same position she wanted me to take with my clients was the position that she was taking with me – she was the expert and

I needed to do as she said. Later, I wrote and published a paper about this experience because it was such a turning point for me. It was from this experience that I discovered the very real difference between my research home which was congruent with my worldview and the clinical training I was getting where I struggled to bring my worldview into practice. I learned that if the space that I need does not exist, I have to create it.

Doris: Sophia ended up writing about this really fraught supervisory experience, published it, and shared it with that white supervisor, which I thought was so brave.

Sophia: It was painful and scary to write that paper but it made our supervision, and our relationship, better. This paper is also an example of what I mean by creating space for myself. I could not speak to this supervisor directly so I found a new way to communicate to her and anyone else that may benefit from what I had to share. I'm still in contact with this supervisor. It didn't destroy us. I brought versions of the paper to her and we talked through it. It was truly an exercise of bridging but also a moment of recognition that what I was going to be learning in school may not be aligned with my spirit.

Linda: **Derek, I'm going to quote a piece from your chapter where you say, "Indeed, I now look back at these painful experiences with a sense of deep gratitude, because they motivated me to find not only 'a way out', but 'a way in'" (p. 144). And I'm interested in that bridge between some of the things you went through, like being thrown on the floor by police and being searched without apology. How did you go from that experience to a sense of gratitude? What was that bridge?**

Derek: When I came into contact with these horrific experiences, I wasn't thinking that I'm going to end up in this wonderful place of revelation, and gratitude. I'm a large Black man so I'm mostly either apologizing for who I am, or trying to bring myself down so that everybody else could feel comfortable. I recall just being slammed to the floor with my stethoscope and other things all over the train station. That's one form of violence but when I put on a white coat, or a stethoscope and I walk in as the doctor, I'm still that Black guy. The Black guy that can have a great idea is the same Black guy that you have to watch. I feel as if those painful experiences were imbibed and I metabolized them. I think I evolved. Pain is a motivator. Once we feel pain, we want to get out of that pain and typically, it motivates us to do something to find relief. And for me, finding relief ultimately meant not just running **away** from my experiences, but running **toward** a new experience.

I needed to create something that would help heal me. I kept looking outwardly for it and wanting somebody to validate me and then I realized that nobody is going to do that. So I started looking inward, thinking about what I really want to do, and I was talking with God. Most of our culture's coping comes through our spiritual and ancestral connections, drawing from what's deep within. I began to have ideas about starting my own practice. And that came out of pain, but you have to go inward first because the answers are not outside. I'm grateful because if I hadn't had those experiences, I would have been comfortable. I actually was looking to be just comfortable, go to work, get paid, and just live a great life. But a great life doesn't really exist for most Black males, Black folks, People of Color. I was able to find a way out by finding a way in, if that makes sense.

Doris: **Several of you referred to this visceral embodied feeling that you couldn't ignore; it wasn't just a cognitive process. It forced you to pay attention in a way that everything else didn't. How do we make space for that part of our experience in these spaces that only want part of us to show up?**

Hector: When systems grounded in white supremacy culture claim they want a part of us, we must question: do they genuinely want any part of us? The violence we often endure in academic spaces suggests they don't want any aspect of us – not our ideas, questions, presence, leadership, or skills. Linda, your question about how we respond to this is critical. Considering whether we internalize this narrative is the initial question for us to consider in addressing your important question. If this narrative becomes ingrained in our beliefs, it will undoubtedly impact our well-being. Likewise, resisting white supremacy culture also takes a toll. You may be wondering, what should you do? One way forward involves resisting the dominant dehumanizing narratives about our community and immersing ourselves in counter-narratives about our people; these stories are all around us. They're in our families, in our communities, and yes, they're inside of us. Our people are not just brilliant; they're so much more. The term "brilliant" hardly scratches the surface of our collective potential!

And I truly believe we would have solved so many problems in the world if we were not too busy fighting, and making meaning out of our pain and the violence that we experience as People of Color. In psychology, we can be hyper-focused on people's resilience and resilience means becoming stronger in the broken places. I'm thinking, just don't break us! Can you just stop doing the breaking?

Derek: I wish I had heard this growing up or during my evolution. Here we are in this group, talking and in its own way, *this* is evidence, *we* are evidence of something, but it won't make it into a journal, right? I think we need to really have our own journals, our own research entities where we are in charge of what comes in and what's being said. I just wanted to put that out there because I feel like this is so valuable, what we're doing right now.

Doris: **One of the audiences for this book is early career BIPOC professionals who are seeking access to the "hidden curriculum" for success that they're not getting through mainstream channels. I'm curious about whether this is scary to speak and write about. So many of you talked about these moments where you started asking questions. How did you do it? Were you scared? How did you deal with that?**

Nayeli: Many of us who have attended PWIs [predominantly white institutions] and programs find ourselves as one of the few People of Color who understand the expectations placed upon us. As E. J. and Derek have pointed out, we may not change the color of our skin, but our thoughts and behaviors have been influenced and socialized by the dominant white culture. We know that we may be perceived as troublesome if we begin to raise concerns. Sometimes, it takes a while to realize because we are so grateful to be at the table. I was one of the first People of Color in my program, and it took me some time to start recognizing what was missing because being in a doctoral program was like a dream, and all I wanted was to learn. I thought that what I was learning was valuable. When I started working with clients of color in the early 2000s, empirically based manualized treatments were popular. I took pride in learning and applying these therapies and interventions effectively. However, what I considered effective did not necessarily translate into healing for the People of Color I was serving. This awareness became particularly evident when I started working with Black children in Southern Illinois. They often asked me about the racist incidents they faced at school, leaving me at a loss for how to respond. I had received no training to support them in navigating their experiences, understanding the racism influencing their lives, and addressing its impact on their mental health. Manualized treatments were designed for someone other than my clients. This was when I began asking questions, but I couldn't find any answers in the training I received. During that time, I feared that if I created too many problems by questioning the training I was receiving, I would close doors to myself and those who came after me since I felt like, in the eyes of many, I represented my entire ethnic group. My mentor used to say that you need to get your ticket punched and get out, but sometimes, I wondered how to do that while being true to my values and my commitment to social and racial justice.

E.J.: A lot of that resonated with me, too. Unfortunately, I think it's going to be a perpetual struggle to think about whether I am still challenging the system, trying to make the system better for other people like me. Or have I become just another brown person perpetuating the system? Am I still doing good work for my communities or am I so enmeshed in the system that I'm just a part of it now? I think that that's the existential fear. And as Nayeli and Hector alluded to, we were taught to be strong and resilient. But where do we draw the line? Or, are we now just simply giving people permission to continue oppressing us, to treat us like shit?

Linda: **I'm hearing a theme about calculating the costs of our choices. Are there other reflections on costs, maybe trade-offs, or benefits to embodying your full self and expressing your voice?**

Derek: I think the benefit for me, now that I have my own independent mental health entity for the past 20 years, is that I find solace in the fact that when somebody comes through the door, I'm not answering to someone else's framework, or trying to fit into someone else's theoretical construct or policy, for handling the individual in front of me. I can blend in critical race theory or pray with a person. It's a trade-off because we can't make massive changes like some large hospital, but for a small practice that is operating within the system, we are making a difference. I was also thinking about Hector's point and the many times I have talked about the "broken places" without thinking about what the hell broke us to begin with.

Doris: One response is to create safe havens, places of refuge, whether it's our research labs, our own clinics, or even in just one relationship within a toxic environment. Hector and Nayeli, you two have a very long history of collaboration, and you've created a lab that pushes out a lot of important public-facing content. Could you speak about how your relationship with one another as collaborators has helped you to find your voice? How has your relationship facilitated your process of being more authentic in your work?

Hector: Thank you for the question. It's crucial to have people you can truly trust, individuals who understand your experiences and are genuinely curious about what you're going through as you navigate the complexities of life with its pains, hassles, surprises, and joys. One of the reasons I continue to be in Chicago is the difficulty of replicating my professional relationship with an academic sister in whose hands I wouldn't hesitate to place my life. Nayeli is that person; together, we've co-created something truly special outside the white gaze of academia. We often say that our ancestors watch over us; it's their plan, we're just listening to their whispers.

Nayeli: Academia is difficult for many reasons, and one of them is that it is hard to find people you can trust completely, people who know and understand what it is like and who truly have your back. And Hector is that for me. I always say that my relationship with Hector is a gift from my ancestors. He calls me his academic sister, and I say my relationship with him is better than being a sibling. We have the same values, mission, and work ethic, and we have created a lab that puts those values into practice. Beyond our academic work together, I deeply admire Hector as a person. He is absolutely beautiful, talented, caring, and a supportive human being. I wish all People of Color were as fortunate as me to have someone like him in their lives.

Hector: Oprah created a billion dollar empire around finding yourself, and what we tell our students is *you are not lost*. The system wants us to think that we're lost, but we're not. So there's nothing to find, but there's everything to create.

Sophia: I immerse myself in Black psychology, where I can wrap myself in the words of people I've never met who remind me that I'm not losing my mind. They give me language that I couldn't otherwise find and they have kept me company while I've journeyed.

E. J.:   I'm not as fortunate as Hector and Nayeli who are working and supporting each other but I have many other things here, and I'm grateful. I just want to highlight one of the things that Sophia shared, that even the validation that you get from people, reminding us that what we experienced was real, that in itself can be powerful. We might not be able to solve the problem, but it allows us to move on.

Doris: I was just thinking that what also sustains me are all of the roles I have outside of academia, because my academic identity is just one slice of who I am. I am sustained by my family, even the patients that I work with, and they remind me that there are other people that see me, that care about me. So it doesn't matter so much what that white colleague or administrator thinks. That is actually a pretty radical act of resistance, just not caring as much as they want you to care, and I feel like that is a kind of liberation from the system.

E. J.:   That's the same thing for me. It doesn't matter how much I mess up at work, I know my kids are still going to accept me as I am. That really helps me. I remind myself and I tell people this – I just work *at* the university, I don't work *for* the University. I work *for* my people.

Doris: **I love that! Our last question is, if you could go back in time and send a message to your younger self, what would you want to tell yourself?**

E. J.:   I would share that today's solutions can become tomorrow's problems so always remain humble and open to changing, growing, learning, and doing better.

Sophia: The message that I would give my younger self is to speak up. I've always been scared to talk. I would tell my younger self to speak anyway, and that is how you find your voice. That's how you learn your heart. You say something.

Hector: I would tell my younger self that they are like a buoy in the ocean, that their role is not to control the sea but to decide on the anchors to navigate the tides and waves without getting carried away and lost in the currents. I would explain that in storms, in their ebb and flow, a fleeting drama always unfolds. That when the final curtain descends, the rain shall cease, the waters shall rest, and you beloved, you will prevail.

Nayeli: I would tell myself that I can find many of the answers to the questions I had in my people's history. I come from a country still experiencing the impact of colonization. If I had looked into history for answers when I started my journey, I would have been better able to understand what was happening to me, my family, and my people. I'd have found the strengths that my ancestors used to survive and thrive, which have been passed on to me. The second lesson I would tell myself is not to buy into the idea of being an imposter or internalize the notion that I do not belong in certain spaces. While it's true that academic settings were not built with people like me in mind, that does not mean we don't belong in them. In fact, given the many barriers we have to confront to gain entry into graduate school, we not only belong there but have earned a place at the head of the table. If anyone is an imposter, it is those who have been allowed to enter these spaces because of the privilege of their skin color, socioeconomic status, or family connections, not their work.

Doris: I would tell my younger self that there's nothing wrong with you. I would tell myself to trust my own intuition because it is such a powerful source of wisdom that is totally unrecognized by the academy.

Linda: I would remind myself that my very presence is a disruption to the status quo and if it makes people uncomfortable, that is not my problem. Try to get along, but don't go along.

Doris: **Thank you so much for being with us. We're so grateful to all of you.**

Linda: **Thank you for literally *being* with us.**

Taking a Leap   **Part II**

In this second part of the book, we delve into career decision points where one chooses a path or combination of paths to pursue (e.g., academia, clinical practice, consulting, organizational leadership).

We begin with three chapters about the process of questioning, unlearning, and ultimately rejecting clinical practice models centered in white supremacist ideologies that separate us from Indigenous wisdom and knowledge, and fail to address the needs of communities of color. In **Chapter 10**, Kenneth V. Hardy, a Black cisgender marriage and family therapist, consultant, and academic, describes his realization that that he had become a "Good Effective Mainstream Minority" (Hardy, n.d.) and his subsequent development of Soul Work, a trauma-informed, racially focused, and holistic approach to healing for communities of color. In **Chapter 11**, Amanda Mays, a queer woman of color, describes her development of a personal brand and journey as a co-founder of a values-driven group psychotherapy practice of Black and Brown practitioners that centers BIPOC/LGBTQIA+ clients, equity-focused clinical and fee structures, and holistic community investment across all structures. In **Chapter 12**, Derek H. Suite, a Black psychiatrist, describes his experiences of structural violence and racial battle fatigue as a Black male physician in a PWI, and his decision to start his own culturally attuned, spiritually sensitive, and holistic group practice.

The next four chapters focus on the importance of building personal and institutional practices to buffer the exploitative, individualistic nature of work in a white supremacist, patriarchal, capitalist society. These practices are essential for restoring a sense of wholeness, balance, and communal

DOI: 10.4324/9781003309796-12

connection. In **Chapter 13**, Robyn L. Gobin, a Black cisgender woman psychologist, presents radical self-care as a powerful form of resistance for BIPOC that can support community-level wellness, freedom, and joy. In **Chapter 14**, Milo Dodson, an African American early career psychologist and senior manager, describes his value-driven, strengths-based approach to promoting diversity, equity, inclusion, and belonging in the tech industry. In **Chapter 15**, Black scholar-activist and social work practitioner Kirk "Jae" James examines the trauma of oppression and its impact on his life and frames restorative practices as tools for liberation. In **Chapter 16**, Helen Neville, Jioni A. Lewis, and Bryana French, three Black woman counseling psychology professors, describe their approach to social justice mentoring that integrates Black feminism, intersectionality, and radical healing frameworks. They close with recommendations for early career professionals engaging in mentoring activities to promote transformative change in academic and institutional settings.

Focusing on specific challenges of an academic career, Chapters 17 to 19 reimagine traditional models of pedagogy, academic publishing, and tenure review and promotion processes to expand beyond narrow definitions of academic success. In **Chapter 17**, Grace S. Kim and Karen L. Suyemoto, two Asian American feminist clinical psychology faculty, consider the challenges and rewards of teaching from a transformative education approach that emphasizes *teaching to* and *teaching as* whole people to foster students' conscientization, community building, and empowerment. In **Chapter 18**, Maryam Kia-Keating, a professor of clinical psychology in an RI research university, offers strategies to guide early career BIPOC scholars in designing a transformative career, both through traditional academic publishing as well as leveraging non-academic outlets for maximum reach and impact. In **Chapter 19**, Karen Jackson-Weaver, an African American leader in global higher education, offers strategies for faculty wellness and advancement for minority scholars in the professoriate.

We close this section with a powerful Community Conversation with Robyn L. Gobin, Ramani Durvasula, Maryam Kia-Keating, and Terrance Coffie about how they are leveraging the power of the media to decolonize psychological science, make mental health education more accessible, and advocate for policies to benefit BIPOC communities (**Chapter 20**).

Soul Work   **10**

A Pathway to Help Heal Communities of Color

Kenneth V. Hardy

Historically, the clinical field has devoted minimal attention to the specific therapeutic needs of clients of color, although fortunately this has begun to change. Despite gradual increasing interest in these issues, our society's commitment to the romantic myth of colorblindness continues to contribute to a massive dearth of knowledge and understanding regarding what is needed to facilitate a healing process for clients and communities of color. Clients of color undoubtedly grapple with many of the same life stressors as their white counterparts, and they must also contend with the stranglehold of living their daily lives within a vortex of racial oppression. In fact, attempting to overcome the devastating effects of racial oppression is a predictable, normal, and necessary developmental task that must be dealt with across the lifecycle for most families of color, regardless of gender, class, or sexual orientation. Unfortunately, it is an ongoing endeavor that is neither negotiable, nor obviated by other social privileges that People of Color might otherwise possess or enjoy. In this chapter, the terms people, clients, or communities of color are primarily referring to Black or Brown people although the approaches presented can be helpful and relevant to other groups.

The racial climate in the United States of America is such that if one is a Black or Brown Person of Color, one is inevitably engulfed in the asphyxiating and soul crushing dynamics of racial oppression. Regardless of the social outcome measured, whether related to educational achievement, health outcomes, prenatal death rates, home ownership, generational wealth, or a host of other issues, Black and Brown people are typically disproportionately located at the lower end of the negative outcomes. All these disillusioning

DOI: 10.4324/9781003309796-13

outcomes are connected to living in a pro-racist society in the firm grip of racial oppression where the impact of the centrality of whiteness is pervasive yet ignored and/or denied.

Throughout the field, scant comprehensive and concentrated attention has been devoted to even attempting to earnestly ascertain what is it that constitutes the centerpiece of a healing process for communities of color. Sadly, this issue was never seriously contemplated at any point during my graduate school education in marriage and family therapy or during two postdoctoral training programs I completed in racially diverse cities with large populations of clients of color. Once again, the myth of colorblindness, and the belief that the process of healing is centered around a universal set of therapeutic common factors, promulgated a "one size fits all" approach to healing.

Unfortunately, I was heavily indoctrinated into this way of thinking, and it greatly influenced my ideas and beliefs, and how I practiced therapy and approached the process of healing. This was nonetheless the case even when my lived experience as a Black man contradicted the premises and principles of much of what I was taught clinically and academically. In my training, there wasn't much space or freedom to assume a *both/and* position, which would acknowledge that both common *and* unique therapeutic factors could and do co-exist. The assumption was that all clients were essentially the same regardless of racial background or identity and that *healing was healing*. There was little to no acknowledgment that the concept of healing and what was necessary to promote it could be powerfully shaped by sociocultural factors such as race, class, gender, sexual orientation, religion, and a myriad of other factors.

On Becoming a *Whitened* Black Therapist

Regrettably, the formative years of my training were steeped in the belief that clinical efficacy was rooted in understanding the fundamentals of human behavior and how to effectively respond to it therapeutically. At best, this view was somewhere between race-neutral and race-oblivious. In other words, there was no substantive attention devoted to race, racial differences, or how the healing process might be defined or altered by the realities of race. All the theories I was exposed to were advanced by white theoreticians. All my professors, supervisors, and instructors were white, as were my internship and dissertation advisors, and neither their whiteness nor my Blackness was ever acknowledged or discussed. These critical issues were treated as though they were irrelevant. Although race, and especially whiteness, was never ever overtly discussed, it didn't have to be because it was deeply and indelibly etched into the culture of the training program, often to the oblivion of those entrusted to be trainers. When whiteness is not explicitly named, and white trainers tend to think of themselves as "trainers" without consideration of their racial identities, it is easy to ignore the pervasive and unexamined ways in which who they are racially impacts interactions, policies, and all dimensions of the training experience.

Whenever I or a liberal white classmate amassed enough courage to mention race, the conversation was often brief, lacking in depth and critical inquiry, and often dismissed as my personal agenda to unnecessarily and inappropriately "racialize issues that were not racial." The terse responses to me were never considered racial microaggressions, indicators of racial bias, or inappropriate. Instead, they were considered testimonials asserting and reasserting the purist, Eurocentric view regarding the universality of the human experience. Adherence to this dogmatic view was necessary to graduate and ultimately to be successful in the field, even when it culminated in the "mis-serving" and under-serving of communities of color. While many of these practices are often challenged in contemporary graduate and training programs, they unfortunately still exist in more sophisticated ways.

After years of training and subsequently entering clinical practice, I quickly and keenly became aware that I was doing so as a well-trained *whitened Black clinician*, and later as a GEMM, i.e., a **G**ood **E**ffective **M**ainstream **M**inority (Hardy, 2008). I was eventually forced to confront my ineptitude in providing the type of racially relevant care that was so desperately needed within communities of color after being challenged by a youth of color, Omar. He was perplexed by an incongruity he saw in me that my training had made it difficult for me to discern. In a state of flustered bewilderment, he stated, with a look of painful puzzlement, "Yo Doc, I been tryin' to figure you out and I just can't get a grip on you, man. I mean, I see your complexion, but I don't feel a connection." He went on to say, "To be honest, I feel Blacker than you and I am only half Black. I'm thinking maybe you should check yourself before you wreck yourself. I'm just sayin'."

Like many of my white counterparts, I had been trained to view the slow or minimal treatment progress of a client of color as evidence of their resistance to the process or an indication that they were probably not working hard enough. Not once did I consider, or was I ever trained to even hypothesize, that maybe what I was generously offering was grossly misaligned with what they needed. My initial reaction to Omar was to dismiss his difficult – but brutally honest and accurate, I might add – feedback as *adolescent resistance*, which it could have been. However, it was also an accurate assessment of how I was showing up in our therapeutic relationship. He needed, as he later indicated, to "feel" me, especially as a Black man, who happened to be his therapist. He wanted and needed to know that he could open up and explore issues that were both central and unique to his life as a Person of Color. In a multitude of ways, and especially prior to his confronting me, I was oblivious to all the barriers that I had created in the process for him to receive what he wanted and needed from me. Interestingly, the barriers were neither intentionally nor consciously created. Instead, they were embedded in my approach to therapy and how I had been trained. My indoctrination and subsequent perfection of becoming a GEMM had earned me tremendous respect in the wider field while also deeming me ineffectual in the consulting room with clients of color. My distant, slightly emotionally detached, "professional" psychologically oriented approach to healing was an impediment to the process, rather than the conduit I wished it to be.

It was my work with Omar that inspired me to begin thinking differently about therapy with clients of color and how it both parallels and departs from therapy with white clients. My in-depth work with Omar, along with my own experience as a client with a white therapist whom I admired and respected, drastically challenged and changed my approach to therapy and began to enhance my understanding regarding what is needed therapeutically for clients of color to heal. While my therapist was empathic, understanding, and insightful, race was always a major barrier in our work. I always had felt that race was a central organizing principle in my life, and I was mystified and chagrined that it was never talked about in therapy unless I raised it. Even then, it was greeted with a polite, superficial, and brief curiosity that lacked traction, authentic interest, or engagement. After a while, I ceased to mention race because it seemed fruitless. I realized how much my experience as a client so closely mirrored what I imagined Omar's early experience was with me as his therapist. It is a major therapeutic dilemma for many clients of color when they work with white therapists who avoid mentioning race for fear of saying the wrong thing, and with some therapists of color who likewise neglect to mention it in any substantive way because they do not wish to be narrowly defined by their race. Mutism about race in therapy often inadvertently denies clients of color the opportunity to participate in a healing process anchored in *soul work*.

Soul Work as Healing Work

Communities of color need the same empathic and insightful care that all clients desire and deserve. They also need treatment that is potently racially attuned. The core of the work that so many People of Color need, regardless of the anatomy of the presenting problem, is essentially *soul work*. It is soul work that begins to stitch, repair, and reconnect all the parts of the human spirit that have been broken, maimed, mutilated, and dispirited by hyper-exposure to racial oppression, and ultimately racialized trauma. Soul work is a racially focused holistic approach to healing that embraces and weaves together the emotional, psychological, spiritual, and relational dimensions of both the psyche and soul. It is predicated on the belief that full engagement of mind, body, and soul are tantamount to the process of healing.

Whether the presenting problem is centered around enuresis or encopresis, adolescents or adults, death or divorce, the therapist must be committed to engaging in soul work. This racially focused work is not intended to ignore or supplant addressing the pressing presenting issue(s) for which clients are seeking assistance, but instead, to augment it. After all, there is no manifestation of pain and suffering experienced among communities of color that is completely segregated from the nuances of race.

A Pathway to Helping Communities of Color Heal

To facilitate healing for communities of color, critical attention must be devoted to the following: (1) acknowledgement and validation; (2) willingness to engage in authentic race talk openly; (3) addressing invisible racial trauma wounds; and (4) embracing and employing racially relevant healing approaches. It is worth noting here that the effective execution of these therapeutic principles does not de facto constitute soul work, but rather creates and provides the foundation for it to occur.

Acknowledgement and Validation

No matter how ubiquitous race is throughout our lives, our societal impulse is to deny the significance of it. Even when communities of color have been openly, directly, and inarguably assaulted by racism and oppression, it is not uncommon for many whites to deny, minimize, or attempt to negate its significance. Unfortunately, the consequence of this common society-wide practice is that many communities of color must live concomitantly with the painful realities of racism and the widespread denial that it is a salient issue. The lack of acknowledgment and validation of these experiences is "crazy-making." It is emotionally and psychologically destabilizing and often leaves individuals drowning in a sea of uncertainty and self-doubt. Many People of Color struggle with recurring and daunting thoughts: "I must be crazy," "Is something wrong with me?" "Is this in my head?" "Am I an imposter?" "Am I being hypersensitive?"

One of the first steps to creating a pathway to healing for communities of color centers around the proactive and public proclamation that race is a legitimate and critical issue that is worthy of consideration. When the issue of race is proactively introduced and pursued by the therapist rather than waiting for the client to do so, it conveys the soul liberatory message that "I want you to **know** that I **know** that race is an important dynamic for us to consider in our work. It is not the *only* dynamic; however, it is an important one!" This is one of many ways ac**know**ledgment can be executed and integrated into the therapeutic process. While this might, at first glance, be reasonably construed as a "clinical strategy," it is so much more and requires more than a commitment to "doing." It requires a commitment to and comfort with "being" and bearing witness. It is the therapist's emotional availability and presence with the client that provides the groundwork for healing. This is an important task for the therapist to implement even if/when the client is seemingly oblivious to race and its widespread effects.

The healing potential of acknowledgment is fostered by the power and audacity it contains in clearly and directly "naming" that which is rarely overtly named throughout our society, and particularly in a context where it is neither contentious nor contested. The process of acknowledgement not only names the unnamable, but it also legitimizes (i.e., validates) the process of doing so. It asserts and affirms that the exploration of race is not just permissible but expected and is an essential component of the work to be done. This positioning paves the way for the second critical step toward promoting soul work and a pathway to healing, which involves transitioning from acknowledging race to supporting and encouraging deep uninhibited conversations that center it.

Race Talk

It is rare that Black and Brown people receive the space and grace to talk openly and uninhibitedly about race, free of threat, reprimand, and/or reprisal.

As such, both their voices and the legitimacy of their race-related stories are either managed by suppression, i.e., the willful and deliberate act of holding back, or repression, i.e., an unconscious act of forgetting or denying. Either way, Black and Brown people are coerced to sit in a cesspool of race-based agony with their voices muted, while fiercely fighting off complex feelings ranging from hopelessness to fury and rage.

Creating a safe milieu where People of Color can tell their stories in their own words – without interruption, edit, or censorship – is crucial to soul work and the process of healing. It is imperative that they do so with the understanding that both what is said and how it is said will be graciously and respectfully received with empathy and validation. Paving the way to talk about race enables People of Color to tell and honor the three pivotal stories that are liberatory and constitute the essence of soul work. These three stories are: 1) Stories of Suffering (which center what happened to me); 2) Stories of Struggle (which center my journey to overcome and reclaim myself); and 3) Stories of Survival (which center how I am overcoming, aspire to overcome, and/or how I overcame). Without sanctioning race talk, expressions of acknowledgement and validation, these critical stories will remain untold, and healing severely thwarted. When the significance of race is acknowledged and talking about it is fully embraced and practiced, it paves the way for the third step of healing, i.e., addressing the invisible wounds of racial trauma.

Addressing the Invisible Wounds of Racial Trauma

It is virtually impossible to be hyper-exposed to racial oppression and not be scarred and injured by racial trauma. Unfortunately, even with the nascent trend emphasizing trauma-informed care, the phenomenon of racial trauma is rarely considered. It is typically excluded in the broader discourse about trauma, and it certainly does not exist in our clinical lexicon. It is unnamed, unacknowledged, and therefore deemed non-existent, even though communities of color are vastly affected by it. The deleterious wounds associated with racial trauma are also essentially unnamed and invisible. There are seven intersecting invisible wounds that must be acknowledged, validated, and addressed as a condition for healing. These wounds are: 1) internalized devaluation; 2) the assaulted sense of self (Hardy, 2013); 3) learned voicelessness; 4) psychological homelessness; 5) survival anxiety; 6) complex loss and collective grief; and 7) rage (Hardy, 2023).

In therapy and beyond, tending to these wounds is vital to promoting healing for communities of color. When the invisible wounds of racial trauma are acknowledged, validated, and treated as a centerpiece to the healing process, the focal point of the work must be designed to accomplish the following goals:

1. Develop and adopt counternarratives that restore dignity and systematically expunge all internalized race-based toxic messages from the psyche and soul;
2. Actively and assertively promote race-based self-love in all its manifestations – physically, emotionally, psychologically, spiritually, and relationally;
3. Overcome voicelessness and learn how to speak for the liberation of one's soul, rather than for the approval of whites and others;
4. Invest in relationships and relational connectedness;
5. Develop and fortify strategies of survival by investing in the power of community and relationships;
6. Make a deliberate effort to acknowledge and embrace loss and to create emotional, psychological, and relational space for mourning. This process also includes expressing grief for losses associated with one's literal self as well as one's symbolic self (e.g., the members of one's tribe); and
7. Embrace rage and identify ways to re-channel it. During this phase, it is important for communities of color to accept that rage is a natural reaction to unnatural and oppressive conditions. Thus, it is critical that they embrace, rather than deny, their rage and understand that doing so is necessary for healing.

These goals are integral to the process of healing but are difficult to achieve if traditional individually oriented talk therapy is the only tool that is used. The type of healing that is desired, needed, and envisioned inevitably requires therapists and aspiring healers to be amenable to using a wide range of racially relevant healing strategies.

Embracing and Employing Racially Relevant Healing Strategies

The healing process needed for communities of color requires the acceptance and application of a variety of therapeutic strategies that extend well beyond what has been historically propagated in mainstream mental health services. For example, music, song, poetry, prayer, and spoken word are all powerful culturally based tools that may foster healing. Dance, drama, movement, and somatic embodiment approaches (Menakem, 2017) are important tools for mending and bridging the Eurocentric-imposed fractures that often exist between mind, body, health, and healing. It is not only important that therapy and other sacred places create ample space for the integration of these varied instruments of healing, but also that they are applied with a communal-relational focus. This is not an indictment of individual work, but rather a testimonial and affirmation of the healing potential of relationships. The type of relationally based work described here is even fundamentally different from traditional group therapy approaches, which often involve working with a collection of individuals often without a shared racial experience, background, or history.

When we adopt a relational approach to healing, it becomes easier to call upon and incorporate immediate and extended family members in the process, as well as peers, religious and community healers, and ancestors. In this work, the boundaries of the healing circle are permeable, expansive, and fluid, facilitating the cultivation of a safe and sacred holding space. The space that is cultivated can offer communities of color the opportunity to counteract devaluation, mend the assaulted self, promote and model self-love, re-ignite and reclaim race-related joy that has been stolen or compromised by racism, transform learned voicelessness to voice, allow space for mourning and grief, develop strategies for survival, purposefully direct and re-channel rage, and perhaps most importantly, create an existential and spiritual home for those of us who are psychologically homeless.

Healing Beyond the Therapy Room

It is widely known within many communities of color that the aforementioned approaches to healing are rarely found in traditional psychotherapy settings, at least in a comprehensive and consistent way. For example, in the African American community, healing routinely takes place in the community barber shop, hair salon, fraternities and sororities, and in the Black church, where song, scripture, spoken word, movement, and "narratives" of suffering, struggle, and survival are acknowledged and validated as a matter of common practice. These are the places where hope is restored and despair defeated, if only momentarily. These community-based resources constitute the epicenter for soul work and healing for many communities of color. Yet, more is needed. While these "healing centers" are vital pillars of the community, many do not offer the depth, continuity, and sustainability to adequately meet the gravity of the need. New and additional pathways for healing communities of color are needed. Expanding the conceptualization of therapy by extricating it from the shackles of white supremacist ideology and being more intentional about attending to the impact of racism and other systems of oppression on all our lives would be an important first step. Such a significant change would inevitably challenge our existing preconceived notions about what constitutes healing and what is required to achieve it. Most of all, embedded in this evolving process would be the unapologetic embrace of soul work as a viable pathway to healing that promotes and restores hope and aims to heal the souls of communities of color in all the hurt places.

References

Hardy, K. V. (2008). On becoming a GEMM therapist: Work harder, be smarter, and never discuss race. In M. McGoldrick & K. V. Hardy (Eds.), *Re-visioning family therapy: Addressing diversity in clinical practice* (3rd ed.). The Guilford Press.

Hardy, K. V. (2013). Healing the hidden wounds of racial trauma. *Reclaiming Children and Youth, 22*(1), 24–28.

Hardy, K. V. (2023). *Healing racial trauma: Clinical strategies for treating invisible wounds.* W.W. Norton & Company.

Menakem, R. (2017). *My grandmother's hands: Racialized trauma and the pathway to mending our hearts and bodies.* Central Recovery Press.

Developing Your Brand

Building a Private Practice

Amanda Mays

Many discussions about therapeutic practice reflect on the centering of white supremacy, the pervasive system to ensure white dominance and control – and the call for diversification of the mental health profession field (Badwall, 2015; Calkins, 2020). Further, there's an increasing visibility of the experiences of Black, Indigenous, and People of Color (BIPOC) social workers (and other mental health professionals) in their educational and professional settings and the significant toll on their well-being, and ability to sustain long- term careers (Onque, 2022).

Our Vision

Deep gratitude to Taryn Crosby, LCSW and Rafael Martinez, LCSW, who along with me – began visioning our practice with a reflection on our own experiences as Black and Brown practitioners in our academic education and as therapists, with opportunities to grow and innovate in our clinical practices. Across the board, we had predominantly white professors and supervisors. We found ourselves regularly dismissed and even punished in the systems that theoretically were supposed to elevate our learning and professional growth, but in reality were daunting and ever changing goal posts that we felt stuck and stagnant within.

DOI: 10.4324/9781003309796-14

Our drive was to begin a journey that was centered in shared values, an acknowledgement of internalized racial trauma, and the historical siloing of our own communities. We did not set out with an idealized outcome or belief that we could "overcome or fix" the historical and current socio-political hold of white supremacy. We situated ourselves in an affirmative position, namely that we DIDN'T know what the full journey would look like, that we had to stay in places of discomfort together – within our differing racial and lived experiences, navigating structures and systems of whiteness – to create a secure enough container for deeper exploration, curiosity, and connection.

We situated ourselves in the joy, strengths, and innovations across BIPOC communities. Our foremost priority was affirmative clinical space for our clients and the early career therapists working in our practice, while also intentionally creating structures that acknowledged disparities in therapeutic access and financial resourcing.

Our Practice

Our practice is solely Black and Brown practitioners, prioritizes BIPOC clients, integrates equitable resourcing and access across all clinical and financial elements and integrates holistic community investment across all structures. We did not want to replicate the exploitative norm of the social work and other mental health fields, and recognized opportunities to create space for the complex narratives (and power dynamics) of BIPOC/LGBTQIA+ communities. Additionally, we created a fee structure that allowed for broader community investment – clients capable of paying higher fees transparently understood and actively wanted to contribute to those with limited financial capacity. This has presented many uncomfortable discussions and challenges as we sit in the fact that broader systems are actively racist, our own internalization of scarcity and protectiveness, along with the very simple truth – that we could NOT fully make up for all the systems outside of our control that limits access to resourcing.

A Little About My Brand

I have had the great fortune of working across professional streams in the social work field and with multiple communities. This is the beginning of my "elevator pitch" in an attempt to make my professional journey legible and exciting. The thing about elevator pitches is that they exclude nuances, fears, and the various existential crises that often come with being a member of our field.

Here come the checkmarks: I am a Queer South Asian cis woman, adoptee (and eventual foster child) with a perceived disability. I say checkmarks, because we know that these labels are extraordinarily important to define our proximity to privilege – both/and are WOEFULLY inadequate in describing the nuance and textures of our journey. Having direct experience growing up in a majority white community and involvement within the social welfare system, I knew from a very young age that I was disposable – meaning that my body, being, and future would always be at the mercy of an exploitative system demanding that I work smarter, harder, and longer than my peers to eek out a survival – I was not entitled to the safety of mistakes, let alone security and stability.

The reality of sustaining a long- term career in social work and other mental health careers requires us to be messy, challenged, deeply uncomfortable, and honest with ourselves in our purpose. I'm going to be a little controversial here when I say that my passion has not been my driving force throughout my 20 plus years in social work – rather, I have found functional values and purpose that I can center whatever my professional role. Passion IS important, however it has been my experience that this word passion gets deeply intertwined in altruism, selfless giving, idealism, and many other adjectives that lead to burnout emotionally, professionally, and financially.

Back to my elevator pitch, or what we'll call my brand. I HAVE had the fortunate opportunity to work in a variety of professional capacities throughout my career – the variety of roles has allowed me a holistic and textured perspective on the social work field as a whole, and has taught me some humbling lessons in my own capacity.

Throughout my journey, my purpose was to create as much space as possible for narratives and voices that go unheard and unacknowledged – this is my center and function as a professional.

Specifically, how do I shift systems that I work within to reflect the meaningful needs of the communities that I have partnered with – in contrast to the common narrative in which people receiving support are asked to pretzel themselves in order to receive services. Further, these same systems have asked me to pretzel myself as a practitioner. Asked over and over again to bring my skill and labor – but please leave my personhood at home. Given the intensity of the work we do in social work, to leave our own humanness and that of the communities we partner with makes for a system that is never equitable.

Autonomy over my clinical ideas and work, and to nurture space for Black, Indigenous, and POC practitioners to have agency over their professional selves, are fundamental to me.

Remember that this is one field – and social workers often feel compelled to categorize (and separate) ourselves by professional titles and areas of work. We get lost in dizzying definitions about what is "true" social work as well as confusing conversations about "serving" those in true need. The way service is used in this context is coded white altruism.

Do You Really Get to Decide Your Brand?

We carry the weight of our identities and lived experience, spanning from the hurt and pain or hopes and dreams from our families and communities to the daily microaggressions and barriers we must navigate. As mentioned above, in the beginning of my career, I felt that I had to prove to my white superiors and peers that I deserved the opportunity to be in the field. And though I knew that my focus was helping marginalized communities, I nonetheless was perpetuating a script of inferiority on myself and worse, my clients.

Our brand is the integration of our values, philosophy, and service offerings displayed through our public presence. We don't fully get to decide what our brand is – it is in part chosen by the ways we are perceived, and what our communities need from us. And many of us choose to carry that representation proudly. We WANT to heal the pain and trauma of our communities and families. We WANT to be the actualization of their hopes and dreams. The problem is that we are at risk of losing our authenticity, or find ourselves at the mercy of others' perspectives and needs.

Capability Versus Capacity

During the immensely powerful Racial Reckoning in 2021, through the present, our practice has had a stream of requests to clinically support BIPOC communities for no cost, and though we cared deeply about the pain that was emanating across our communities, and provided support that aligned with our capacity, we knew that overextending ourselves and burning out is not a value – it's a trap.

As a professor, I've discussed the distinctions between Capability versus Capacity. In the context of ableism, we can see that many folks have the capability of doing just about anything. However, the built environment and social oppression render an individual without the capacity of doing these things. Capabilities are infinite; humans grow and learn and are able to do so many things. Capacity is more finite; if there is not enough resourcing – we burn out.

Now I want to flip this analogy. So many of us in the BIPOC communities can't reflect on our capacity because whiteness requires us to do double time to prove our capabilities. A reflection or decision about our capacity feels in direct conflict with our communities' survival. I want to do so many things, provide support wherever I can and to whoever needs it, yet I can't. I am a mere mortal. And dear reader, you are also a mere mortal.

We also get stuck in the binary of "success/failure" which are terms that feed white supremacy, making it stronger in fact. As long as we are using binary definitions of our personhood and professional capacities, the system can stay intact and undisturbed. Allow our journey to be about depth instead of destination, and truly give ourselves the deserved space to try, and try again, as many times as we need. And within that journey, we must give ourselves the permission to adapt and change our vision, our capacity – and do the dreaded: say no.

Your Brand

So, when beginning to think through what you want your brand or public presence to be, it may help to answer these questions:

1. What are my fundamental values? How does this translate into a functional purpose?
2. Who am I really doing this for? Why am I doing this for myself (does not involve anyone else's needs)?
3. Where am I most at risk of overextending myself?
4. How do I feel about saying no? Being in healthy conflict with others?

Now take these answers to someone you trust, and ask them to give you honest feedback. From there you have the basis of your brand as you start, and allow it to evolve over time.

You Are Going to Make Mistakes

I feel the need to say this out loud for all to hear: PERFECT is not a real thing, there is no such composite of perfection. It doesn't exist. My experience is that the internalized definition of perfection is just us criticizing ourselves as a way we can "feel" in control, and though a sense of safety is necessary, we don't want to limit our ability to learn and grow.

This internal sense of control is deeply impacted and compounded by the structures of whiteness that withhold resources, knowledge, and affirmation from our communities. I have often felt that all I did automatically had very high stakes attached. What if I represent my identities in the "wrong" way? What if I am not able to do all the things another may need. And most critically, what if I can't do everything myself?

Healthy rigor allows for an iterative internal and external process – repeat the act, remember lessons from before and work through it again. This does take courage to risk not knowing something, or having mastery of a skill readily available to us.

My largest lessons throughout my career have been attached to my hubris, when I thought that I SHOULD be doing something to HELP others. The pressures I put on myself involved me not engaging in uncomfortable humility – asking others about their perspectives and needs, calibrating my actions and expectations to a partnered perspective. In the whirl of my hubris, I made decisions for others based on my own narratives of my role.

Humility is a gift leading to a place where safe curiosity can flourish. Instead of a punishing "I messed up, I should have done better," you can transform into "what was going on for me that I moved too quickly, or had that reaction?" Doing a self-inventory of your own processes and needs is fundamental to sustaining your practice:

1. What is my authentic learning style and process?
2. How do I feel when I don't know something?
3. How do I feel when asking for help?
4. What have my experiences taught me about being fallible or making mistakes?

Again, share your answers with someone you trust for their feedback and refine what you need to allow yourself a paced and caring learning curve.

Let's Talk About MONEY

In my experience, this is one of the most uncomfortable topics for us to have with each other, and then with our clients. It is also a central trauma that we must support ourselves and our clients in navigating. To better understand this discomfort, we need to situate ourselves in a normalizing context before going any further:

Black, Indigenous, and POC communities are intentionally and deeply under-resourced. Within the oppressive structures of white supremacy and our intergenerational trauma, it is common for our feelings about money and resourcing to be centered in fear, scarcity, abusive and exploitative power dynamics, and an inherent lack of security. And the capitalistic structures centered in whiteness actively create barriers and unnecessary gate-keeping to keep us in an insecure place.

Not a single mental health degree program requires, or consistently integrates, any education about the mechanics of the business and financial systems that are involved in providing mental health care. We may learn about the history of social policy systems – but not the specifics of Medicaid, Medicare, and private insurance funding and disbursement. We are actually taught that "money and business" is irrelevant, or even antithetical to providing "good" mental health care.

We are taught a very limited perspective about ourselves and clients of color regarding financial resourcing and decision making.

To have our own business, to own our work, is **actively discouraged**. Yet managing your own business requires you to get comfortable with the discomfort of finances very quickly and you need to make sure you are prepared for this tumultuous process. Ask yourself:

1. Was money discussed in my upbringing? My academic education? In what tone was it discussed?
2. What are the work ethics or traits I have been taught connected to money?
3. What comes up in sharing my financial experiences with others?
4. What are the conflicts and discomfort I have about charging clients for services?
5. How do I feel about seeking support about areas of financial and business literacy I don't have knowledge in?

Share these answers with someone you trust and get honest feedback to begin to create a plan of support for yourself.

Don't Go It Alone

There are many complex and interconnected elements to running your own private practice and it can be lonely and daunting. It is required that you create a network of professional and personal support to ensure you can remain focused on your work while also sustaining yourself. I intentionally chose to create a private practice business with partners because I understood enough about myself to know that I couldn't do it all, and that I wanted to be in a continuous state of learning and growth. I sought out colleagues in my professional network that:

- I LIKED – folks that I could build interpersonal along with professional relationships with;
- I admired and respected in terms of their clinical perspectives and experiences;
- Had skills and strengths that I did not have;
- I could be in safe and generative conflict and difference of opinion with.

You may choose to start a solo practice as well. Either way it's important that you have a network of support you can access as you go along your journey. The roles of therapist, business owner, and, if you so choose, clinical supervisor or employer often carry inherently conflicting responsibilities. Ensure that you are giving yourself time to scaffold implementing elements of your practice so that you can have secure and sustainable growth.

Let's start with YOU, and identify areas of support:

- Your personal therapeutic space;
- Your supervision (or clinical support) space;
- Peers and colleagues you can share experiences with – preferably in a formal structure;
- People in your personal circle of community that are not mental health professionals. It's important to keep balance in our perspectives and "talking shop" all the time can be quite harmful;
- Individual activities that are just for you! Things that are containing and bring pleasure / comfort – again, non-"work" activities.

It may feel like going against the "do it ourselves" values within our communities to seek professional help in areas we are not as familiar with such as business concepts. As I mentioned above when discussing money, shame, scarcity, and fear can drive these decisions – please hear me when I say, the money and legal elements of running your business are things you SHOULD and DESERVE to get assistance with.

Below are some business and client elements that are helpful to have in place.

- Business structure and accounting systems – A certified public accountant (CPA) can assist in advising on, and setting up these elements. There are many complexities to navigate and I strongly recommend you find a CPA that has experience working with direct service businesses.
- Client agreements, fee range, and billing structures – Ask professional peers not only their range of fees, but also what that materializes into monthly. There are guides for the legal requirements of treatment agreements and insurance panel credentialing, and now third party entities that you can sign up with to accept insurance.
- Advertising and public presence – Investing in a website where clients can learn about you and your practice is critical. Additionally, you should seek out listservs and groups that have a similar niche as you – most referrals come from word of mouth in your professional networks and clients.

Let's Wrap Up

First, let me say Thank You! Thank you for caring about yourself, about the trajectory of your career, for your courage to try new things – for being YOU! I've heard the adjective RADICAL ascribed to our practice with regularity, and I feel ambivalent about this description. And I recognize that I feel urgency. We NEED BIPOC practices to become commonplace for our communities to access the affirming care we deserve and for our practitioners to have ownership and agency in our professional selves and ways we approach our communities' health and well-being. This creates a significant ripple effect to move social and clinical work beyond the limits we are currently constrained by, to the deep and meaningful ways our communities' wisdom is central and the catalyst for abolition of the current structure.

Throughout my journey, both ups and downs, I have loved my work, and I hope this guide gives you a useful framework to think about, and move forward with your love, values, and vision.

References

Badwall, H. K. (2015). Colonial encounters: Racialized social workers negotiating professional scripts of whiteness. *Intersectionalities: A Global Journal of Social Work Analysis, Research, Polity, and Practice, 3*(1), 1–23.

Calkins, H. (2020). *Increasing the visibility of providers of color.* American Psychological Association, September 1. www.apa.org/monitor/2020/09/increasing-providers-color

Onque, R. (2022). *Why therapists of color are leaving the profession.* CNBC, September 28. www.cnbc.com/2022/09/28/heres-why-therapists-of-color-are-leaving-the-profession.html

Combating Racial Battle Fatigue and Navigating and Challenging Predominantly White Institutions

12

Derek H. Suite

Racial battle fatigue (RBF), coined in 2003 by social psychologist, Dr. William Smith, was originally used in reference to the race-related responses of Black men to the cumulative and ongoing effects of microaggressions, insults, slights, and invalidations associated with racism. Over the past decade, RBF has been amplified to describe negative racial experiences of all People of Color (POC). It is in the amplified context of RBF that I present this retrospective analysis and reflection on my personal and professional journey as the co-founder of Full Circle Health (FCH), a culturally competent, spiritually sensitive psychiatric group practice that has served over 350,000 People of Color since its inception.

In addition to sharing racially charged challenges involved in navigating a predominantly white mental health system as an independent, Black-owned mental health practice, I will share personal and professional strategies of innovation, adaptability, resistance, and resilience that have helped me fashion FCH as a beacon of hope and healing for individuals at risk for the negative and debilitating outcomes of RBF. I trust this reflection will provide ideas, insights, and inspiration as you contemplate your relationship with

DOI: 10.4324/9781003309796-15

racism and think about how you currently navigate and possibly challenge institutional or structural racism within the context of your professional journey.

Challenging Circumstances Give Birth to Positionality, Perspective, and Purpose

Looking back at my childhood and early schooling in Trinidad, nearly everyone I encountered was a Person of Color, and the widely shared values of education, hard work, and achievement were the overarching priorities and influencers of my worldview and self-esteem. I had no real appreciation of racism and its effects in Trinidad. In fact, the national motto of Trinidad, *"together we aspire, together we achieve,"* only reinforced in me an idealistic, and perhaps naïve, sense of the collective power of unity and diversity. My naiveté quickly changed within the first few months of my acculturation to the United States at age 11, where white students would make fun of my accent and my skin color. Through repeated exposure to overt and subtle racism within the United States, I learned that I had to fight for my self-confidence and find ways to preserve my self-esteem. Throughout my medical education, residency training, and early career, I relied heavily on the values that were instilled in my childhood to cope with various racist experiences and the ensuing RBF, which were perpetually shaping and reshaping my psyche, positionality, and perspective, and simultaneously influencing my trajectory and destiny as a Black male physician.

In retrospect, RBF, though ever-present, had become an unspoken part of my medical school experience, which I subsequently learned was not unique to me as a Person of Color. Indeed, research studies confirm the negative impact of RBF on Black male identity and belonging in medical education (Strayhorn, 2020). Indelible memories of racially charged incidents in medical school and residency training still haunt the recesses of my mind. In 1990, as a medical student, I was on an Amtrak train back to medical school from New York, after visiting my parents. Upon arriving at the 30th Street train station in Philadelphia, I was suddenly surrounded by several individuals who forced me to the ground, pointing guns at my head, while they emptied my travel bag and rummaged through my belongings. After a thorough search of my travel bag and my body revealed nothing suspicious, the mostly white police force eventually told me that I fit the description of a Black male transporting narcotics, and walked away. There was no apology, no helping me up off the floor, and no assistance gathering my personal items.

This harrowing 30th Street incident would haunt me for years, but it was just the beginning of what would be an immersive, multilayered experience of racism littered with microaggressions and micro-insults during medical school and residency, including being complimented because I spoke English so well, or being mistaken for a food services staffer when entering a patient's room despite wearing a white coat, a stethoscope, and physician's identification badge. It also included being asked to produce additional identification when walking into the hospital after hours with white colleagues (who would vouch for me to no avail), or having my on-call room searched by hospital security while working overnight shifts at the hospital.

As an early career doctor, I would receive memos asking me to cease and desist from prescribing and incorporating spiritual and other holistic approaches into clinical practice because there was no "credible, conclusive, or evidence-based" research to support a spiritually driven approach to health and well-being. Silenced by the ruling majority and prevailing authorities, I succumbed to the institutional pressure and stayed silent – just as I did with the cops at the 30th Street station. I recall once breaking my usual "Black man silence" to share my observations about the hospital's apparent biased pattern of automatically screening Black patients (not *all* patients) to be ruled out for substance use, even if they deny any prior history. To my surprise, my observation was called "irresponsible, inconsiderate, and ridiculous" by an attending physician in front of the predominantly white hospital staff. In a word, I felt "trapped" by these belittling experiences. I realized that I could no longer navigate and survive in an institution where I felt powerless to stop the systematic, implicitly biased policies and practices that targeted individuals based on race.

After many soul-searching nights filled with prayer, meditation, and reflection, I understood that my disillusionment was tied to my inability to find synergy and congruence for my vision on what healthcare should look like for People of Color. In m0y h0eart, I knew the only way out was to create a culturally competent and spiritually sensitive psychiatric practice.

Seeking Solid Foundation: The Power of Theories, Frameworks, Structures, and Constraints

Many of my white colleagues working in predominantly white medical and mental health institutions repeatedly warned me that the notion of starting a "culturally and spiritually driven" psychiatric practice was unrealistic and that the chances of it surviving on its own were remarkably slim.

They seemed genuinely unaware that heavily factoring a clients' race and racialized narratives vis-à-vis their cultural and spiritual experiences and practices could significantly affect their health, well-being, and response to treatment. RBF was not in their calculus because race and racism were not critical to the healthcare equation for them. Like my colleagues, I was educated in predominantly white institutions that did not teach racism as a critical contributor to the expression of illness – even though it is well-documented that race significantly influences how people think, behave, and function (Roberts & Rizzo, 2021). Most theoretical frameworks (and the institutions that accept, teach, and implement them) are overwhelmingly represented by white scientists and researchers who historically have not incorporated race-related stress as a significant risk factor for mental illness and, as has been documented, a potentially more powerful risk factor than stressful life events for psychological distress (Utsey et al., 2008). Not surprisingly, my colleagues were not fully aware of the impact of the legacies of scientific and structural racism that contribute to People of Color's ongoing mistrust of medical and mental health systems (Sharma & Kuper, 2017; Suite, La Bril et al., 2007). Without this context, they were unable to integrate the historical experiences of racism with People of Color's current (and often daily) experience of structural and institutional racism (Franklin et al., 2014).

Against the prevailing winds of institutional and structural racism, I forged ahead to establish Full Circle Health using a blended and integrative framework that combined major tenets of Critical Race Theory (CRT) combined with elements of Biopsychosocial-Spiritual (BPSS) and Narrative Therapy (NT) frameworks. Because CRT examines race as a pervasive social (as opposed to a biological) construct that permeates American society, it appealed to me based on my personal experiences with racism as a Black male, and structural racism experiences as a Black male physician (Serafini et al., 2020). Unlike many of the theoretical frameworks that were part of my medical and psychiatric training, CRT acknowledges that racist ideologies have been historically practiced and perpetuated in mental health and offers a critical lens through which Eurocentric, ethnocentric, and race-related inequalities could be deconstructed and examined (Moodley et al., 2017).

Amplifying CRT using a narrative approach allowed for an expansion of the FCH theoretical framework because of narrative therapy's strong emphasis on mutuality, respect, and collaboration between the provider and client and the creation of a safe storytelling space where multiple viewpoints and perspectives can emerge and co-exist in the context of openness and optimism (Edwards & Walker, 2019). Another advantage of the narrative approach that can be very appealing and helpful to People of Color is the importance narrative therapy places on examining words and their meaning (Carr, 1998). Terms such as "doctor," "supervisor," "therapist," and "noncompliance" are meticulously scrutinized (or avoided) because of the implicit power and control implications and potentially pejorative connotations. Additionally, narrative therapy does not involve challenging and opposing clients by persuading or coercing them to change, or minimizing their unique stories (Edwards & Walker, 2019). Instead of cheerleading and exhorting, the narrative facilitator stays "a step behind," acknowledges the clients' problem-saturated perspectives, and helps them externalize these internalized perspectives in their own voice and make choices about who they will be and how they want to live (Edwards & Walker, 2019).

To complete the FCH theoretical foundation, I saw value in the integration of the BPSS model over the traditional Biopsychosocial (BPS) approach that permeated my training. I moved past the BPS to the BPSS model because of its ability to consider multiple dimensions of wellness and aid in differential diagnosis, and how it aligned with my personal conviction that a person's spiritual beliefs factor significantly into their understanding, compliance, and response to treatment. Interestingly, ample evidence supports that most Americans believe in God or a higher power and want their religious beliefs and spirituality included in their healthcare (Lee & Newberg, 2005; McCauley et al., 2005). Despite this evidence, fewer than 20% of healthcare providers regularly incorporate spirituality in the treatment process (Suite, Rollin et al., 2007).

Within the confines of this integrated framework, FCH clients effectively tackle RBF by working through the fear, anxiety, frustration, burnout, disillusionment, anger, and depression that People of Color so often experience living in and navigating historically and predominantly white spaces. Our clients struggling with RBF continue to report feeling a sense of deep relief and validation because they could share their presenting histories in the context of their racialized experiences of environments and encounters (CRT context). Clients repeatedly expressed feeling empowered by sharing (and externalizing) their traumatizing experiences, while exploring potentially alternative stories (NT context). They also shared their immense satisfaction that the FCH approach also incorporated a traditional "scientifically oriented" examination of how their experiences connected to their biological, psychological, social, *and spiritual* (BPSS) concerns. This multi-layered and blended theoretical approach, derived from my personal experiences, field research, and informal feedback from hundreds of racial trauma survivors, served as the culturally informed, spiritually sensitive foundation on which FCH still stands today.

Personal Reflections on the Personal and Professional Journey

My journey to the creation of FCH in spite of racism and RBF serves as a personal reminder that inspiration draws power from adversity. Indeed, I now look back on these painful experiences with a sense of deep gratitude because they motivated me to find not only "a way out" but "a way in" – a way to extricate myself from constraints of institutional racism, yet, at the same time, be inspired to "be the change I wanted to see" by reinventing my life as a founding member and leader of an independent healing resource in the broader, societal context of racism and mental healthcare.

Imagination Can Take You Anywhere: Show the World You've Got Pride

Though small in comparison to many traditional mental health institutions, FCH has become a force for culturally and spiritually sensitive healing; a place where faith and love abound; a place where dignity and pride in one's culture and beliefs are welcomed. The September 11, 2001 tragedy was a watershed moment when FCH was called upon to lead a multidisciplinary team of mental health clinicians to provide stress management services to mission-critical federal employees, using the FCH model of care. This launched FCH into becoming a trusted provider to several government officials and entities. Beyond providing services to government entities, FCH has won recognition for its work with underserved populations and is an approved graduate and postgraduate clinical internship site for psychology and social work programs of many leading universities. Furthermore, FCH also provides mental health support for numerous community agencies, including those that serve justice system-involved and foster care youth.

Fighting Dragons and Slaying Monsters with Courage and Creativity

In the early days of FCH, my wife Darcel and I would wake up each morning, turn to each other, and one of us would say, "Are you ready to fight some monsters and slay some dragons?" Although we have won many battles, we are acutely aware that the war rages on given the significant amplification of mental health concerns in the wake of the recent reckoning around social injustice sparked by the horrific murder of George Floyd and others in the middle of the devastating twin pandemics of COVID-19 and social injustice. FCH continues to navigate the challenge of staying financially profitable as a private, Black-owned small business that depends heavily on reimbursement from medical insurance or the rare funders willing to help FCH expand its work by investing in an anti-oppressive and social-justice-oriented mental health practice.

Lessons Learned: Self-Care Means Putting Your Oxygen Mask on First

Given an opportunity to do it all over again, I would change little because the negative experiences associated with my RBF, though mentally and physically exhausting, ultimately served a higher purpose by giving birth to FCH – which stands as a protest to inequities, disparities, and racism in mental healthcare. Moreover, without the FCH experience, hundreds of children and families may have had no opportunity to heal from the emotional and psychological wounds of racial trauma and RBF and have no culturally informed, coping, or mental recovery strategies to effectively navigate forms of racialized trauma. In hindsight, I would share this advice with my younger self:

> Brother, pay more attention to your self-care through this journey and build in more time for the things that you are sacrificing along the journey – your sleep, nutrition, exercise, mental recovery, and giving yourself permission to have fun. Because one day, you will look up and you will be older – and perhaps very successful – but paying a steep price for your lack of self-care and wondering was it worth it.

That said, finding evidence-based recommendations specifically for RBF self-care within the context of healthcare continues to be a vexing challenge with no substantive research findings in extant healthcare literature, nonetheless powerful RBF self-care concepts such as "unplugging" from people and places, connecting with community, prioritizing holistic approaches to physical health, finding or creating "safe spaces," and considering counseling have emerged within the social sciences (Quaye et al., 2019).

Your RBF Plan: Practical Wisdom and Recommendations for the Journey Ahead

Ironically, my encounters with racism as a Black male and my failure to meaningfully impact institutional racism in mental healthcare as a Black male psychiatrist, though quite painful, presented an unanticipated opportunity for me to critically reflect and reexamine my core values, highest priorities, and ultimate life purpose. I trust that you, too, will find and benefit from unanticipated opportunities as you reflect and embark on your professional journey. As you move forward, here are some practical recommendations to keep in mind:

1. **Take a moment and reflect on your past (or current) experiences with RBF and be honest with yourself.** Have you talked yourself out of opportunities based on RBF? Are you angry, resigned, cynical, hopeless, or bitter? Wherever you are on the professional journey, please appreciate that RBF is a very real "thing" and will be an integral (and intrusive) part of navigating predominantly white spaces. It should be fully anticipated and not ignored. Having a personalized RBF plan makes the journey navigable, reducing the risk of being either blindsided or worn down by the effects of institutional racism.

2. **Identify a mentor or an elder who has traveled a similar path and can serve as a guide, confidant, and sounding board during the more challenging times.** If you cannot find someone in your field of endeavor, consider someone who is in a mission-critical or battle-tested leadership position who has faced and successfully managed the challenges associated with RBF (and has copious "war stories" to share). I encountered several spiritual elders and advisors (mostly pastors) along my journey and took full advantage of their wisdom because they had such a broad understanding of the vicissitudes of the "RBF-life" and could be counted on for an optimistic perspective.

3. **Equip yourself by reading as much as you can on RBF as there is a wealth of credible information online.** One empowering and instructive resource to add to your RBF library, whether you are just launching out or have been at it for a while, is *Black Founder: The Hidden Power of Being an Outsider* by Stacy Spikes. Spikes employs an unfiltered and unflinching approach to confronting the forces that contribute to RBF and shares several strategies for overcoming its potentially debilitating effects.

4. **Connect with, or establish, a community of support with friends, colleagues, or like-minded individuals who share similar experiences.**

This will provide a reservoir of collective strength and resources to help you combat the isolation and loneliness that RBF too often imposes. Ultimately, RBF self-care, especially for healthcare providers working in predominantly white institutions, should seek to not only include "unplugging" but also eventually incorporating one's values, culture, tribe, and re-claiming joy, pleasure, peace, and rest and not being bashful about setting limits and challenging norms vis-à-vis a "legacy of oppression" (DeAngelis, 2022).

You may be surprised to learn that, despite over 20 years in professional practice, I feel as if I am only just beginning to appreciate the immense importance and true value of having a bona fide RBF plan to my overall well-being and success. Honestly, I am still working on incorporating the above recommendations into my ever-evolving RBF plan as a Black male navigating not just predominantly white institutions but the community at large. I have learned that it takes conscious and deliberate intention, unwavering commitment, and unbridled courage to construct, implement, and live by a personalized RBF plan and would urge you to strongly consider building or refining your RBF plan now. It's never too early or too late. Remember the old saying: *"The best time to plant a tree was 20 years ago, and the next best time is now."*

Shalom and blessings.

References

Carr, A. (1998). Michael White's narrative therapy. *Contemporary Family Therapy, 20*(4), 485–503. https://doi.org/10.1023/a:1021680116584

DeAngelis, T. (2022). *For psychologists of color, self-care is much more than that.* Monitor on Psychology, July 1. www.apa.org/monitor/2022/07/news-psychologists-self-care#:~: text=Self%2Dcare%20for%20psychologists%20of,being%20a%20strong%20 Black%20woman

Edwards, T. M., & Walker, M. (2019). Enhancing transformation: The value of applying narrative therapy techniques when engaging in critical reflection. *Journal of Transformative Education, 17*(4), 337–352. https://doi.org/10.1177/1541344619847142

Franklin, J. D., Smith, W. A., & Hung, M. (2014). Racial battle fatigue for Latina/o students. *Journal of Hispanic Higher Education, 13*(4), 303–322. https://doi.org/10.1177/15381 92714540530

Lee, B. Y., & Newberg, A. B. (2005). Religion and health: A review and critical analysis. *Zygon, 40*(2), 443–468. https://doi.org/10.1111/j.1467-9744.2005.00674.x

McCauley, J., Jenckes, M. W., Tarpley, M. J., Koenig, H. G., Yanek, L. R., & Becker, D. M. (2005). Spiritual beliefs and barriers among managed care practitioners. *Journal of Religion and Health, 44*(2), 137–146. https://doi.org/10.1007/s10943-005-2772-2

Moodley, R., Mujtaba, F., & Kleiman, S. (2017). *Routledge international handbook of critical mental health* (1st ed.). Routledge.

Quaye, S., Karikari, S. N., Allen, C. R., Okello, W., & Carter, K. D. (2019). Strategies for practicing self-care from racial battle fatigue. *JCSCORE, 5*(2), 94–131. https://doi.org/10.15763/issn.2642-2387.2019.5.2.94-131

Roberts, S. O., & Rizzo, M. T. (2021). The psychology of American racism. *American Psychologist, 76*(3), 475–487. https://doi.org/10.1037/amp0000642

Serafini, K., Coyer, C., Brown Speights, J., Donovan, D., Guh, J., Washington, J., & Ainsworth, C. (2020). Racism as experienced by physicians of color in the health care setting. *Family Medicine, 52*(4), 282–287. https://doi.org/10.22454/fammed.2020.384384

Sharma, M., & Kuper, A. (2017). The elephant in the room: Talking race in medical education. *Advances in Health Sciences Education, 22*(3), 761–764. https://doi.org/10.1007/s10459-016-9732-3

Strayhorn, T. L. (2020). Exploring the role of race in Black males' sense of belonging in medical school: A qualitative pilot study. *Medical Science Educator, 30*(4), 1383–1387. https://doi.org/10.1007/s40670-020-01103-y

Suite, D. H., La Bril, R., Primm, A., & Harrison-Ross, P. (2007). Beyond misdiagnosis, misunderstanding and mistrust: Relevance of the historical perspective in the medical and mental health treatment of People of Color. *Journal of the National Medical Association, 99*(8), 879–885.

Suite, D. H., Rollin, S. A., Bowman, J. C., & La Bril, R. D. (2007). From fear to faith: Efficacy of trauma assessment training for New York-based southern Baptist church groups. *Research on Social Work Practice, 17*(2), 258–263. https://doi.org/10.1177/1049731506296678

Utsey, S. O., Giesbrecht, N., Hook, J., & Stanard, P. M. (2008). Cultural, sociofamilial, and psychological resources that inhibit psychological distress in African Americans exposed to stressful life events and race-related stress. *Journal of Counseling Psychology, 55*(1), 49–62. https://doi.org/10.1037/0022-0167.55.1.49

Radical Self-Care for BIPOC

13

Robyn L. Gobin

One of my favorite poems is Lucille Clifton's *Won't You Celebrate with Me*. The woman portrayed in Clifton's poem overcame obstacles to becoming the most authentic version of herself. She relied upon her intuition and good sense to guide her. Her mind was liberated from the lies that tempted her to throw in the towel. She was aware of the oppressor's goal, yet unwavering in her faith and will to thrive. Her confidence motivated her to celebrate her triumph publicly and proudly. I love this poem because, in many ways, I aspire to be like the woman Clifton wrote about. I have learned that thriving, as Clifton's poem illustrates, requires radical self-care.

I stumbled upon self-care at a time when I was approaching life in a manner that looked nothing like the woman Clifton wrote about. I was mentally, physically, and spiritually exhausted, disillusioned, and out of touch with my values. As a Black cisgender woman born and raised in the South, the idea that I needed to work ten times as hard to get half as far as my white counterparts was deeply ingrained. Grinding non-stop was the only way I knew how to approach life. My worth was entirely intertwined with my work. Fueled by perfectionism, imposter syndrome, and an insatiable need for external validation, my sole focus in life was constantly producing more and more work, with the hope of one day finally feeling worthy.

I was the epitome of the superwoman schema (Woods-Giscombé, 2010): strong, self-sacrificing, fiercely independent, emotionally suppressed, success no matter the cost, undeterred by physical and emotional pain, and prioritizing everyone else's wishes and needs at the expense of my own. All the while, I was unfulfilled, because in all the busyness, I had lost sight of my

DOI: 10.4324/9781003309796-16

power and ability to choose a different approach. I ran around aimlessly on autopilot, going with life's current rather than choosing my life's direction. I was flourishing financially, educationally, and socially on the outside, but inside, I felt empty.

I remember waking up one day after completing my first year as a tenure-track assistant professor and feeling so underwhelmed, uninspired, and trapped in a life that was supposed to be "#goals." That day, I was finally at my breaking point. All the years of high achievement, hustling to look good in the eyes of others, and mass producing solely for the benefit of the academy had taken its toll. I knew something needed to change. I vowed to take back control of my life. I yearned to reclaim joy, excitement, purpose, and pleasure. I wanted to slow down and give myself permission to rest, but I was deathly afraid of being perceived as lazy or wasting my potential. Deeply rooted ancestral trauma caused me to fear the consequences of not constantly jumping through hoops to prove my value to others. I desperately wanted someone to come save me; to give me permission to pump the breaks. The day I stopped waiting to be saved and gave myself permission to begin exploring self-care was the day my life changed.

Positionality

Any discussion of self-care as it relates to BIPOC folks is incomplete if race-based stress and Audre Lorde are not mentioned. Race-based stress has been defined as "emotional or physical pain or the threat of physical and emotional pain that results from racism" (Carter, 2007, p. 88). These experiences often have psychophysiological effects that can be life threatening (Mays et al., 2007).

Audre Lorde let us know how vital self-care is to our existence when she wrote, "Caring for myself is not self-indulgence, it is self-preservation and that is an act of political warfare." She acknowledged how self-care allows us to resist the toxicity of existing in an environment where discrimination, systemic inequalities, and oppression constantly threaten our well-being and survival. Because this environment leaves us depleted mentally, physically, and emotionally, our survival, as a BIPOC community, demands that we acknowledge the impact of the environment and replenish ourselves. The very act of BIPOC practicing self-care in an environment "we were never meant to survive" (Lorde, 1978) is radical. What makes radical self-care "radical" is acknowledgement of the historical, social, and political context that makes practicing self-care challenging for BIPOC. As Michaeli (2017, p. 53) explains,

"Self-care in a world that denies you care means revolting against the unequal distribution of life and death, health and illness, well-being and suffering, of care-giving and receiving roles, as fixed by patriarchy, white supremacy, global capitalism, and other systems of domination and exploitation." In alignment with liberation psychology (Prilleltensky & Prilleltensky, 2003), I see radical self-care as a resistance technique for BIPOC communities. This conceptualization of self-care differs from the standard discourse around self-care in the literature.

Critical Commentary on the Self-Care Literature

The self-care literature has historically conceptualized self-care as behaviors that individuals engage in to improve or sustain health, prevent disease, cope with stress, or restore balance to a life that has become unbalanced (Levin & Idler, 1983; Evans-Hudnall et al., 2014; Miller et al., 2019). One of the major limitations in the literature has been its primary focus on the individual to the exclusion of environment, context, and cultural forces. Furthermore, there is a dearth of literature that discusses intersectionality (Crenshaw, 1991) and how the connection between an individual's identities and social locations result in different needs, capacities for, and access to self-care.

As a remedy to the limitations in self-care literature and discourse, drawing on Miller et al.'s (2019) model of self-care, Wyatt and Ampadu (2020) offer a conceptual framework of radical self-care that centers intersectionality, environmental factors, and social justice. I find this framework extremely beneficial in its conceptualization of self-care as extending beyond behavioral actions. More than a mere coping strategy, Wyatt and Ampadu (2020) frame self-care as a "process and practice that moves us closer to health, wellness, and liberation" (p. 218). Their model identifies five factors or layers of self-care: self-care support, self-care orientation, self-care motivation, self-care skills, and self-care behaviors. Each factor considers internal and external factors that have the potential to motivate or discourage self-care. While this model was designed with Black communities in mind, given their similar experiences of oppression and race-based stress, other communities of color are likely to benefit from this framework.

Self-care support includes the knowledge, resources, initiatives, and community-building that is necessary to meet the needs of BIPOC. It is important that BIPOC are sufficiently educated about self-care and provided with opportunities to practice self-care in ways that are sustainable and meet their unique needs.

Self-care orientation refers to one's beliefs about self-care and how those beliefs impact one's willingness to make self-care a priority. The orientation toward collectivism and community values among BIPOC and the caretaking role that women of color frequently occupy may create a barrier to self-care. Therefore, it is important that self-care awareness initiatives address feelings of guilt and connect self-care with overall community wellness.

Self-care motivation refers to the internal driving force that motivates self-care behaviors. The multiple demands that BIPOC contend with daily can cause motivation for self-care to diminish over time. Moreover, Wyatt and Ampadu (2020) assert that attitudes that frame self-care as a self-indulgent act that makes one lazy and less productive can be a barrier to self-care. Self-care is more sustainable among BIPOC when stereotypes are intentionally opposed, and local opportunities are available to engage with other community members as an act of self-care.

Regarding *self-care skills*, Wyatt and Ampadu (2020) describe, "Knowing when and how to execute self-care behaviors is a skill set that requires self-awareness coupled with practice" (p. 217). The authors suggest mindfulness practice can increase awareness of self-care needs, which in turn allows BIPOC to create tailored self-care plans that meet their unique needs.

Lastly, *self-care behaviors* are the actions individuals take to nurture themselves holistically. Wyatt and Ampadu (2020) assert that attending to self-care support, orientation, motivation, and skills can position BIPOC to engage in self-care behaviors that are truly nourishing. They stress the importance of identifying barriers to self-care behaviors and BIPOC having agency in choosing both individual and community self-care practices that support them in several areas of wellness (e.g., physical, emotional, social, financial, etc.).

Personal Reflections and Unlearnings

If I had to summarize my self-care journey, I would describe it as an ongoing process of unlearning unhelpful habits and thoughts I have believed about myself and about the possibility of creating a mental health career that is affirming, healing, inclusive, and truly transformative. The more I practice self-care, the more authentically I show up. Authenticity coupled with giving myself permission to dream has allowed me to shape a career that reflects my passions, values, and moral compass (like the woman in Clifton's poem).

Unlearning #1: There Is Only One Right Way

In her 1982 speech at Harvard University, Audre Lorde proclaimed: ". . . if I didn't define myself for myself, I would be crunched into other people's fantasies for me and eaten alive" (Lorde, 1984, p. 137). An integral part of my self-care journey has been freeing myself from the colonialist belief that there is one right way to be a psychologist. In graduate school, we are told there are certain ways to practice, do research, and affect change at community and national levels. We are told that we need to choose a theoretical orientation and a singular career path. When it comes to professionalism, we are told there is a certain way to speak and write. Over time, I have found many of academia's rules restrictive and misaligned with my goals and larger purpose. My self-care practices have given me permission to be myself, embrace multiple roles, and shape a multi-pronged career that includes classroom instruction, advocacy, consulting, clinical practice, research, training, mentoring, public speaking, contributing as a mental health expert for media outlets, and writing for public audiences.

Unlearning #2: Pull Yourself Up by Your Own Bootstraps

Growing up, the saying "If you want something done right, you've got to do it yourself" was consistently taught and modeled by the matriarchs in my family. Naturally, I adopted this self-reliant mindset. In graduate school I remember being petrified to go to office hours or ask clarifying questions during class. In my mind, asking for help or admitting I did not understand something could jeopardize my standing in the program. As the only Black woman in my graduate program, I had to prove that I belonged there and asking questions was in opposition to my goal. Self-reliance led me to mask my struggles and suffer through challenging coursework in silence unnecessarily. As I began to meet other BIPOC students on campus, I learned the benefits of vulnerability in one-on-one interactions. It led to deeper connection and lessened my sense that I was alone in the fight. Eventually, I sought community spaces outside of my university that embraced a collectivistic orientation toward mental health research and practice. Being in community with others who see all of me and give me permission to show up as my authentic self has fostered self-awareness, self-acceptance, and self-trust. I have learned to accept my limited capacities as a human being. I have learned my strengths and weaknesses, and I have grown comfortable asking for help, viewing it as an act of grace toward myself, rather than a sign of weakness or incompetence.

Unlearning #3: Rely on Others for Validation

When I was in graduate school, my dependence on external validation and approval led me to hold back my honest thoughts and perspectives for fear of offending others. Dependence on external validation also led to me attaching my worth and value to how other people responded to me. As BIPOC, reliance on external approval and validation can be intensified by being "the only" in predominantly white spaces. Through practicing self-care, I have honed the habit of self-validation. This has freed me from depending on others to assess my status in life or tell me what to do next. While I have strong mentors whose opinions I value, self-care has helped me grow comfortable with making my own decisions and having the final say.

Unlearning #4: Perfection Is Achievable and Required

For as long as I can remember, I have been a high achiever. Growing up, my straight A's got me praise, attention, and adoration from my family and community. In elementary school, whenever I would earn a "needs improvement" in conduct or (God forbid) get a "B" on my report card, I was met with questions and disappointment from my parents, with the overarching message that they knew I was "capable of more." Pleasing my parents and making my family proud became a way of life and along with it came perfectionism.

In graduate school, my perfectionist tendencies gave way to imposter syndrome. As the only Black woman in (not just my cohort but) the entire graduate program, I felt the weight of the world on my shoulders to represent the Black community well. Convinced that I was inadequate for the job of representing the entire Black community, I became terrified that one day people would discover that I did not belong in one of the top clinical psychology programs in the country; that one day I would screw up badly and be revealed as a fraud. Carrying the entire Black community on my back daily was draining. Once I discovered self-care, I slowly relieved myself of this burden. Self-care helped me realize that it is not my job to make sure none of the white people I interact with leave our interactions with a negative perception of Black people. No person has the power to change others' perceptions of an entire community. Nobody should bear the weight of representing an entire community. Self-care helped me to see that showing up as the best imperfect version of myself is enough. Through practicing self-care, I have learned to give myself permission to make mistakes, change my mind, let go of goals and dreams that no longer serve me, and be okay with tasks remaining on my to-do list at the end of the day.

Unlearning #5: Rest and Self-Care Are Unproductive

The inclination toward productivity, hustle, and grind culture are in direct opposition of a self-care ethos which invites us to slow down, check in with ourselves, and reassess our goals, and reconnect with our values and dreams. While grinding will get you far in terms of career achievements and status, if we get in the habit of pushing ourselves beyond our limits, we risk burnout and compassion fatigue. Many BIPOC enter the mental health field driven by a larger purpose that, to some extent, involves pouring back into their communities. For me, it is important that the services I offer my community come from the best part of me, not what's left of me after I am depleted. To offer my best, I must take time for rest, rejuvenation, and joy. I cannot afford to wait to rest until I feel like I have earned it. Though it can be difficult to prioritize, I have never regretted taking time for self-care. Self-care and rest have helped me access greater creativity in my work, and they help me allocate my precious time and energy into activities that are most aligned with my values.

Practice-Based Recommendations

A number of wide-ranging self-care practices have been integral to helping me create a life and mental health career that I desire. A holistic wellness perspective on self-care compels me to nurture not only my physical health, but to incorporate self-care practices that address my social, emotional, vocational, intellectual, and spiritual needs. I will conclude this chapter by sharing a few self-care practices that have supported my unlearning and overall wellness. I hope they plant a seed that might benefit you on your self-care journey. Space limitations prevent an in-depth discussion of the self-care strategies. For a more comprehensive guide on self-care practices,

I recommend my book, *The Self-Care Prescription: Powerful Solutions to Manage Stress, Reduce Anxiety, and Increase Well-Being* (Gobin, 2019).

Practice Mindfulness Meditation

Mindfulness meditation has helped me embrace my emotions and see myself more clearly. While leading a meditation practice, my teacher once offered the following guidance: "We can be soft without collapsing, upright without rigidity." As a Black woman who is prone to morphing into a strong Black woman, it has been useful to remind myself of my teacher's advice daily: Being soft and vulnerable doesn't make me weak. I can feel my feelings without fear of falling apart. At the other end of the spectrum, I can be strong, taking action to protect those I love and uphold my boundaries without becoming cold and rigid. There are several YouTube videos and apps that provide audio guidance to support you in beginning or reengaging a mindfulness practice. Liberate Meditation app offers audio meditation practices by BIPOC for BIPOC. Shine and Insight Timer are excellent apps as well.

Cultivate Self-Compassion

Self-compassion involves cultivating a kinder and gentler relationship with yourself, particularly during times of personal failure, struggle, or pain. It also involves recognizing that you are not alone in your struggles. Self-compassion has helped me take unnecessary pressure off myself and supports me in managing the self-criticism that often accompanies perfectionism. For BIPOC, practicing self-compassion can be powerful in helping us to care for the people and communities we care about without abandoning ourselves. One self-compassion practice that has been particularly helpful for me is *Compassion with Equanimity*, which, in part, involves inhaling as a signal of compassion for yourself and exhaling in the spirit of sending compassion and well wishes to loved ones or community members who are suffering.

Give Your Best "Yes"

As multi-talented, multi-passionate, highly skilled folks, BIPOC are often pulled in several directions and face competing demands for limited time and energy. Learning to say "no" (sometimes to very good opportunities) is vital for our self-care. One strategy I have found helpful in determining when to say "yes" and when to say "no" is asking myself three questions: How will saying "yes" benefit me? How important are these benefits to me (in other words, are they aligned with my values)? What will this "yes" cost me in terms of time, energy, or other areas of life? Sitting with these three questions provides me with the clarity needed to set appropriate boundaries around my time, avoid overcommitting myself, and give only my best "yes."

Connect with BIPOC and BIPOC-Affirmative Spaces

Navigating graduate school and a career in the mental health field can be isolating experiences. I have found it essential to connect with like-minded BIPOC and BIPOC-affirmative spaces to sustain and uplift me throughout the various phases of my career. As a graduate student, I sought out BIPOC graduate student groups both on campus and through national associations (e.g., Association for Black Psychologists, National Black Graduate Student Association). I found it useful to diversify my network such that it includes people who I could connect with academically, spiritually, and vocationally.

Create Margin in Your Day

The varied personal and professional responsibilities we have as BIPOC can make 24-hours seem insufficient to put a dent in our to-do list. We can be tempted to pack our days to the brim leaving us vulnerable to exhaustion, overwhelm, and ultimately resentment. Lately, I have been giving myself the gift of creating margin throughout my day – little pockets of space where I don't have anything planned. This reduces stress by helping me feel less rushed and it makes space for self-care practices like a five-minute break between appointments, carving out time for a screen-free lunch break, or taking a walk outside. I would be remiss if I did not mention working to the point of burnout here. In resistance to capitalism and exhaustion culture, I set firm boundaries around working hours, and I reserve weekends for family, rest, play, and ease.

Cultivate Joy and Gratitude

In an episode of OWN Network's *Queen Sugar*, one of the main characters, Aunt Violet, remarked: "You know, sometimes we get so caught up striving for our dreams that we forget we're living inside of them. We human beings always want more and more. Sometimes we just have to sit with people that we love and take it all in." This quote reminded me of the importance of creating moments of joy and being thankful for how far we've come while we are still in pursuit of our dreams. We don't have to wait until we fully arrive to experience joy and pleasure. We can sing, dance, laugh, play, access pleasure, listen to music, and gather in community right now. We face many barriers to joy as BIPOC. We may feel like there is too much important work to do to be joyful. We may have internalized the belief that we don't deserve joy. Race-based stress may crush our desire for joy. Yet, let us remember that being joyful amid oppression is an act of resistance (Lu & Steele, 2019). Our ancestors sacrificed so we can live a good life – one where we can intentionally access joy while still in pursuit of liberation for ourselves and our communities.

References

Carter, R. T. (2007). Racism and psychological and emotional injury: Recognizing and assessing race-based traumatic stress. *The Counseling Psychologist, 35*, 13–105. https://doi.org/10.1177/0011000006292033

Crenshaw, K. W. (1991). Mapping the margins: Intersectionality, identity politics, and violence against women of color. *Stanford Law Review, 43*, 1241. https://doi.org/10.2307/1229039

Evans-Hudnall, G. L., Stanley, M. A., Clark, A. N., Bush, A. L., Resnicow, K., Liu, Y., et al. (2014). Improving secondary stroke self-care among underserved ethnic minority individuals: A randomized clinical trial of a pilot intervention. *Journal of Behavioral Medicine, 37*(2), 196–204. https://doi.org/10.1007/s10865-012-9469-2

Gobin, R. L. (2019). *The self-care prescription: Powerful tools to manage stress, reduce anxiety, & enhance well-being.* Althea Press.

Levin, L. S., & Idler, E. L. (1983). Self-care in health. *Annual Review of Public Health, 4*(1), 181–201.

Lorde, A. (1978). *The black unicorn.* Norton.

Lorde, A. (1984). *Sister outsider: Essays & speeches by Audre Lorde.* Crossing Press.

Lu, J. H., & Steele, C. K. (2019). "Joy is resistance": Cross-platform resilience and (re) invention of Black oral culture online. *Information, Communication & Society, 22*(6), 823–837. https://doi.org/10.1080/1369118x.2019.1575449

Mays, V. M., Cochran, S. D., & Barnes, N. W. (2007). Race, race-based discrimination, and health outcomes among African Americans. *Annual Review of Psychology, 58*, 201–225. https://doi.org/10.1146/annurev.psych.57.102904.190212

Michaeli, I. (2017). Self-care: An act of political warfare or a neoliberal trap? *Development, 60*(1–2), 50–56. https://doi.org/10.1057/s41301-017-0131-8

Miller, A. E., Green, T. D., & Lambros, K. M. (2019). Foster parent self-care: A conceptual model. *Children and Youth Services Review, 99*, 107–114.

Prilleltensky, I., & Prilleltensky, O. (2003). Synergies for wellness and liberation in counseling psychology. *The Counseling Psychologist, 31*(3), 273–281. https://doi. org/10.1177/0011000003031003002

Woods-Giscombé, C. L. (2010). Superwoman schema: African American women's views on stress, strength, and health. *Qualitative Health Research, 20,* 668–683. https://doi. org/10.1177/1049732310361892

Wyatt, J. P., & Ampadu, G. G. (2020). Reclaiming self-care: Self-care as a social justice tool for Black wellness. *Community Mental Health Journal, 58*(2), 213–221. https://doi. org/10.1007/s10597-021-00884-9

Putting People First
14

Promoting Diversity, Equity, Inclusion, and Belonging in Industry Settings

Milo Dodson

Let me tell you something right from the beginning: I feel insecure writing this chapter. I would be doing you a disservice and not being my authentic self if I did not explicitly state this up front. It is not that I have ever felt an ounce of pressure from the editors, other contributors, or my employer about this chapter. In fact, it was co-editor Dr. Doris Chang's compassionate invitation to open my chapter with this authentic vulnerability (thank you, Dr. Chang!).

Rather, my insecurity is linked to variations of the same, reoccurring conversation about professional identity I had while pursuing my PhD in Counseling Psychology. I frequently received messages about what I was "supposed to do" upon graduation and was told – mostly by peers – that I "had" to choose one of two pathways: 1) be a researcher/professor, or 2) be a therapist. Over and over as we walked across campus. That's it. One or the other. I did not realize it at the time, but this nauseating repetition led to consistent emotional activation within me and a desire to prove them wrong even if I ultimately chose one of the two pathways. I felt defensive. I felt defiant. I felt my future being disrespectfully limited, priming me to develop an insecurity that in order to do what we are "supposed to do" as counseling psychologists, I could not be my full self. I could not pursue what I was most interested in. I had to become someone else.

DOI: 10.4324/9781003309796-17

Hearing that I "had to choose" a single professional pathway felt all too familiar to my lived experience at that point in my early twenties. Being biracial (African American and Italian American) and navigating the world primarily as a Black man, I had to avoid so many sources attempting to socialize and influence me to choose one racial identity over the other. This was more than just another instance of "you can't tell me what to do." This was exactly what Carl Rogers (one of my clinical heroes) described as an incongruence between the perceived self and actual self, functioning as an internalized, "How dare you try to tell me who I can be?" Thus began my realization of how inextricably linked our personhood is with our professional perspective. The researcher as the instrument of analysis. The therapist as the instrument of healing. In all professional endeavors, I would be an instrument of change: I would always be a person first. Whether publishing research in peer-reviewed journals, teaching in a classroom, or providing individual/group therapy, I like to think I have always been critically aware that all my professional endeavors are informed by my multicultural identities, worldview, and lived experiences.

Due to the high degree of variance across industries and companies, no single text can convey a one-size-fits-all approach to starting an industry career doing diversity, equity, inclusion, and belonging (DEIB) work. So please note: This chapter is not meant to be an exhaustive overview of Dos and Don'ts. Rather, with cultural humility and a heart filled with gratitude, I offer this chapter as an informed reflection of my professional journey (Pro Tips included), hoping that it will ultimately spark professional inspiration and catalyze systemic change. Before we get there, allow me to answer the question I know a few of you may be asking yourselves: What does DEIB work actually involve and how do you do it as someone with training in a mental health field? While approaches to DEIB vary across companies, this chapter describes the approach to promoting DEIB in industry settings that I have personally developed in my role as Senior Manager for Diversity, Inclusion, and Community Outreach at Belkin International. Belkin is a tech accessories company with global headquarters in El Segundo, California. To be clear, while I am discussing this work through my personal perspective as a counseling psychologist, this is not work that I have done in isolation or without collaboration from colleagues across all departments. This is actually my first Pro Tip: Regardless of DEIB practitioners' backgrounds, we cannot effectively be agents of change without prioritizing collective growth over personal accomplishment and without focusing more on the *we* than the *me*. No one can or should do this work on their own and I am grateful for the support of my colleagues, knowing that we are committed to doing this work together.

DEIB in Action: Walking the Talk

From my perspective, the primary driver of DEIB work should be research-based and data-informed Education and Awareness. Not only is this a DEIB commitment (more on that later) at Belkin, but also one of four DEIB Focus Pillars to drive action. It is the core of our DEIB programming and we offer an average of 2–3 voluntary opportunities (e.g., panels, discussions, workshops) per month in addition to facilitating tailored conversations with teams, departments, and senior leaders and conducting annual required DEIB training in our Learning Management system. Pro Tip: For folks who may be interested in entering the field, providing DEIB-related trainings and talks in industry settings is a recommended starting point. It was my personal entry point years ago when friends at various companies were looking for a speaker. Part of my inspiration came from Dr. Anneliese Singh (see also Singh et al., this volume), who once told me at a convention that (paraphrasing) "the core of diversity and inclusion work is teaching." So, who better to lead with Education and Awareness than a psychologist?

The second DEIB Focus Pillar that organizes our work at Belkin is Talent Recruitment and Retention. Since diverse representation does not automatically create inclusion in the workplace, recruitment and retention efforts are strongly connected. In other words, we would be doing employees from underrepresented communities a disservice if retention efforts to build inclusion did not match recruitment efforts to increase representation. As an example, on a daily/weekly basis, I a) hold multiple conversations with our Talent Acquisition team to plan outreach opportunities to universities and community organizations and b) strategize with leaders/hiring managers related to enhancing the overall employee experience. Pro Tip: Common factors of therapy (e.g., collaboration, empathy, positive regard) also apply to industry.

The third DEIB Focus Pillar in our model is Connection and Collaboration. On a regular and ongoing basis, we collectively connect with one another from a stance of empathetic curiosity to see how we are doing as people, not just employees. We have also established seven employee resource groups (and counting) focused on creating connection and community for Belkin employees, as well as professional interest topics (i.e., sustainability and a leadership-development-focused book club). Pro

Tip: Community building is what counseling psychologists and other mental health professionals do, so this is another meaningful opportunity for folks with similar backgrounds to lean into our training and education. As a Black man doing DEIB industry work, I am simultaneously creating supportive spaces for others while also building support for myself. I am both a group facilitator and a group participant, which as you can imagine is both rewarding and challenging.

Belkin's fourth DEIB Focus Pillar is Professional Development. Whether offering an educational assistance program, a global mentorship program, or professional development plan, investing in the professional growth of our people (not just as employees) is paramount. I work closely with our Training and Development Manager to offer workshops (i.e., psychological safety, growth mindset) to colleagues around the globe. Pro Tip: I have often drawn from my vocational psychology course when thinking of new professional development opportunities for colleagues. When transitioning from my position at the University of California, Irvine Counseling Center to Belkin, I utilized many resources for my own professional development including a) LinkedIn's Top Voices in Diversity and Inclusion such as Ruchika Tulshyan, b) books by Howard J. Ross and Lily Zheng, and c) podcasts by Brené Brown (e.g., Brown, 2022). Lots of Brené Brown.

Building My Own Path to "Both/And"

Fortunately, even though I was told I "had to choose" between research and clinical experience and nothing else, I was still able to gain research and clinical experience, both of which inform my DEIB work. In my previous research, I frequently adopted a transformative-emancipatory paradigm. This paradigmatic approach provides space for social justice work (Mertens, 1999), and social justice is at the core of all (good) DEIB work. I believe that a primary purpose of constructing knowledge is to help inform and improve society (Banks, 1993, 1995). As a researcher, I assume that knowledge is influenced by human interests, is not neutral, and by extension, "the data never tell you what to do because it's really your judgment" (Hill, *Dare to Lead Podcast*). Furthermore, knowledge "reflects the power and social relationships within society" (Plano Clark & Creswell, 2008, p. 73). Generally speaking, a transformative-emancipatory paradigm argues for using data to help shape social justice inquiry, in hopes that the data can subsequently be used to decrease social inequalities. Recognizing the societal influences that affect how we collect and interpret data is just as critical for industry as it is in rigorous and robust academic research.

My Pro Tip for recognizing societal influences within industry is that companies must adopt a "people first" mentality for all policies, procedures, and business decisions. "People first" is a term I believe I first read via Madison Butler, Founder of Black Speakers Collection, on LinkedIn. To me, "people first" means that the DEIB work we do within industry to improve society must start with recognizing and validating that employees are people, first. This applies to my colleagues as well as to myself. The principle of "people first" allows for employees to receive both comprehensive professional development opportunities and emotional support. "People first" means that employees are not told that their professional growth should follow a binary "either this or that" trajectory like my peers attempted to impress upon me in graduate school. How could I possibly trust and want to be led by someone who does not take the time to get to know me as a person and learn what I find meaningful? How could I possibly want to invest more time and energy in a company whose leaders do not take the time to even ask how I am doing? Consistent with the person-centered approach I previously adopted in my clinical work, I believe that the most effective work between an employee and manager is accomplished when a dyad addresses power dynamics and builds a trusting relationship supported by congruence, unconditional positive regard, and empathy.

Looking Back to Move Forward: Combining Experiences for More

Combining my transformative-emancipatory approach to research, a person-centered clinical orientation, and an ever-evolving self-awareness is critical to my DEIB work in industry. Being transparent about my identities and positionalities is core to my approach, beginning with how I introduce myself. Personally, I am not interested in learning about DEIB practitioners' credentials, certifications, or degrees if I do not know a) how their multicultural identities intersect and are positioned within their work and b) their motivation for facilitating deeply emotional, life altering behavioral changes in their clients. In the words of my esteemed mentor, counseling psychologist Dr. Thomas Parham, "Degrees and credentials do not equate to competence." So, before we continue any further with this chapter, allow me to re-introduce myself beyond the brief introduction, LinkedIn profile, or headshot caption you may have previously read about me.

My name is Milo Laurenz Jerome Alexander Dodson. I am a biracial man of unequaled resilience. I am the unexpected yet successful and proud product of a K-12 public school education system and a single parent household. I am the annihilator of any stereotype that is set upon me. I am the stone that was once rejected now serving as the cornerstone. I am the voice for every forgotten inner child. I am the mystery meat that is never understood but always enjoyed. I am tenacity, compassion, and humility incarnate. I am my only true obstacle. I am a walking contradiction of low self-esteem and grandiose dreams. I am the thirst that neither Gatorade nor Sprite can quench. I am the cool on the other side of the pillow. I am a raging bull with a china shop attached. I am everything naysayers wish I was not. I am what happens when you begin to believe and become who you are.

My privileged identities harmonize with my marginalized identities. At the time of writing this chapter, I am 37 years old and approximately two years, six months into my current management position at Belkin. I identify as a newly married, cisgender heterosexual male, able-bodied Catholic, from and currently living in a middle-class home. As previously mentioned, I provide context about my cultural identities to demonstrate that I recognize my identity as a Black man doing DEIB work within the tech industry that has historically seen low representation of Black people. I am tragically aware that even as an instrument of change, I am in ongoing need of multivariable healing while also being the healer.

But this opportunity was almost over before it started. When I was 15 years old, I was assaulted by the police in front of my mom while riding our bikes home from the movies. The officer did not care to listen to my mom's plea to stop, nor did he care to listen to hear me talk about my 4.0 GPA and multiple Advanced Placement classes. He saw that I was Black and that was enough to warrant the assault. The experience of going back to school a few days later, still traumatized, shaped my worldview. This was also one of my earliest lessons that healing was necessary for me to turn my trauma into triumph. Moreover, it served as a salient example of why a "people first" approach to performance is necessary. If my teachers and the administration did not take the time to fully see me, validate my pain, and ask how they could support me, then I easily could have failed my classes. When you take the time to focus on the person, performance improves.

Starting my undergraduate education as a first-generation college student two years later, I knew I needed to find a support network. Thankfully, Notre Dame's Balfour-Hesburgh Program – a summer program that provides a supportive learning community to high-achieving students from underrepresented populations – became my home away from home. I began learning about research and enrolled in business marketing, psychology of business, and industrial/organizational courses while pursuing my undergraduate and graduate degrees. These experiences put me on the path to DEIB consultation work, beginning with an opportunity to co-lead a teambuilding and leadership development retreat for Red Stripe's Jamaican-based Human Resources Team. I cannot say that I was leaning toward doing full-time DEIB consulting at this point in my life, but I knew I wanted to somehow incorporate it into my professional repertoire.

Then there was the Examination for the Professional Practice of Psychology (EPPP), our discipline's licensing exam. Whew. I almost want to leave this last piece out, #IYKYK ("if you know you know"), but let me clarify why this emotionally wounded me so deeply as it also adds to my aforementioned insecurity regarding writing this chapter. It took me multiple attempts to pass the EPPP. Approximately two years after I passed the exam, I discovered that there are statistically significant racial differences in pass/fail rates. Compared to the EPPP failure rates for white s (14.07%) and Asian Americans (24.0%), the rates for African Americans (38.5%) and Hispanics (35.6%) were far higher, meeting the criteria for disparate impact outlined in Title VII of the Civil Rights Act of 1964 (Sharpless, 2019).

But why is this important, you ask? Am I just "making this about me?" Yes, actually, but not in the self-centered way you may be thinking. Based on research conducted by the American Psychological Association, "Black psychologists comprised just 3% of the psychology workforce. Black male psychologists made up just 0.87% of psychologists" (APA, 2021). So as I'm doing this DEIB work in the tech industry, I am acutely aware that I am not only an employee within an industry that has historically not employed many people who look like me, but I am simultaneously representing an entire discipline of professionals that also have not historically looked like me.

Motivate with Love, Not Fear

If I know anything as a counseling psychologist, it is that a strengths-based approach will yield more effective and sustainable results. I am (Pro Tip) wholeheartedly invested in motivating others out of love with zero interest in motivating others out of fear. Case in point: When stating that racism is a problem for white people, not Black, Indigenous, and other People of Color (BIPOC), to solve and that sexism is a problem for men, not women, to solve, my goal is to educate and inspire rather than to shame. Specifically, I share research about peer-group interventions to show that there is a path forward.

Psychoeducation based on shame is not a tool for social justice because shame does not put people first. It prioritizes fear and disregards humanity.

If there was ever a field that needed a strengths-based approach, it is DEIB training and consulting. Historically housed within Human Resources, DEIB practices were often focused on limiting liability and protecting the company's interests, rather than focusing on employees' well-being, professional development, and success. People, myself included, are often surprised that sex discrimination has only been illegal in the US since the Civil Rights Act of 1964 and that it took another 16 years for the Equal Employment Opportunity Commission to define sexual harassment as a form of sex discrimination. Additionally, the Americans with Disabilities Act was not passed into law until 1990. Even within the field of psychology, I remember feeling shocked to learn how long it took to formally adopt the Guidelines of Multicultural Education, Training, Research, Practice, and Organizational Change for Psychologists (APA, 2003). Knowing this multifaceted history, I am not surprised that DEIB work started from a deficit-based approach, and needless to say, not a "people first" philosophy.

In my first few months at Belkin, I knew that the global DEIB roadmap we were formalizing needed to include operationalized definitions for diversity, equity, inclusion, and belonging. Fortunately, we were guided by one of our corporate North Stars, Community and Education, which has been part of our DNA since the company was created in 1983. We define *diversity* as representation (e.g., Who is in the room across multiple levels of leadership?), *equity* as opportunity (e.g., Who has not been let into the room and who does not have equitable resources to do their job while feeling emotionally supported?), *inclusion* as engagement (e.g., Whose ideas in the room have not been heard and whose ideas may not be taken seriously because they are underrepresented in the room?), and *belonging* as connected to well-being (e.g., Does being in the room create a sense of empowering, meaningful purpose and promote a healthy and connected community?) Our five DEIB Commitments are a) shared responsibility, b) education and awareness, c) cultural humility, d) active listening, and e) accountability. As a collective, we want liberation and to dismantle societal inequities. We do not want to have to stand on crates to see over a fence, but to tear the fence down for an unobstructed view of justice in the workplace. We want to work together to collectively liberate ourselves from oppressive barriers that block our progress, not just enhance performance and productivity.

Our Core Values form the backbone for our DEIB trainings. Belkin's five Core Values (Be Positive Active, Pursue the Ideal, Maintain Your Edge, Recharge, and Succeed as a Team) were in place well before my arrival in

January 2021. An example of how we have integrated Belonging into the company's *Recharge* core value is through collaboration with our benefits team and creating the monthly "Mindfulness with Dr. Milo" series. If you were to attend, you would hear me regularly say, "Recharge is a requirement, not a reward." Because this is a core value, we intentionally create time to recharge, for ourselves first as people, not making it contingent upon completing a certain amount of work. Supporting employees means supporting their mental health. Our *Succeed as a Team* core value is also evident throughout our interdepartmental and collaborative approach to DEIB work. As mentioned earlier, this is not about me, but we.

As DEIB work evolves as an industry itself, especially in response to the changing norms and expectations in the workplace as a result of the COVID-19 pandemic, I do not see a path forward that does not include and center on workplace well-being and work–life harmony. What has become even more apparent is how much potential for growth and improved workplace well-being we have when we work together. If someone says they are not responsible for DEIB because it is "something HR does," they are not doing their job. Period. From an entry-level position all the way up to the CEO, DEIB must be prioritized and integrated into all business units, practices, and policies, not simply as a stand-alone sector of the company that will become tokenized for commercial gain. I am so incredibly personally and professionally grateful to receive this supportive prioritization and integration at Belkin. Otherwise, historically excluded, marginalized, and underestimated groups within industry settings will continue to receive performance feedback that is weaponized (e.g., "she is always angry" or "he always tries to play the race card") and used to perpetuate workplace inequities.

DEIB is about cultivating opportunity and a pathway to our shared liberation. By nature, this shared liberation focuses on marginalized and underrepresented identities but also extends to all multicultural identities, including privileged identities. To assert that the "new" positions "targeted" toward underrepresented groups (i.e., BIPOC and women) are "taking away opportunities" from majority groups (e.g., Florida's 2023 Immigration Law or Texas' 2023 law banning DEI offices and initiatives across state colleges) implies and assumes the positions were originally made for white men. Anecdotally, I have even seen this fallacy surface in conversations around new superhero TV shows and movies. For example, questioning "why are all new superheroes women?" implies that superheroes were not meant to be anything other than men. In other words, this is not only a man's world, but a man's Marvel Cinematic Universe.

To all who read this, please hear me well: Regardless of what people tell you, you do not have to create your professional identity based on an arbitrary binary of one choice over another. You can be both Pema Chödrön and Kendrick Lamar in your emails and meetings. Bring your full selves to all spaces, your beautiful awareness, knowledge, and skills, like Dr. Joseph White, Common, and Dr. Elisabeth Kübler-Ross. You are not "crazy" for feeling insecure in professional settings at times. We belong wherever we are. Take a breath, recharge, and listen to that insecurity because it is trying to give you the ultimate Pro Tip: Put people (including yourself) first.

References

American Psychological Association. (2003). Guidelines on multicultural education, training, research, practice, and organizational change for Psychologists. *American Psychologist, 58*(5), 377–402. https://doi.org/10.1037/0003-066x.58.5.377

American Psychological Association. (2021). Demographics of US psychology workforce [Interactive data tool]. www.apa.org/workforce/data-tools/demographics

Banks, J. A. (1993). The canon debate, knowledge construction, and multicultural education. *Educational Researcher, 22*, 4–14. https://doi.org/10.3102/0013189x022005004

Banks, J. A. (1995). The historical reconstruction of knowledge about race: Implications for transformative teaching. *Educational Researcher, 24*, 15–25. https://doi.org/10.3102/0013189x024002015

Brown, B. (Host). (2022). Brené Brown with Dr. Linda Hill on leading with purpose in the digital age (No. 53) [audio podcast episode]. In *Dare to Lead with Brené Brown*, April 18. Parcast. https://brenebrown.com/podcast/leading-with-purpose-in-the-digital-age/

Mertens, D. M. (1999). Inclusive evaluation: Implications of transformative theory for evaluation. *American Journal of Evaluation, 20*, 1–14. https://doi.org/10.1016/s1098-2140(99)80105-2

Plano Clark, V. L., & Creswell, J. W. (Eds.). (2008). *The mixed methods reader*. SAGE.

Sharpless, B. A. (2019). Are demographic variables associated with performance on the Examination for Professional Practice in Psychology (EPPP)? *The Journal of Psychology, 153*(2), 161–172. doi:10.1080/00223980.2018.1504739.

Restorative Practices are Liberatory

15

An Open Letter to BIPOC Scholar-Activists and Practitioners Committed to Anti-Oppressive Practice

Kirk "Jae" James

Peace!

Colleagues, brothers, sisters, co-conspirators, and comrades: Whether it is proclamations about diversity, equity, and inclusion, social justice, or anti racist/anti-oppressive practice, social work, and other helping professions have a long history of efforts to appear more equitable and aligned with their organizing values. However, based on my lived experiences as a Black male social worker, exposure to research that pathologizes BIPOC clients, and repeated witnessing of harm directed at colleagues and students (past and present), I can emphatically say that the social work profession is *often* not a safe place for Black, Indigenous, and other People of Color (BIPOC) (Abrams & Dettlaff, 2020; Jema l, 2022; Ocampo & BlackDeer, 2022).

Like many helping professions rooted in white supremacist ideologies and practices, social work oscillates between introspection, growth, reckoning, evolution, and dissonance. So when the opportunity arose to write a book chapter sharing pertinent advice with the next generation of scholar-activists and practitioners, thoughts of James Baldwin immediately came to mind because of his commitment to love, truth, and narrative shifting as tools of change. There is also a strong parallel between Baldwin's (1962) "A letter to my

DOI: 10.4324/9781003309796-18

nephew" and the conversation we must have today as BIPOC practitioners. In the letter, Baldwin struggles but ultimately shares the horrors that await his nephew as a young Black man coming of age in Harlem during the Civil Rights era. However, Baldwin knows that for his nephew to have any opportunity to dismantle the racial nightmare that is the United States, he must be prepared to survive! Baldwin's letter is a grim foreshadowing of what his nephew and others will continue to face simply because they are BIPOC. However, Baldwin is not resigned to what is, but knows that by guiding his nephew to the truth, he will find knowledge, gain tools, heal, and be better prepared to bring about a new world *not* rooted in the ethos of white supremacy.

Like Baldwin and his nephew and my experiences *surviving* more than four decades in a racialized world, I know that the mere presence of *hope* is a liberatory act (James, 2021). So I will continue to imagine, believe, and put action toward the "promised land" – a world without police, jails, prisons, and poverty. A world in which every human being can self-actualize! However, while hope is a powerful tool, my work in academia for the last 15 years has focused on advancing praxis, by which I mean the embodiment of values, knowledge, and theory toward eradicating injustice – something that my ancestors sacrificed, cried, bled, and died for.

Before I had heard the term "scholar-activist," my practice as an educator was inseparable from my practice as an activist. A big part of that is the knowledge that academia, with the power to shift minds and shape practices, is also a bastion of white supremacy and oppression. So from the outset, I saw my role in academia as a disruptor of the banking system of education and the dissonance of white supremacy. However, on my journey as a scholar-activist, I have seen too many students, colleagues, friends, family, and comrades get sick (mentally and physically), burnout, and quit because they enter the academy and other predominantly white spaces expecting them to actualize their proclamations of inclusivity, diversity, and safety for BIPOC practitioners (Azhar & McCutcheon 2021; Freire, 1996; hooks, 1994; Ocampo & BlackDeer, 2022). In fact, this chapter is written at a *moment* when the labor to exist within the academy, coupled with the violence of the world and the toll of this work on my family, friends, and personal well-being, feels frankly overwhelming!

I often ponder if we can truly do liberatory work, in such violent and dissonant systems, without destroying ourselves? I think the answer is yes, and it begins with *truth*. It begins with naming the atrocities we have and are experiencing in predominantly white spaces while demanding actual change and action toward their purported values (Eads et al., 2023). But to show up for change, whether in the academy, not-for-profit institutions, marginalized communities, or the world, we must also survive and actively participate in their transformation.

Anti-Oppressive Practice

A core component of anti-oppressive practice (AOP) is the understanding that oppression is traumatic and that alleviating oppression requires a trauma-informed lens (James, 2021) which calls to mind Audre Lorde (2017), a black queer scholar, writer, and feminist activist who proclaimed, "Caring for myself is not self-indulgence, it is self-preservation, and that is an act of political warfare." I am not sure how much Audre Lorde knew about the science of trauma, but I suspect she knew on a deeper level that taking care of herself and our communities was of paramount importance in liberatory work. Audre Lorde's proclamation *may* have more relevance in a world still trying to quantify the impact of the COVID-19 pandemic, which will take decades and longitudinal research to understand empirically. However, what we do know is that social isolation, fear, microaggressions, loneliness, gaslighting, hate crimes, transphobia, anxiety, depression, economic insecurity, patriarchy, legal injustices, global uncertainty, and watching Black people get murdered by police officers are trauma-inducing and have a significant impact on our collective health, especially as BIPOC practitioners and communities with pre-existing trauma histories.

Oppression Is Trauma

We live in a traumatic world, and social workers and other helping professionals are often on the front lines of the work (Brown, 2020). The root understanding of trauma comes from war and is often conceptualized by clinicians through the lens of post-traumatic stress disorder (PTSD). But what happens when the traumatic stressors in our personal and professional lives are not PTSD, but an endless series of wars – in the form of racism, micro microaggressions, poverty, geopolitical conflicts, police violence, and the internalization of centuries of white supremacy to name a few. These are the questions we must ask ourselves, our organizations, our educational systems, and our communities to understand the impact of trauma holistically and intersectionally.

As BIPOC practitioners, we are often not taught to care for ourselves; or consider how histories of trauma, coupled with doing AOP work, impact our health, our window of tolerance, and thus the ability to fully show up as our best selves. I had almost a decade working in varied helping professions before I learned about trauma during the first year of my doctoral program. And while I was ecstatic about this knowledge, I initially felt ashamed knowing that my trauma history impeded numerous personal and professional relations. I was mad at myself for the times I felt depressed, triggered, or angry, and lied, screamed, or was unable to listen to others, and far from the person I professed to be. However, I learned how trauma impacts 1) the amygdala, which helps us with emotional regulation; 2) the hippocampus, which aids memory and learning; and 3) the corpus callosum, which enables left and right brain coherence. I learned how prolonged trauma tells our body's central response system to produce cortisol, which is vital for singular traumatic stress, but toxic and even deadly when overproduced in response to unrelenting trauma. These learnings helped to engender self-compassion and grace, and fostered a deep commitment to individual and collective healing (Bremner, 2006; Van der Kolk, 2014).

My growing understanding of trauma changed how I viewed myself as a scholar-activist and practitioner (James, 2021). Slowly, I realized that the work was not just *out there* in marginalized communities but *here* with my family, my friends, and my own trauma history. So with therapeutic support and the knowledge that *my* right to healing, joy, and safety would directly correlate to my ability to show up for and advocate for my community (Hadi, 2020), I slowly began to unpack experiences that I didn't even know were traumatic. This exploration began with my childhood in Jamaica, and its beautiful beaches and magnificent sunsets, which Reaganomics turned into a battlefield of social, political, and economic violence, almost overnight. I unpacked growing up amidst food shortages, tear gas, assassinations, dead bodies, and machine guns that went off all day and night.

Decades later, I realized how traumatic it was to leave my country of birth, family, and friends behind when Mom and I migrated to New York City in February of 1986 – having never before experienced winter, much less minus-degree temperatures – in search of a better life. And while there were undoubtedly more opportunities in the United States, there also was more violence and more trauma in the form of racism, classism, forced assimilation, police brutality, and a long history of anti-Blackness. Furthermore, as a Black man who came of age in the era of "mass incarceration," I learned firsthand the trauma of police, jails, and prisons when I was arrested in Brooklyn on April 13th, 1994, and charged with multiple counts of conspiracy to sell drugs and guns under the Rockefeller Drug Laws, which mandated a life sentence akin to murder for possessing or attempting to sell as little as four ounces of cocaine (Drucker, 2002). So despite being only 18 years old with no prior arrests, I was denied bail, sent to Rikers Island with poor legal representation, and sentenced to *seven years to life* in prison six months later.

My experiences with oppression and the carceral system inspired me to be a social worker, but my journey within social work has been far from utopian. In more than two decades in the profession, I have been underpaid, unfairly fired, lied to by deans and administrators, lacked mentorship, been "ghosted" in the hiring process, told that my research was too "radical" and not fundable, assigned the most demanding classes, had white colleagues with seniority say and do extremely harmful things, and did work that wasn't compensated or acknowledged, among other hardships. Even the good parts of the job – like helping to reallocate resources to marginalized groups, sharing and learning in intentional communities, and mentoring students of color who have never had a BIPOC instructor – can be emotionally overwhelming without appropriate institutional support (Choi, 2023).

My childhood, adulthood, and professional experiences continue to shape me. It would take decades for me to learn and acknowledge without shame that my lived experiences as a Black man in a racialized world were indeed traumatic – and that there is a parallel process in showing up for myself, that allows me to show up with my family, friends, students, colleagues, and others who depended on me. However, when I did learn, a whole world opened up.

As BIPOC social workers, mental health professionals from other disciplines, academics, and scholar-activists, we are the instruments of our liberation. Our minds and bodies are the tools that will learn, develop, and implement AOP. However, trauma is the drama that affects the efficacy of our tools and, thus, our ability to do the work we intend. However, mitigating the impact of trauma is possible. The brain and the body can heal! I cannot promise that the work will be easy. But I cannot overstate how important trauma awareness and intentionality toward healing have been to me (Ahmed, 2021).

Restorative Practices

A few years ago, I taught a class on trauma and healing at Sing Sing Maximum Security Prison. I began the class by defining trauma and discussing its impact on the brain and body. I then asked people who had experienced trauma to raise their hands. No one did! I then asked how many people had been shot? And maybe a quarter of the class raised their hands. I then asked who had been stabbed? And maybe another quarter of the students raised their hands. I then asked who had been jumped or beaten up? And almost all the hands went up. For a second time, I asked the class to raise their hands if they had experienced trauma, and they all laughed. After the laughing ceased, I asked what were some of the ways they took care of themselves while incarcerated? The answers ranged from taking college classes, reading, playing chess, writing letters, weightlifting, and working out in the yard, to meditating, creating art, and staying up late at night listening to music and having solo dance parties in their cells. Finally, I asked the class how they *felt* when participating in what I termed: "restorative practices"? There was a pause for a minute before one of the men blurted out, "Joy," which made everyone laugh.

Finding *joy* in our lives during challenging times is restorative to the mind and body, and is one of the greatest mediators of trauma (Brown, 2019). It is how my ancestors and other oppressed people have survived the horrors of this world. It is also something that is not commodified, dependent on someone else, or can ever be taken from you. My students at Sing Sing have shown me this. Many of them will never see their families or communities again and are destined to die in a human cage. But they continue to maintain hope and cultivate joy in their lives.

Mitchell and Binkley (2021) identified *self-care* as an ethical imperative for AOP education and practice. While I agree, I believe the COVID-19 pandemic has made the term "self-care" analogous to other capitalistic slogans designed to profit from our collective trauma (Kisner, 2017). As a result, in my communities, I have begun utilizing the term *restorative practices* (RPS), which is often associated with "restorative justice," and the utilization of intersectional frameworks to understand, create accountability, and repair harm (Sedillo-Hamann, 2022).

RPS are not prescriptive, not a one-size-fits-all model. Rather they are intentional and consistent activities you and your community engage in to mediate trauma and restore health. RPS should be analyzed and tailored to one's specific circumstances, needs, and areas of growth. For example, I love to cook, run, do yoga, lift weights, get massages, get acupuncture, meditate, soak in claw foot tubs, listen to live music, collect vinyl albums, read, take unplanned trips, spend time in the Islands, peruse the internet for vintage BMWs, shop in thrift stores, buy mid-century furniture, and spend time with children, family, and friends. I am also a believer and proponent of Indigenous spiritual practices that include plant and herbal medicines which have demonstrated efficacy in treating people with severe trauma histories (Orsolini et al., 2019; Perkins et al., 2023).

On a professional level, RPS begins by cultivating awareness of the systems, triggers, and unique challenges we face as BIPOC professionals and identifying activities that soothe and restore our minds and bodies. Such practices include saying "no," conducting self and community check-ins, utilizing supervision, cultivating mentoring relationships, setting boundaries, and building communities of praxis with friends and colleagues who share similar values. In the classroom and other educational spaces, intentionally addressing trauma, power, positionality, and privilege – for example, through co-creating expectations, ground rules, and collective accountability – has been restorative and invigorating!

RPS are our tools of healing, but as with any tool, it is essential to carefully assess the problem and use the right tool for the job. For example, my first few semesters working in the academy would often conclude with my back out of whack and immobilized for weeks. After repeating the same pattern for years, I consulted numerous specialists who saw nothing physically wrong with my body. Finally, through readings like *The Body Keeps the Score: Brain, Mind, and Body in the Healing of Trauma* by Van der Kolk (2014), I learned about the Psoas muscle, which connects our upper and lower body, and contracts when we experience trauma. However, prolonged and acute trauma (the story of my life), makes the Psoas muscle tight and unable to release, which in turn causes numerous physical ailments, including my back pain.

While the pathways to healing and restoration are numerous, yoga and specific poses like "pigeon," which targets the Psoas muscle and hips (where I often hold tension), have been healing for my body. While academic semesters still feel like a set of back-to-back marathons, I am happy to report that it has been more than three years since I have been shut down by back pain.

Conclusion

bell hooks (1994) wrote, "All of us in the academy and in the culture as a whole are called to renew our minds if we are to transform educational institutions–and society" (p. 34). Our minds and bodies are one, and white supremacy is the disease, the trauma that is destroying us from within. As a BIPOC practitioner, my personal and professional journey has been littered with trauma, some of which I never thought I would survive. But against all odds, I am here! My life today is a direct result of social workers and helping professionals like you – who came into dark spaces, saw my humanity, fostered hope, and gave me the tools to survive, thrive, and utilize my power, positionality, and privilege toward our collective liberation!

I am a scholar-activist and social worker who believes in abolition as a theory of change. I believe in the collective of human beings that I have met – in the schools, the streets, the barrios, the jails, the prisons, the projects, the wards, the garrisons, and the ghettos throughout the world – who continue to abolish, imagine, co-create and give of themselves to free us from the grasp of white supremacy. However, colleagues, brothers, sisters, co-conspirators, and comrades: the change we desire starts with us, not in theory, but in praxis, meaning you must become trauma-informed and utilize RPS to survive!

As BIPOC practitioners and scholar-activists, you are the love, hope, and dreams of the ancestors. You are the hope of this world, but the journey will be tough. I will leave you with a few of the last words that James Baldwin (1962) shared with his nephew:

> It will be hard, James, but you come from sturdy peasant stock, men who picked cotton, dammed rivers, built railroads, and in the teeth of the most terrifying odds, achieved an unassailable and monumental dignity. You come from a long line of great poets, some of the greatest poets since Homer. One of them said, "The very time I thought I was lost, my dungeon shook and my chains fell off."

Forward Ever!

References

Abrams, L. S., & Dettlaff, A. J. (2020). Voices from the frontlines: Social workers confront the COVID-19 pandemic. *Social Work, 65*(3), 302–305. doi:10.1093/sw/swaa030.

Ahmed, Z. G. (2021). Leading from the inside out: Contemplative practice as radical self-care for BIPOC activists. *Journal of Women, Politics & Policy, 42*(1), 73–90. doi:10.1080/1554477X.2021.1874186

Azhar, S., & McCutcheon, K. P. D. (2021). How racism against BIPOC women faculty operates in social work academia. *Advances in Social Work, 21*(2/3), 396–420. doi:10.18060/2411.

Baldwin, J. (1962). A letter to my nephew. Progressive.org, December 1. https://progressive.org/magazine/letter-nephew/

Bremner, J. D. (2006). Traumatic stress: Effects on the brain. *Dialogues in Clinical Neuroscience, 8*(4), 445–461. https://doi.org/10.31887/DCNS.2006.8.4/jbremner

Brown, A. M. (2019). *Pleasure activism.* AK Press.

Brown, M. E. (2020). Hazards of our helping profession: A practical self-care model for community practice. *Social Work, 65*(1), 38–44. doi:10.1093/sw/swz047.

Choi, M. (2023). BIPOC women faculty in community colleges and the expectations of emotional labor. *New Horizons in Adult Education and Human Resource Development, 35*(2), 104–107. https://doi.org/10.1177/19394225231171592

Drucker, E. (2002). Population impact of mass incarceration under New York's Rockefeller drug laws: An analysis of years of life lost. *Journal of Urban Health, 79*(3), 434–435. doi:10.1093/jurban/79.3.434.

Eads, R., Bright, C. L., Lee, M. Y., & Franke, N. D. (2023). Promoting diversity and inclusion in social work doctoral programs through mentoring: Perceptions and advice from BIPOC students. *Journal of Ethnic & Cultural Diversity in Social Work.* doi:10.1080/15313204.2023.2200985.

Freire, P. (1996). *Pedagogy of the oppressed* (revised). Continuum.

Hadi, S. A. (2020). *Take care of yourself: The art and cultures of care and liberation.* Common Notions.

hooks, b. (1994). *Teaching to transgress.* Routledge.

James, K. J. (2021). Black lives, mass incarceration, and the perpetuity of trauma in the era of COVID-19: The road to abolition social work. In C. Tosone (Eds.), *Shared trauma, shared resilience during a pandemic.* Essential Clinical Social Work Series. Springer. https://doi.org/10.1007/978-3-030-61442-3_29

Jemal, A. (2022). Critical clinical social work practice: Pathways to healing from the molecular to the macro. *Clinical Social Work Journal.* https://doi.org/10.1007/s10615-022-00843-1

Kisner, J. (2017). The politics of conspicuous displays of self-care. *The New Yorker, 14*(3). www.newyorker.com/culture/culture-desk/the-politics-of-selfcare

Lorde, A. (2017). *A burst of light: And other essays.* Courier Dover Publications.

Mitchell, M., & Binkley, E. (2021). Self-care: An ethical imperative for anti-racist counselor training. *Teaching and Supervision in Counseling, 3*(2), 5. https://doi.org/10.7290/tsc030205

Ocampo, M. G., & BlackDeer, A. A. (2022). We deserve to thrive: Transforming the social work academy to better support Black, Indigenous, and Person of Color (BIPOC) doctoral students. *Advances in Social Work, 22*(2), 703–719. https://doi.org/10.18060/24987

Orsolini, L., Chiappini, S., Volpe, U., De Berardis, D., Latini, R., Papanti, G. D., & Corkery, J. M. (2019). Use of medicinal cannabis and synthetic cannabinoids in post-traumatic stress disorder (PTSD): A systematic review. *Medicina, 55*(9), 525. https://doi.org/10.3390/medicina55090525

Perkins, D., Ruffell, S. G., Day, K., Pinzon Rubiano, D., & Sarris, J. (2023). Psychotherapeutic and neurobiological processes associated with ayahuasca: A proposed model and implications for therapeutic use. *Frontiers in Neuroscience, 16*, 879221. https://doi.org/10.3389/fnins.2022.879221

Sedillo-Hamann, D. (2022). Trauma-informed restorative justice practices in schools: An opportunity for school social workers. *Children and Schools, 44*(2), 98–106. https://doi.org/10.1093/cs/cdac004

Van der Kolk, B. A. (2014). *The body keeps the score: Approaches to the psychobiology of posttraumatic stress disorder.* Guilford Press.

Integrating Social Justice, Black Feminist, and Radical Healing Mentoring

16

Lessons for Transformational Change

Helen Neville, Jioni A. Lewis and Bryana French

For students of color, mentoring serves as a vital support system, determining their ability to access higher education, persist in doctoral programs, and thrive in their chosen professions. Similar to positive models of well-being within communities of color, mentoring transcends individual guidance and includes a deliberate transformation of harmful environments that impede growth to environments that foster healing and belonging. In this chapter we present ten recommendations for future and current early career mentors. The recommendations emerged from an intergenerational conversation among the three of us about our mentoring approaches. The discussion was informed by our dynamic and evolving professional-personal relationship spanning over 15 years – moving from a traditional mentoring relationship (with Helen in the role of mentor), to collaborators, to intergenerational peers.

To provide context for our recommendations, we first discuss our positionality, including our backgrounds and mentoring approaches. Next, we highlight the core aspects of social justice mentoring, while integrating aspects of a Black feminist and radical healing approach. Then, we provide

DOI: 10.4324/9781003309796-19

our recommendations organized from individual to institutional levels of transformative change.

Positionality Statements

Helen Neville

In terms of my own positionality, I am Black woman counseling psychology and Black studies researcher. I adopt a social justice mentoring approach. I believe that capitalism undermines human development and thriving, and that capitalism has shaped racial and gender oppression. Because these forces are working against the common good, I see it as my responsibility as a human being and as psychologist to help dismantle these interlocking forms of oppression. A key piece of this work is naming injustices and the root causes of those inequities. I try to *model social justice values and practice* in all aspects of life. In this way my personal values and ethics around justice and equity feed into the way that I approach teaching and mentoring.

Jioni Lewis

As a Black woman from a working-class background and a first-generation college graduate, my lived experiences with interlocking systems of racism, sexism, and classism have shaped my critical race and feminist consciousness. I am an associate professor of counseling psychology who studies interlocking systems of oppression, intersectionality, and Black women's health and well-being. My identity as a Black feminist psychologist serves as the foundation of my research and praxis. Thus, I strive to ground my research and mentorship approach in a Black feminist and intersectionality framework.

Bryana French

My intersectional lens and radical healing approach to mentoring is a reflection of my identities and life experiences. I am a Black mixed woman, mid-career counseling psychologist. I work full time as an associate professor and have a small part-time private practice. I am the first person in my immediate family to graduate from college and was raised by divorced parents in loving homes. I am a cancer survivor and amputee and a survivor of sexual violence.

Thus, I value intersectionality; practice self-reflection and authenticity; take a relational approach to teaching, research, and practice; and aim to confront the impacts of systemic oppression in everything I do.

Core Aspects of Our Integrated Mentoring Approach

While a social justice orientation is at the core of each of our mentoring approaches, we each bring unique elements to our approach. Helen adheres to a social justice mentoring framework (Neville, 2015) that she has modeled in her mentoring relationship with Jioni and Bryana for the past 15 years. Jioni incorporates a Black feminist and intersectionality lens into her mentorship approach (Lewis & Williams, 2022). Bryana weaves aspects of the psychology of radical healing framework into her approach (French et al., 2020).

According to Neville (2015), social justice mentoring encompasses five key areas: identifying core dimensions of social justice (i.e., defining what social justice practice involves), clarifying one's social justice stance (i.e., describing your personal perspective on social justice and understanding root causes of inequity), modeling social justice values and practices (i.e., living your values openly and consistently), actively working to transform learning and training environments (i.e., providing valuable and purposeful educational experiences), and encouraging students and trainees to establish mentoring networks (i.e., building supportive personal networks for growth and collective action).

Incorporating a Black feminist and intersectional approach to mentorship draws on core feminist principles, such as valuing the relational process of mentoring, building a collaborative relationship, striving to share power in the relationship, and empowering students to feel a sense of agency and self-efficacy in their academic training and career development (Enns & Sinacore, 2005). Another key aspect of our Black feminist mentorship approach is to cultivate a collaborative and supportive community of support among our doctoral students (Lewis & Williams, 2022). When we (Jioni and Bryana) were graduate students at the University of Illinois, we had the opportunity to be trained in a social justice-oriented research lab working under Helen's mentorship. When we first began our careers as assistant professors, we had a desire to carry on a similar tradition of building a Black feminist and social justice-oriented research team, modeling how to cultivate a supportive and collaborative community of scholars and providing a nurturing space for students to thrive. Cultivating a collective space for students, particularly marginalized students, to grow, learn, and support each other throughout their doctoral training has been integral to our mentorship approach.

Integrating radical healing into our social justice and Black feminist approach to mentorship incorporates an understanding of the role of healing from racial trauma in the lives of students of color. Radical healing is a multi-systemic approach to healing racial trauma that involves becoming whole in the face of identity-based wounds (French et al., 2020). It is the process of sitting in the dialectic space between resisting interlocking systems of oppression and envisioning possibilities for a socially just future. A radical healing approach to mentoring incorporates the five core anchors of our model into the way we mentor students of color, including helping students to develop (a) critical consciousness (i.e., developing a critical understanding of oppression through reflection and action), (b) cultural authenticity and self-knowledge (i.e., connecting with one's cultural roots and developing one's own self-definition), (c) radical hope (i.e., fostering hope and envisioning possibilities for a better future), (d) collectivism and social support (i.e., connecting with one's cultural values and community for support), and (e) strength and resistance (i.e., relying on cultural strength and resisting oppression as a form of healing; French et al., 2020).

Emerging from our dialogue, we offer ten recommendations for early career professionals as they engage in mentoring activities to promote transformative change in academic and institutional settings. We categorized the recommendations into three interrelated areas where we believe change can take place: individual, settings, and institutions.

Actions to Nurture Personal Change (Individual Level)

1. **Prioritize Student Needs:** Transformative change begins at the individual level. Our collective commitment to social justice and Black feminist mentoring underscores the importance of focusing on students' needs, setting aside personal or program agendas. This includes listening and providing opportunities for students and trainees to unearth their own path, which many times is different from our hopes for them (e.g., choosing to provide mental health services over an academic profession). Prioritizing student needs translates to getting to know trainees as people, to understand their interests and their personal and professional goals.

This counters the work climate in many mental health professions where the priority is to increase productivity in self and others. Placing student needs first, we have modified what and how we mentor. For example, we have worked with students to secure emergency funds to help with life expenses or found creative ways to offer students time away from their training program so that they can heal or grieve. By attending to student needs, we send a signal to trainees that there is another way of operating that is more humane and holistic.

2. **Model Personal Integrity:** We believe that it is more effective to model ethical ambition than to talk in the abstract about being a justice-oriented mental health professional. Thus, we emphasize the importance of upholding personal integrity and values, even when there are costs associated with challenging the prevailing norms or existing policies impacting the most marginalized students and communities. A trusted mentor's actions, both within and outside the mentoring relationship, can carry significant weight. Our ongoing efforts to model an alternative way of being, both individually and in collaboration with others, aim to promote growth and foster respectful relationships, while challenging oppressive systems. Students keenly observe such efforts. Each of us has received feedback expressing gratitude for modeling courage, taking a public stance for justice, and inspiring students to authentically live out their values.

3. **Expand Traditional Boundaries:** Redefining conventional boundaries within the institution may be essential to cater to the diverse needs of marginalized students and trainees. Many marginalized students lack the social capital and resources available to their privileged counterparts. Adopting a holistic mentoring approach necessitates respectfully engaging with students to create nurturing spaces where they feel a sense of belonging and receive necessary support. This can range from providing emotional support during personal challenges to advocating for their rights in formal settings to creating personal connections. During our conversation, Bryana shared a story about inviting a student to a family holiday meal. She was anxious about her decision and whether it crossed boundaries of professionalism – but ultimately, she realized that communities of color often have a wrap-around approach to supporting each other and expand rigid notions of boundaries. There is always a tension between negotiating boundaries that help students while acknowledging appropriate boundaries that are set in place to protect students from harm. This includes respecting students' boundaries and

not expecting them to divulge personal information about their lives that they choose to keep private.

4. **Acknowledge Resistance and Internalized Oppression:** Acknowledge and address the resistance and internalized oppression experienced by students, particularly within toxic environments. Working with students of color in hostile spaces presents additional challenges, as racism within mental health training spaces can mirror society as a whole and permeate all aspects of training. As Black women, witnessing students internalize this oppression while we advocate for them in private is disheartening. Internalized racism may present itself in a range of ways, including publicly disrespecting faculty of color through demeaning or harsh criticism, such as challenging the person's competence. Navigating this complex dynamic requires understanding the nuances of these challenges and supporting students through them, ensuring they recognize us as allies even amid adversity. Each of us has had some form of "come to Jesus" conversations with students of color to shine a light on internalized oppression and how it manifested in the mentoring relationship.

Actions to Facilitate Transformative Spaces (Setting Level)

5. **Promote Flexible and Understanding Spaces:** Strive to create adaptable, humane, and understanding environments within classrooms, labs, and other settings that arewithin our control. Over the years, we have come to understand the need to recognize the diverse needs of students and offer flexibility to accommodate those needs. During the COVID-19 pandemic, like many faculty across the country, we remained flexible about assignments, class activities, and research projects. We invited feedback from students about learning expectations and provided space to discuss healing and self-care.

6. **Empower and Encourage Student Voices:** Cultivate a supportive atmosphere where students feel empowered to voice their concerns and address microaggressions or inequalities in their academic spaces. One of our important roles as mentors is to nurture critical consciousness, including increasing an awareness of root causes of inequities at the training site, developing a sense of self-efficacy that they can take action to impact change, and encouraging individual and collective action to

create shifts in policies and practices. As an example, Bryana developed and facilitated a student of color group on her campus to fill a gap in graduate student support. This group offered a platform to discuss experiences with racism, seek advice on practice-oriented challenges, and explore topics like liberation psychology. She focused on empowering students to develop self-efficacy and personal agency, encouraging them to speak up and assert themselves in addressing issues within their academic spheres, be it in the classroom, program, or university department.

7. **Infuse Social Justice Advocacy in the Curriculum:** Collaborate with colleagues to embed social justice advocacy training into academic curricula, addressing themes related to social justice, diversity, and equity. Our commitment to intersectionality, self-reflection, authenticity, and a relational teaching approach is central to this work, aiming to confront the impacts of systemic oppression in all aspects of education and practice. Helen exemplifies this approach in her community-based research projects and classroom activities, such as consultation projects with community partners. Our recent efforts involve incorporating healing practices into training spaces and amplifying student voices within those environments. In addition, Jioni has collaborated with colleagues to design a social justice practicum course, which helps students to develop social justice advocacy and consultation skills and to partner with a community-based organization to work on systems-level change (Hage et al., 2020).

Actions to Help Create Institutional Change (Institutional Level)

8. **Advocate for Compassionate Approaches:** Encourage policies and practices that adopt a compassionate stance when dealing with students facing challenges. Mentors should consider individual circumstances, advocating for nuanced policies that cater to students' diverse needs. For instance, we all shared situations when we have advocated for students of color facing unique challenges and tried to help our colleagues understand the impact of discrimination and microaggressions on their experiences. Our role as mentors is to help transform spaces and to humanize our students and their experiences. By doing so, we can create desired changes in cultural norms.

9. **Raise Awareness and Foster Dialogue:** Engage in open conversations with colleagues and peers to illuminate the limitations and biases inherent in existing institutional practices. Promote discussions about the impact of these practices, particularly on marginalized students. By fostering awareness, we can collectively address these issues and advocate for change.

10. **Promote Equity Through Intersectional Advocacy:** Actively confront racial, gender, and other biases within the institution, engaging in collaborative efforts to dismantle discriminatory practices. Raise awareness about intersectionality and its impact on students' experiences, advocating for inclusive policies that recognize intersecting forms of discrimination. Work collaboratively to implement structural changes within the institution, ensuring that policies and practices align with principles of equity, diversity, and social justice, fostering an inclusive and equitable environment for all. This includes creating changes in admissions and hiring committees. Each of us strives to recognize the structurally embedded aspects of our training. For example, in our roles as directors of doctoral training programs or other administrative positions, we have each worked to identify policies and practices that could disproportionately negatively impact students of color and other marginalized students. We have worked with colleagues to implement changes that will lead to greater equity, whether in program handbook policies or by enhancing transparency in decision-making processes.

In this chapter, we presented ten lessons drawn from our mentoring experiences, with a specific emphasis on guiding students of color. While our approaches may vary, they all encompass a social justice perspective infused with elements of Black feminism and radical healing principles. Four of these lessons we outlined were geared toward actions that early career professionals can take when working with students of color to facilitate personal and professional growth. Three of the lessons provided practical advice for mentors to create more equitable lab, classroom, and other learning spaces. The remaining three lessons were aimed at promoting institutional change, enabling students of color to not only access these spaces but also thrive within them. Collectively these lessons were based on the premise that mentoring involves viewing students of color holistically, treating them with care and compassion, and establishing equitable personal and learning environments where they can flourish.

References

Enns, C. Z., & Sinacore, A. L. (Eds.). (2005). *Teaching and social justice: Integrating multicultural and feminist theories in the classroom.* American Psychological Association. https://doi.org/10.1037/10929-000

French, B. H., Lewis, J. A., Mosley, D., Adames, H. Y., Chavez-Dueñas, N. Y., Chen, G. A., & Neville, H. A. (2020). Toward a psychological framework of radical healing in communities of color. *The Counseling Psychologist, 48*(1), 14–46. https://doi.org/10.1 177/0011000019843506

Hage, S. M., Miles, J. R., Lewis, J. A., Grzanka, P. R., & Goodman, L. A. (2020). The social justice practicum in counseling psychology training. *Training and Education in Professional Practice, 14*(2), 156–166. https://doi.org/10.1037/tep0000299

Lewis, J. A., & Williams, M. G. (2022). The promise and perils of conducting intersectional feminist research. In. K. Richmond, I. Settles, S. Shields, & A. Zelin (Eds.), *Feminist scholars on the road to tenure: The personal is professional.* Cognella Academic Publishing.

Neville, H. A. (2015). Social justice mentoring: Supporting the development of future leaders for struggle, resistance, and transformation. *The Counseling Psychologist, 43*(1), 157–169. https://doi.org/10.1177/0011000014564252

Antiracist and Anti-Oppressive Pedagogy

Putting Theory into Action

Grace S. Kim and
Karen L. Suyemoto

17

Education, like other cultural endeavors, is deeply rooted in the values and norms of a given society. US education reflects the normalization of inequities and oppression in our culture, privileging the voices and values of people who are white, cis-hetero-patriarchal, middle to upper class, and non-disabled. US education not only reflects these inequities; it has often socialized students into an ideology that maintains this oppressive status quo – what Noam Chomsky calls education for indoctrination (Chomsky, 2012). But education has also been a means to resist legacies of oppression – what Chomsky refers to as education for liberation and enlightenment (Chomsky, 2012). But how and why does one become the kind of educator who strives to teach from an antiracist and anti-oppressive stance? And what does that teaching praxis actually look like? For almost two decades we have been reflecting on those questions, though we still don't have complete answers. This chapter is an invitation to think with us about possibilities of more fully integrating anti-oppression into the content and practice of your teaching, to join our exploration of questions and possibilities, rather than prescriptions and certainties.

DOI: 10.4324/9781003309796-20

Locating Ourselves in Teaching

When we teach, we share our positionalities with students, inviting them to consider how their education has been affected not only by the dominant US culture but also by their teachers' intersectional experiences of privilege and oppression. We acknowledge that like all of their teachers, we have made curricular and pedagogical choices (including what *doesn't* get covered). And we name that we are sharing our positionalities so that they may actively consider their effects on our teaching and their learning. Our positionalities and related experiences affect our writing, as well as our teaching – they affect all that we do, of course. So we also want to share with you, so you can also consider what we say in the context of "where we are coming from."

I (GSK) identify as a 1.5 generation[1] Korean immigrant, Asian American, middle-class, non-disabled, bicultural and bilingual, heterosexual woman. I am trained in Clinical Psychology, and am a clinical associate professor in the Counseling Psychology program at Boston University. While I have enjoyed teaching and interacting with students since my first course, I never actually received formal training in how to teach from an antiracist and anti-oppressive lens. When I first started teaching full time as a faculty of color and one of few Asian American faculty, I tried to infuse diversity and social justice topics into all my courses. I kept asking myself how I might do this effectively, a question I continue to ask myself. I learned a lot from my colleagues who are excellent teachers, and from Karen, by observing them teach, and through a lot of conversations that often started with, "I have a teaching dilemma."

I (KLS) identify as a multiracial Sansei (third generation Japanese American), as Asian American, queer, middle class, currently non-disabled. I am trained in Clinical Psychology and am currently a tenured full Professor at University of Massachusetts Boston (UMB), which is a Department of Education designated Minority Serving Institution. I have been at UMB for over 20 years, with a joint appointment in Clinical Psychology and Ethnic Studies. When I started at UMB, I really wasn't qualified to be teaching Ethnic Studies, but I was seeking a position that would encourage, even require, me to grow into more fully living my social justice values. When I first started teaching, I was passionate, idealistic, and wanted to change the world. I was also pretty naïve and ignorant. I'd never

---

1 The 1.5 generation term was first used in the 1970's to describe immigrants who came to the US as children or adolescents, whose experience is in between that of their parents, born in Korea, and children born in the US who may feel more American.

taken an Ethnic Studies class, and my graduate program had almost no content about race or ethnicity. But I benefited from a few supportive and generous colleagues who helped me figure out teaching and mentoring generally.

We've known each other for over 20 years. In fact, Grace (as a graduate student at UMB) interviewed Karen (as a prospective faculty member). I (Grace) often think "Thank goodness that the department followed through and hired Karen!" She taught me about being an ally and an advocate, and modeled what it means to teach from a transformative education (TE) lens. Also, through sharing her own life experiences as a multiracial Asian American, Karen created opportunities for honest and meaningful conversations, which led me to reflect on my own privilege even within the Asian American community. I (Karen) often also reflect on the many things that I learned from Grace – not only about mentoring and academia, but also about being Asian American as monoracial and as an immigrant. Grace (and my other mentees) taught me so much about what I didn't know, about the knowledge I took for granted, about the joy of being trusted to hold a student's growth and well-being, and about the kind of connections that could be possible but also about the importance of boundaries and awareness of power differences, especially while still in institutional (academic) roles influenced by the white supremacist system.

Transformative Education

For us, integrating anti-oppression into our teaching is rooted in both our own and our students' process of conscientization, reflecting the praxis of TE philosophy and critical pedagogy – informed by scholars such as Friere, hooks, and Anzaldua. To participate in the process of liberation is the goal of TE. The teaching praxis to support this goal needs to step away from the usual practices of emphasizing abstract "objective" content, cognitive learning and pedagogy characterized by hierarchical dynamics where the teacher is the expert knower, students are supposed to absorb the wisdom, and learning assessment emphasizes memory, basic understanding, and (possibly) application. This traditional model pays scant attention to analyzing, critiquing, or creating knowledge for change.[2] Coupled with commercialization of education, where

---

2 In addition to critical education and critical theory more generally, the kind of praxis we are talking about is central to good learning and expanded on within education, psychology, and adult learning more generally – see, for example, work building on Benjamin Bloom's taxonomy of educational objectives and Jack Mezirow's transformative learning.

educational institutions run like businesses, this traditional model educates students to maintain the status quo. For students who are marginalized, the approach is akin to gaslighting, as it often leads them to question their own experienced reality and maintain (or deny) their own oppression. Minoritized faculty also struggle as they push against the system that continues to reify inequity in the academy (see the books *Presumed Incompetent I and II*).

In contrast, when conscientization and liberatory skills are central goals, then our teaching needs to fully engage students (and professors) as whole people. By conscientization, we mean the process of building critical consciousness related to justice and equity, raising our own and students' awareness of sociopolitical and cultural histories and contexts that shape their current world; encouraging students to ask critical questions about all knowledges; and providing skills so that they can make active choices about using knowledge and skills to maintain or to change our systems and cultures to become more equitable and just for all people. Engaging students as whole people means considering and actively engaging students' values, histories, emotions, relationships, and positionalities within oppressive hierarchies in the classroom – in content and discussions and interactions. It means welcoming students' complex experiences and responses, embracing and exploring both differences and similarities in power, privilege, and oppression that affect the production of knowledge *and* the process of learning.

This whole person approach is not the teaching or learning approach most of us have experienced in our own education. Most of us have rarely, if ever, experienced a classroom that actively engages ideological, internal, interpersonal, and systemic power, privilege, and oppression. This means that we need to begin with questioning and likely unlearning at least some aspects of our own experience of education. And we need to also consider how our own experiences of oppression and privilege, pain and resistance, ignorance and fragility have shaped us, our own understanding of our material, and our views of the students we are teaching.

Reflections and Recommendations

Centering Motivations and Beginnings (and Overcoming Doubts and Fears)

One of the biggest challenges of TE praxis is being able to envision what transformation through education might actually look like – in the curriculum, in the classroom, for the students, and for the teacher. It is still (sadly) the case that most of us have very limited in vivo experience of TE. Most often, minoritized people simply know that what they have experienced or what is "mainstream" hasn't really worked for them. They may not even know this consciously – maybe it is just a sense of dissonance, of distance, of dis-ease. For me (GSK), as an immigrant I rarely questioned education before graduate school, even when what I was taught was not remotely close to my lived experiences. While I did well, I felt disconnected, like I didn't belong. It was only much later that I realized the issue was not me, but the ways in which whiteness is centered in the curricula, and white cultural values were upheld in pedagogy.

Some of us may have experiences of how traditional education has more actively damaged us. My (KLS) earlier experience of education was much like Grace's – a sense of disconnection but little conscious awareness of that. But unlike Grace, graduate school was an actively oppressive experience for me, one that pathologized my experience as a queer Person of Color, while also enacting passive oppression in its almost complete inattention to race, culture, or ethnicity in the curriculum. When I started teaching and mentoring students, my most pressing goal was for students to *not* experience what I had. It wasn't until later that I developed a more proactive (versus reactive) understanding of how education could be a means to empower students to challenge the oppression that existed in the world, and in the field of psychology.

For both of us, our interest in TE was rooted in our own experiences of oppression and our social justice values. We wanted students to have a radically different experience than we had, to provide a type of education that was not characterized by the depersonalization, marginalization, gaslighting, and psychological violence we had experienced. We also wanted students to see themselves in the curriculum, to believe that they belonged in psychology and in the academy. This goal of positive experience was – for us – a beginning that grew into a fuller understanding of the possibility of TE to provide active skills for healing, and for resisting oppression and promoting social justice. This latter goal is centrally founded in conscientization – the development of critical consciousness not only for positive personal experience or healing, but as the basis of liberatory practice. Thus, understanding the ideological foundation of oppressive systems and one's own socialization into that ideology is not the goal, but is instead the foundation for developing motivation, skills, and critical assessment of possible actions to resist oppression (Hochman et al., 2022).

As a goal, the conscientization that is the foundation of TE seems overwhelming to many educators. This is especially true because if we have engaged in even initial explorations of our own racial, ethnic, and intersectional awareness and understanding, we are aware of how much we don't know. Even if we have a general sense of what we want to accomplish and the content we want to cover, and even if we have been lucky enough to have found critical theory and education authors (e.g., Friere, hooks, Harro) so that we might be able to put language to our educational goals (e.g., transformative education, conscientization, critical consciousness, liberation), it is still so challenging to figure out *how* to teach to this goal. We usually lack models or guides to even consider the questions we should be asking to figure out that "how."

But consider: we can learn and grow in our own journey of conscientization *through* our teaching. If we can let go of the idea that we (the professor) must be *the* expert who knows everything and has an answer for everything; if we can let our own humanity into the room (including our fear and anxiety, at least internally); if we can open to the possibility of learning and growing *with* and *from* our students, then we can start incorporating TE ideas and approaches into our teaching almost immediately. Transparency is important here: to share with students that you, too, are learning and growing. This can be anxiety provoking as well as a learning opportunity, if we are willing to invite them to see our full humanity as well. Our experience is that mental health fields actually have a lot to offer educators in terms of proactively and positively meeting these challenges (see the next section).

Recommendation 1: Connect your own conscientization to your TE teaching approach. Recognize that conscientization is a life-long journey and that you will always need to grow and expand your social justice knowledge and skills. This means taking risks and making mistakes. While the values and aims of TE may be clear, the process of how to bring these values into practice is always a work in progress. It is never going to be perfect. You will likely continue to feel anxious about teaching from a TE lens, and you will probably not feel that you have "mastered" this or are truly "expert." We still get anxious when we teach about oppression and social justice, and we expect it. So, return to the question of your values. What makes you want to teach from the TE lens? Ultimately, why do you want to teach in antiracist and anti-oppressive ways? Teaching for justice is an intention, an attitude, and a value that will shape how you think about every aspect of your teaching.

Recommendation 2: In your TE teaching, start *somewhere* and grow from there. It is not all or nothing. We encourage you to work against perfectionism and make small and active steps, focusing on growing a little bit each day and each year. Some suggestions for beginnings:

- Get started, even if it is only a single class session or a single assignment. While an "add-on" approach of addressing diversity or oppression in one class session is not best practice, it is a step forward from not addressing it at all! Be honest with yourself about what you are ready for and be prepared to teach yourself things that you didn't have the opportunity to learn in school, though yes, it is unfair that your education didn't prepare you to teach in ways that are not oppressive and you now have to invest in your own remedial education about diversity, oppression, and systemic injustice. Remember, this is the experience you are trying to address for your students!
- Choose the content of your course, textbooks, and readings to reflect your own values and goals for education. If you have to use an established text, supplement it with content that fosters a critical view and aligns with your values.
- Consider the issue of epistemology. As you look at your courses, ask yourself whose experiences and voices are centered? Whose are marginalized? These questions apply not only to content but also to assignments and assessment.
- Make a clear distinction between "diversity, multiculturalism, and inclusion" versus equity and justice. We are not interested in simply respecting differences. Rather, consider how you can include critical analysis of the effects of power, privilege, and oppression in your content area, and offer students models of how to challenge inequity.

Connecting Your Psychological Knowledge and Skill Sets with Teaching Practice

While you may not feel it sometimes, your training in psychological theories and counseling processes has already given you tools for effective teaching. Our training as clinical psychologists has been of benefit to us in our TE teaching, because that training has included theories and skills focused on the process of change, resistance to change, development over time, and relational process. Conscientization involves shifts in worldviews that also relate to shifts in feelings (e.g., anger and empowerment rather than helplessness and despair), and shifts in relationships as we come to see that structural power and privilege permeate our interactions through processes like internalization and gaslighting. We were struck by how conscientization and transformative education are so rarely explicitly considered as a *psychological* change process, with similarities to a developmental arc of psychological change over time.

Our psychological training can help us understand and effectively address dynamics in the classroom. We can, for example, use our training and understanding of psychological and interpersonal dynamics to proactively address barriers to TE. When people feel threatened and emotionally overwhelmed, for example, they often experience a fight/flight/freeze response. And we know that change is hard, that people often *do* feel psychologically threatened, and that people often use a range of "defenses" to protect themselves against recognizing the pain that often catalyzes change and the pain involved in the process of changing. If we think about these responses in relation to a course or discussion focused on diversity, race, or racism, we might have a different understanding of students who may appear to be "disengaged," "defensive," "resistant," or even "aggressive." And we might try different approaches to help students maintain engagement in a process of change that is emotionally and interpersonally challenging.

Consider the dynamics of "difficult dialogues." I (GSK) taught at a PWI for many years, and often noticed hesitancy, avoidance, and silence among students during difficult conversations about racism, even though the same students seemed talkative and connected to each other when we discussed other issues (e.g., culture and ethnicities). When I attempted to learn more about their difficulty talking about racism (i.e., asking "What makes it so challenging to talk about racism?"), responses trickled out. These responses illustrated the complex feelings students were having internally, and how frustrated they were at the larger systems. Many white students shared that they were worried about others' judgments and feared that they would say the "wrong thing" and offend others. Many students of color talked about how they were protecting themselves from another potential hurt, so they were reluctant to say much in class. In such situations, understanding the cognitive and emotional challenges students may experience while learning about racism (e.g., new knowledge about racism challenging white students' self-views about being good people), and understanding the group dynamics when students from different positionalities and contexts interact with each other can be extremely helpful.

I (KLS) noticed that students would sometimes seem emotionally worked up so that they had a hard time engaging the material or hearing each other. Alternatively, they would sometimes make concepts so abstract and intellectualized that the issues seemed devoid of feeling or connection to real human beings. I started to think about how to manage emotion in the classroom. I didn't want to "tone it down" too much, since oppression is *painful* and confronting that pain is part of moving toward a liberatory process. From my experience as a therapist, I thought about the emotion in the room and "holding" it. I conceptualized both the class session and semester as having an emotional "arc" – similar to a therapy session. I started developing strategies to "titrate" emotions – to help students hold and name their own and each other's emotions, such as having students name their hopes and fears about the course at the very beginning, shared by our co-author, Roxanne Donovan.

When faculty think about changing teaching practice to focus more on social justice and antiracist teaching, they often focus first on changing the syllabi, especially readings. This can be a good first step, but conceptualizing your teaching in light of TE allows you to take a whole-person perspective and long view toward change, moving beyond the shifting of content. Remember that change is hard and happens most often in supportive interpersonal relationships.

Recommendation 1: Bring the assessment skills that you learned in clinical training to examine your own teaching. Ask yourself whether your course materials, plans, and assessments reflect liberated, strength-based views of individuals rather than pathology-focused ones. If you were to come up with a "treatment plan" of sorts to promote positive change in your teaching practice, what steps might you take? What specific environment and relationships would you need to create, what work would you personally need to do, and what would you need to introduce (and when) to your students? Draw on your strengths and think developmentally and systemically.

Recommendation 2: Consider your course an emotional, relational, and intellectual experience. The change process is relational and dynamic, and it has a developmental trajectory. We did not start out knowing this; we learned over time, and the learning process was not only cognitive. Often it involves intense emotions, processing relational issues, and learning from other people.

- Consider the developmental arc of your course and how students may move through developmental stages. You will need to build a shared understanding of concepts and of increasing conscientization, while being supported, encouraged, and caringly challenged in a community. This takes time, and there will be times during the course when emotions will be particularly activated or certain topics will become more salient. Having a general sense of what things may come up or what might be particularly vulnerable points for students could be enormously helpful in proactively addressing potential challenges.

• Teaching is a group process and interpersonal dynamics loom large in any classroom (even in online teaching contexts). Develop strategies for engagement and growth using, rather than resisting, group dynamics (e.g., group formation, maintenance, conflicts). A key task of a TE educator is creating a learning community where each student feels supported, commits to supporting others' learning and growth, and feels encouraged to take relational and intellectual risks, while accepting accountability for their actions.

Conclusion

Teaching from a TE lens with a focus toward justice and equity is *personal*. You are engaging students in difficult dialogues, encouraging them to see things that are painful and "hidden" and *that matter to YOU*. Most likely you won't see immediate results. Taking care of your physical and mental health, knowing your limits, and being in a community that brings you joy are ways this long-term work can be sustained. At the same time, there are substantial rewards, both in the moment and in the long term. What I (GSK) feel most proud of is the longer-term impact of what I taught and the community we have created in the classroom. When students email me about how they are using their knowledge in their clinical practice or in their own work, I feel joyful. I (KLS) love the moments where I can see a new perspective just beginning to emerge in a student. I also find joy in the moments where students trust me (and each other) to be vulnerable, to share a fear, to "look real, not good" (Butler, 1998). These are moments of authentic connection that give me hope for change. And, like Grace, the longer term impact keeps me going, particularly when I see how students bring their conscientization to how they educate and counsel others, promote policy or organizational change. I believe that I have contributed to changes that mean that fewer students will experience the oppression and marginalization I struggled with. I can see how students expect and demand more, and how this "entitlement" is rooted in a social development, within the field and our larger society, toward liberation.

It helps to know that we are not alone in this work. We stand on the shoulders of antiracist and anti-oppressive educators who modeled persistence and hope. We invite you to this community of educators, because education, whether in classrooms or clinics, can be a tool for liberation.

References and Resources

Anzaldúa, G. E., & Keating, A. (Eds.). (2002). *This bridge we call home: Radical visions for transformation*. Routledge.

Butler, S. (Director) & World Trust (Producer). (1998). *The way home* [documentary]. United States: Available from World Trust: www.world-trust.org/the-way-home

Chomsky, N. (2012). The purpose of education. Presentation at the Learning Without Frontiers Conference, London (LWF 12), January 25. www.youtube.com/watch?v=DdNAUJWJN08

Friere, P. (1993). *Pedagogy of the oppressed*. Continuum International Publishing.

Harro, B. (2000a). The cycle of liberation. In M. Adams, W. Blumenfeld, R. Castaneda, H. Hackman, M. Peters., & X. Zuniga (Eds.), *Readings for diversity and social justice*. Routledge.

Harro, B. (2000b). The cycle of socialization. In M. Adams, W. Blumenfeld, R. Castaneda, H. Hackman, M. Peters., & X. Zuniga (Eds.), *Readings for diversity and social justice*. Routledge.

Hochman, A., Suyemoto, K. L., Donovan, R. A., & Kim, G. S. (2022). Understanding and enacting resistance to oppression: Developing as an ally and advocate. In *Unraveling assumptions: A primer for understanding oppression and privilege*. Routledge. https://doi.org/10.4324/9780429059599-14

hooks, b. (1994). *Teaching to transgress: Education as the practice of freedom*. Routledge. https://doi.org/10.4324/9780203700280

Kim, G. S., Donovan, R. A., & Suyemoto, K. L. (2022). *Teaching diversity relationally: Engaging emotions and embracing possibilities*. Routledge. https://doi.org/10.4324/9780429059582

Suyemoto, K. L., Donovan, R. A., & Kim, G. S. (2022). *Unraveling assumptions: A primer for understanding oppression and privilege*. Routledge. https://doi.org/10.4324/9780429059599

Broadening Your Reach

18

Disseminating Science and Knowledge for Maximum Impact

Maryam Kia-Keating

Early career scholars navigate institutional structures and pressures that uphold historical inequities. Systemic conditions within academia can work to constrain scholars' flexibility, preferences, and personal and family needs. There are calls to increase diversity, equity, inclusion, and belonging in the Academy, due to long-standing inaccessibility and barriers to entry and retention for BIPOC scholars; nonetheless, empirical findings demonstrate the enduring privileged demographics of the professoriate (Morgan et al., 2022; Wapman et al., 2022). While understanding individual experiences is helpful, an overhaul at the systemic level is clearly needed. A reimagining and expansion of the meaning and measure of successful scholarship within the Academy has many potential benefits for both researchers and communities, ensuring that scientific knowledge is poised for impact.

In this chapter, I describe some of the pressures that can arise within academic research career paths, and the institutional structures and constraints that BIPOC scholars may face. I share my own experience and make an argument for diversification of one's portfolio. I offer three domains to consider when deciding how to balance publishing academic work and leveraging non-academic outlets for maximum reach and impact.

DOI: 10.4324/9781003309796-21

My Journey

My personal background gave rise to my sense of purpose in my professional pursuits. When socio-political violence erupted, my family and I were forcibly displaced from our home in Iran and, after multiple moves across countries and languages, we eventually resettled in the United States. As I grew older, I saw that this problem was rapidly increasing around the globe, dispossessing millions of innocent people of their homes, a huge percentage of which were children under the age of 18 (Kia-Keating et al., 2018). With the growing prevalence came my sense of responsibility to prioritize work related to communities facing upheaval. So, when I began graduate school, my commitment to research and service to benefit refugee and immigrant communities invigorated my desire to forge a unique path despite the fact that there was no one in my department pursuing that line of research. Ultimately, I was fortunate enough to find ways to work within traditionally accepted structures, as well as to push the boundaries outside the sheltered walls of higher education to reach communities in their own neighborhoods and homes.

Throughout my professional trajectory, I took steps to prepare for a research-focused academic position, as well as to become a licensed clinical psychologist. I moved from the island of O'ahu to attend Dartmouth College and study psychology. I worked as a psychiatric assistant at the inpatient psychiatric unit at The Queen's Medical Center on O'ahu, where the diverse array of patients in crisis provided me with long hours of their life stories, rich multicultural backgrounds, and painful histories of chronic and racial trauma and adversities. I was keenly aware of their strengths and potential for healing, and simultaneously concerned that many of the field's existing approaches didn't adequately support empowerment or resilience. I dedicated substantial time to training and foundational experience in traumatic stress and resilience studies, through positions at the Yale Center for Traumatic Stress and Recovery, McLean Hospital, and the Center for Medical and Refugee Trauma at Boston Medical Center.

After obtaining my master's from Harvard University, I earned my doctorate in clinical psychology from Boston University, and completed a predoctoral clinical internship at the University of California, San Diego (UCSD) Consortium / Veterans Affairs. I moved from a postdoctoral position at UCSD to secure a tenure-track assistant professorship at an R1 public university. The designation of R1 indicates that an institution is a doctoral university with the highest level of research activities. In accordance, the primary expectation for my position is research productivity, while excellence in teaching, professional activities, and service are also critical domains to achieve tenure and promotion. Notably, I also became a parent, having two children during my pre-tenure years. Navigating motherhood at the same time as urgent academic pressures, both of which were literally ticking down "on a clock," created a limited window within which I needed to accomplish certain goals. At the same time, having children also gave me personal meaning and motivation to ensure that my work led to both immediate positive impact, and long-term potential to improve social conditions for the next generation.

I sometimes challenge, and sometimes work within, traditional structures to pursue opportunities to extend my reach both within academic outlets, as well as non-academic ones, with hopes to increase the direct impact for communities. In addition to publications in scientific, peer-reviewed journals, I pursue a variety of collaborations, outreach, consultations, advocacy, and direct service activities. I regularly incorporate ways to achieve community-based impact to my overall portfolio, within a fruitful academic career as a full professor of clinical psychology.

Evaluations in the Academy

Academic research institutions place a heavy emphasis on evaluation. Highly coveted academic positions require tireless work and many sacrifices. In these contexts, it can be difficult to envision activism and impact on the world when that vision is overshadowed by the pressures of a loudly ticking "clock" (i.e., the tenure clock); a metaphorical hourglass from which sand begins rapidly draining the moment after graduation. Contradictions between academic freedom and true liberation are rampant (Guillaume & Apodaca, 2022).

Although academics are evaluated on the reach of their scholarship, the focus is on scholars' impact in the scientific literature. Algorithms, mathematically determining impact based on variables like number of citations in peer-reviewed journals (e.g., h-index), have proliferated as indices of "success" in recent years. Academics are also appraised based on achieving national or international recognition from other scholars, rather than the public. In other words, the basis for evaluation is purportedly a jury of one's peers. However, noted inadequacies of diversity, equity, and inclusion in the Academy beg the question as to who one's "peers" are when centering the experiences of BIPOC scholars (see also Zárate et al., 2017). In fact, recent research has pointed to the high levels of exclusivity making up the institutional origins of a majority of professors; specifically, one in eight tenure-track faculty in the United States are drawn from just five universities where they received their doctorates (Wapman et al., 2022). In truth, the system relies on a contained network of so-called "peers," who reflect only a narrow scope of backgrounds, experiences, or perspectives, and may not understand, accept, or cite work that does not fit within their ideologies (Kozlowski et al., 2022).

"Do more secondary data analyses," advised one well-intentioned and highly successful mentor from the rooftop of a New York City building. I had just finished explaining my deep passion for working with communities experiencing forced displacement. I expressed my plan to build and, most importantly, earn trust and to work in partnership toward immediate and direct benefits to children and families. I was searching for advice and support on how to achieve my goals. But the mentor shook her head at me, smiling wryly. "You can't be naïve about how you use your time." She recommended fast data and fast turnaround, urging me to find a good dataset that we could use to publish together. I walked away from that meeting feeling puzzled and frustrated. The conversation had been one-directional, and I didn't feel heard. She was preaching the "old" rules to me, perhaps with the intention to help me "play the game" and succeed, but without considering the ways this might perpetuate harms, inequities, and injustices.

In fact, I was already steeped in work with communities for whom no secondary datasets, with large, "representative" samples, existed, as in the case of many refugee and immigrant communities. For example, Middle Eastern North African (MENA) research is dangerously deficient in understanding of physical and mental health among these communities and leading to critical research gaps and public health disparities (Awad et al., 2019). If I only prioritized my speed and quantity of publications, it would keep me from engaging in important efforts and could perpetuate inequities of which I was all too aware. Thus, I stayed firm in my resolve to work with and for minoritized communities, regardless of the time and energy it might take.

Fortunately, I was able to garner funding from the National Institutes of Child Health and Human Development (NICHD) to use participatory methodologies with a focus on creating partnership and setting a foundation so that the communities can take the lead in determining their own research priorities and desired social action (Henderson et al., 2023; Kia-Keating & Juang, 2022). My steps were deliberate, and required collective investment and agreement, activities which could not be rushed. Acquiring a federal grant gave my work an acclaimed level of external validation, that aligned with the timing of an academic career path without sacrificing the integrity of the methodologies that I knew were needed.

Diversifying Your Portfolio

It may be tempting to focus either on the number of publications in your early career, or on activities that fulfill your deep investment in meaningful community work, advocacy, and teaching and mentorship. However, neither extreme is as beneficial as finding balance. Balancing your career across domains that meet personal, community, and institutional goals is an approach that is consistent with financial recommendations to "diversify your portfolio." There are a number of benefits in achieving some diversification in the activities you pursue.

1. Diversification keeps your options open in a changing job market. When you have multivaried experiences, interdisciplinary training, and skill sets, you can design your portfolio to showcase your potential fit for different kinds of positions and work settings.
2. Diversification can provide you with multiple income streams. You can engage in additional work, including many direct service activities like private practice, and consultation, where you can easily regulate the amount of time spent. If you are on a nine-month academic salary, you might want to pursue opportunities to augment your salary during the summer months, when you have more flexibility with your schedule.
3. Diversification also keeps things interesting and flexible. Over the course of your career, it can be more meaningful, and enjoyable, to follow your creativity, imagination, and motivations. You can prioritize your preferences, and your family's changing needs.
4. Diversification allows you to build on your passions and knowledge. You can use your multifaceted experiences, identities, and talents to inform the work you do.
5. Diversification increases opportunities for reach and impact. Responding to socio-political contexts, engaging with communities in change efforts, and disseminating scientific information in diverse outlets create avenues to increase your impact.

I made active efforts toward diversification at every phase of my journey, but also did only a little bit at a time. Slowly but surely, I gained strong clinical experiences from diverse settings (e.g., community-based, medical, outpatient, and inpatient) across geographies of peoples and places (e.g., Hawai'i, Boston, Southern California, and the many immigrant and refugee communities resettled in these locations). I embraced and nurtured my multidisciplinary interests through degree programs and certificates in women's studies, and English (Bachelor's degree), education and prevention science (Master's degree), and clinical psychology (doctorate). I incorporated participatory approaches and mixed methodologies in research, including and incorporating cultural strengths and rituals, non-verbal expressions of experience such as photography, art, dance, and music, and providing multiple forms of nourishment (literal, such as sharing cultural food dishes, and figurative) in outreach and programming. Over time, I have and continue to participate in podcasts, engaged with media outlets (i.e., *Psychology Today*), consult to children's media creators (e.g., Disney+, DreamWorks Animation, YouTube Kids), provide pro bono care to communities in the aftermath of crises, create guided meditations with music (ReachandShine.com), and other activities that help to reach communities directly.

Writing Your Own Rules for Reach and Impact

Although there are structural constraints, institutional pressures, and naysayers, it is possible, and perhaps vital, to forge a path that satisfies your spirit. Three key areas are helpful to consider, as you assess and plan your own career path: expertise, activities, and timing.

Build Out Your Areas of Expertise

There are early demands to develop an "expertise," traditionally defined as a signature area that encompasses your "research program." Despite the pressures to narrow your attention to a limited scope, there are still compelling reasons for diversification of your expertise. It may be a matter of necessity to draw on various strengths in order to gain employment, maintain it, and create financial stability. With limited openings in any given year, breadth of experience as well as depth of expertise can be beneficial. Building out your areas of expertise over time helps you to develop a portfolio with products for both academic and non-academic outlets which provide future opportunities. Some products can be variants of an academic paper, social media threads, infographics, marketing campaigns, or other forums within which summarized findings are accessible to broader audiences.

For example, drawing from the latest findings on adversity, protective factors, and the science of resilience and using a participatory co-design process with community health workers, parents, and youth, I offer the HEROES program, a parenting and child program online (www.theheroesprogram.com/) in both English and Spanish. My consultations to children's media on topics such as child development, mental health, identity, representation, and restorative justice, help to bridge the connection between the latest science and engaging storytelling. Finding ways to apply your knowledge to develop, test, and deliver empirically supported health tools and information directly to consumers and benefit communities extends and deepens your expertise over time, while contributing to conversations about critical issues.

Engage in Activities That Matter

What "counts" in the Academy is not always what counts in life. In other words, it's important to reflect on your personal values and priorities, rather than to blindly follow institutional forces. Unquestioningly, scientific, peer-reviewed journal articles reflect incredible time and effort, and play an important role. However, there are notable limits on who accesses, reads, understands, and integrates single-paper findings to social action and real-world change. Scientific work is also methodical, cautious, and often slow to affect public transformation. Researchers have an important responsibility to ensure that empirically supported findings are communicated properly and coherently to communities. Widening your lens to incorporate advocacy, public health campaigns, op-eds, documentaries, podcasts, fiction, and non-fiction for the public increases your potential to engage many more people in a topic of importance, in a timely way.

Within the areas of scientific and community impact, your voice and perspective matter: topics such as disparities, immigration, mental health, and discrimination are impacted by representational diversity among scholars (Kozlowski et al., 2022). Being the person to take on these meaningful, but also weighty and difficult, topics takes courage, strength, and stamina. Seniority, experience, and even awards don't always reflect the best understanding of communities, nor best intentions. In fact, the notion of someone drawn to who they perceive as victims, in order to be viewed as a savior, has been described as "an all-too-familiar pattern of white people of privilege seeking personal catharsis by attempting to liberate, rescue, or otherwise uplift underprivileged people of color" (Aslan, 2022). Despite not having the necessary knowledge base, some people will suddenly start responding to diversity initiatives when they come with funding support or other gains. Teju Cole astutely points out, "The white savior supports brutal policies in the morning, founds charities in the afternoon, and receives awards in the evening" (Cole, 2012). Authentic sources and representation matter. Critical self-reflection is a key step that offers personal growth and accountability in the field (Henderson et al., 2023). It can uncover needs, so that you can embark on collaborative projects with partners who represent the nuanced facets and constituencies to help advance knowledge and create a strong scientific presence on topics and methodologies that align best with community priorities.

Timing Is Everything

Timing pressures created by institutions and organizational structures include the tenure clock, promotion timelines, and time-since-degree cut-offs for eligibility for early career awards. Personal timing pressures may also arise, impacting your family life, parenting, care for older parents or relatives, and other such critical windows that can rapidly close if you don't attend to them. Major decision points and demands often happen within a short span of time, and BIPOC academics, particularly women who bear children, can experience a disproportional cumulative load (e.g., Myers et al., 2020). During my pre-tenure years as an assistant professor, I juggled pregnancy and parenting, while contending with serious family illness and death, amongst other hurdles and challenges.

Mindfulness and yoga were activities where I found solace and strength, sometimes when there was no other space for it in a hectic and difficult day. The best benefits came with daily practice of finding intention, gratitude, and acceptance. I developed Reach and Shine, to share what I have found most useful with others, creating guided meditations set to music that could center and offer grounding. Rather than a quick fix, it creates a space where struggle abates, even if only for a moment, and safety arises, creating the necessary conditions to rest one's nervous system and engage in a practice of radical self-love; in addition to peace and calm, Sonya Renee Taylor argues that is when wisdom has the space to come through (Taylor, 2021).

Concluding Thoughts

Diversifying your portfolio is not only a benefit to your own career longevity and satisfaction, but it creates opportunities for impact and reach, disseminating your research to wider audiences and directly benefit communities. As an early career scholar, time is limited and precious. Designing your own individual path will benefit you both in the short- and long-run, and help you to stay true to your values and priorities.

Ultimately, academic institutions need to make structural changes to adequately address diversity, equity, inclusion, and belonging. True transformation will require shifts in practices and priorities when evaluating research, creative works, and the activities in which BIPOC faculty choose to engage (Suarez-Balcazar et al., 2021). Such changes will help to recruit and retain a strong body of BIPOC scholars in the Academy and build a stronger bridge between scientific knowledge and public interest. In order to truly achieve health equity, scholars must pursue a wider range of outlets for broader impact, and these practices must become the norm, rather than the exception. An exciting vision for the future of the Academy imagines scholars as changemakers, offering their strengths and insights to communities in multiple and varied ways, reducing global disparities, guiding public policy, informing public discourse, offering cures and paths to wellness, and making the world a better place.

References

Aslan, R. (2022). How to avoid the "White savior industrial complex." *The Atlantic*, October 20. www.theatlantic.com/books/archive/2022/10/howard-baskerville-persian-constitutional-revolution/671787/

Awad, G. H., Kia-Keating, M., & Amer, M. M. (2019). A model of cumulative racial–ethnic trauma among Americans of Middle Eastern and North African (MENA) descent. *American Psychologist, 74*(1), 76–87. https://doi.org/10.1037/amp0000344

Cole, T. (2012). The white-savior industrial complex. *The Atlantic*, March 21. www.theatlantic.com/international/archive/2012/03/the-white-savior-industrial-complex/254843/

Guillaume, R. O., & Apodaca, E. C. (2022). Early career faculty of color and promotion and tenure: The intersection of advancement in the academy and cultural taxation. *Race Ethnicity and Education, 25*(4), 546–563. https://doi.org/10.1080/13613324.2020.1718084

Henderson, Z., Kia-Keating, M., & Woods-Jaeger, B. (2023). Reimagining traumatic stress as a participatory science grounded in critical self-reflection: A call to action. *Journal of Traumatic Stress, 36*(4), 665–667. https://doi.org/10.1002/jts.22952

Kia-Keating, M., & Juang, L. P. (2022). Participatory science as a decolonizing methodology: Leveraging collective knowledge from partnerships with refugee and immigrant communities. *Cultural Diversity and Ethnic Minority Psychology, 28*(3), 299–305. https://doi.org/10.1037/cdp0000514

Kia-Keating, M., Liu, S., & Sims, G. (2018). Between the devil and the deep blue sea: Refugee youth in resettlement. *Emerging Trends in the Social and Behavioral Sciences.* doi:10.1002/9781118900772.etrds0460.

Kozlowski, D., Larivière, V., Sugimoto, C. R., & Monroe-White, T. (2022). Intersectional inequalities in science. *Proceedings of the National Academy of Sciences, 119*(2), e2113067119. https://doi.org/10.1073/pnas.2113067119

Morgan, A. C., LaBerge, N., Larremore, D. B., Galesic, M., Brand, J. E., & Clauset, A. (2022). Socioeconomic roots of academic faculty. *Nature Human Behaviour.* https://doi.org/10.1038/s41562-022-01425-4

Myers, K. R., Tham, W. Y., Yin, Y. et al. (2020). Unequal effects of the COVID-19 pandemic on scientists. *Nature Human Behaviour, 4,* 880–883. https://doi.org/10.1038/s41562-020-0921-y

Suarez-Balcazar, Y., Kia-Keating, M., & Jackson, T. (2021). Navigating participation and ethics with immigrant communities. *Qualitative Psychology.* doi:10.1037/qup0000216.

Taylor, S. R. (2021). *The body is not an apology: The power of radical self-love* (2nd ed.). Berrett-Koehler Publishers.

Wapman, K. H., Zhang, S., Clauset, A., & Larremore, D. B. (2022). Quantifying hierarchy and dynamics in US faculty hiring and retention. *Nature.* https://doi.org/10.1038/s41586-022-05222-x

Zárate, M. A., Nagayama Hall, G., & Plaut, V. C. (2017). Researchers of color, fame, and impact. *Perspectives on Psychological Science, 12*(6), 1176–1178. https://doi.org/10.1177/1745691617710511

The Politics of Promotion and Tenure

19

Tips for Navigating the Process While Staying True to Your Values

Karen Jackson-Weaver

Over the last 20 years, I have worked in higher education to support faculty in achieving tenure and promotion from the assistant to the associate rank, and from the associate to the full professor rank. As I have observed this landscape in the academy, many tenure decisions have neither been precisely formulaic nor approached with the sense of keen empiricism that I expected. That is not to say there have not been metrics applied to publications, research, service, or teaching. However, tenure processes vary by institution and the criteria for promotion to associate or full professorship is often unclear. In recent years, more colleges and universities have created handbooks or guides about the tenure and promotion process to provide greater transparency. Unfortunately, institutional and systemic racism, coupled with sexism, have been huge barriers to increasing the number of Black, Indigenous, and tenured associate and full professor Faculty of Color and women faculty in particular.

I am extremely grateful to Dr. Linda Lausell Bryant and Dr. Doris F. Chang for their leadership in assembling this volume, and for their vision to create a robust repository of advice and strategies for historically underrepresented faculty. My hope is that my educational and professional experiences coupled with my perspectives I have shared here will be a tool to leverage as each of you chart your career plans and create a path to success.

DOI: 10.4324/9781003309796-22

Welcome to the Ivory Tower: Reflections on My Learning Journey

From the time I was in kindergarten until 6th grade, I played school. Every. Single. Day. And I loved it! To my older brother and sister's misfortune, I would ask them, " Please play school with me." Every. Single. Day. Their response was mostly "no" or "I'm busy," but they always encouraged me to "have fun and be imaginative," advice I relished and still apply each time I enter the classroom or any learning environment.

Once I started 7th grade, I became very involved in a myriad of after-school activities so while I was not able to "play school" in the same way, I was still very interested in what it meant to be a first-rate teacher and learner. I graduated with a 4.0 GPA from high school and gained early admission to Princeton University. No one was surprised when I decided to major in history and earn a certification in Teacher Education. I called my mother almost every day and told her and my grandmother about my lectures with some of the most brilliant intellectuals in the world, including Dr. Cornel West, Dr. Nell Painter, and the late Nobel Laureate Toni Morrison.

I was also fortunate enough to work with Dr. Ruth Simmons. She was a Vice Provost at Princeton while I was an undergraduate and her influence has been an inspiration to me. Her appointments as President of *three* colleges and universities – Smith College, Brown University (where she was the first African American President in the Ivy League), and Prairie View A & M University, where she recently retired – are legendary. Ruth's humility, administrative prowess, and commitment to excellence deeply resonated with me and are traits I have tried to embody throughout my professional career.

As an undergraduate on Princeton's campus, I always tried to remember that my mother, my grandmother, and all of my ancestors were with me whenever I entered a room. I was physically there, but I also believed they were with me in spirit. Being a first-generation college student, as well as an African-American young woman from the American South, being away from home was a *huge* adjustment. However, the sense of community that I embraced and strived to create became a cornerstone of my personal identity and how I went about my administrative work – intentionally working to create community and belonging wherever I went.

After graduating from Princeton University, I immediately pursued a Master's degree at Harvard University Graduate School of Education. My experience at Harvard was dynamic and transformative. It not only created the foundation for my professional career, but it affirmed my commitment to teaching, research, and public service. I learned from towering legal giants such as Judge A. Leon Higginbotham and Professor Charles Ogletree, and other renowned intellectuals such as Dr. Sara Lawrence-Lightfoot as well as Dr. Chester Pierce (who originally coined the term microaggressions).

These undergraduate and graduate professors modeled transformative teaching and research excellence, and provided me with the theory and scholarly praxis I needed, while exposing me to the work of other practitioners and experts such as Lisa Delpit, Paulo Freire, bell hooks, and many others who shaped my consciousness, practices, and ideological approach. After graduating from Harvard, I worked to save money and gain more experience before pursuing my PhD at Columbia University. While pursuing my doctoral studies in American History, I worked in the Dean's office under Sharon Gamble during Dean Eduardo Macagno's tenure.

One of the highlights during my doctoral studies was having three African-American women professors: Dr. Farah Jasmine Griffin, Professor Kimberlé Williams Crenshaw, and Dr. Edwina Wright, who passed away in 2007. I was a teaching assistant for Dr. Gina Dent as well as a member of an innovative graduate seminar led by Dr. Judith Weisenfeld. To top it off, I was also counseled and advised by Union Theological Seminary faculty like Dr. Emilie Townes. All of them are tenured faculty and leaders in their field. Furthermore, they are all African-American women, a group that is severely underrepresented in the professoriate. Their brilliance and wisdom were priceless to me. The lessons I learned from them about the academy, some verbal and explicit, while some lessons were non-verbal, are very much why I believe I have been successful and have been a conduit in making sure others were also poised for success in the academy.

My dissertation committee included the renowned historians Dr. Eric Foner, Dr. Manning Marable, and Dr. Robin D. G. Kelly. Another highlight was being nominated for the Columbia University Graduate Student Teaching Award. Upon reflection, the faculty and administrators I worked with and their teaching and mentoring excellence had much more of an influence on me than I realized at the time. I am grateful for each of them in ways that I still have not been able to fully articulate.

Even after two decades of being in higher education, whenever I enter the classroom, I harken back to the timely advice from my siblings: "Have fun and be imaginative." My childhood and my educational experiences and mentors shaped my understanding of the academic landscape and prepared me to be a leader and advocate for faculty success and advancement.

As you reflect on your own learning journey as an early or mid-career academic, consider:

- What experiences and resources from your background (e.g., people, educational experiences, etc.) can you leverage to prepare for the rigors of the academy and the tenure/promotion process?
- What skills and approaches have you learned from your undergraduate and graduate experiences that will serve you in the tenure and promotion process, and your ability to thrive and flourish in higher education more generally?
- What tools are in your "tenure" toolkit? As you evaluate your current status, what no longer serves your needs, and can be released? What do you need at this stage of your career and who can assist you in securing what you need for the next stage of your professional journey?

Go Where You Can Grow: Understanding the Politics of the Professoriate

Before finishing and defending my dissertation at Columbia University, I interviewed for and was selected for an executive role in the New Jersey state government. Rather than immediately pursuing a position in the professoriate, I decided to take a detour into the political arena. This was one of the best decisions I ever made.

After working under three gubernatorial administrations as the inaugural Executive Director of the New Jersey Amistad Commission under the Commissioner of Education, Secretary of State, and Governor, I was ready to transition to a leadership role in academia. Trust me when I say that the politics of state government prepared me well for the politics of the academy. Dr. Bill Russel, the Dean of Princeton University's Graduate School at that time, hired me and convinced me that if I could be successful in the political arena, my transferable skills would be an asset to me in academia. He was right!

I was hired as an Associate Dean at Princeton University's Graduate School during Dr. Shirley Tilghman's presidency. Working under her leadership was inspiring and refreshing. In addition to my administrative role, I conducted research and taught in American Studies, African-American Studies, and the Gender and Sexuality Studies programs. I represented the graduate school on university-wide committees, task forces, and working groups to solve a variety of complex problems. In my capacity as an

Academic Dean, I worked closely with the President, the Provost, and all 44 departments and programs as well as with directors of graduate studies and graduate program administrators.

After my tenure at Princeton, I served as the Dean of Students and Senior Associate Dean at Harvard University's Kennedy School of Government from 2014–2017. David Ellwood hired me and was the longest serving, most senior Dean at Harvard on the Presidential cabinet. He along with my direct supervisor, John Haigh, were very supportive of my leadership. While at Harvard, I led over 60 staff members (with seven direct reports) and was responsible for a student population that represented over 165 countries. I oversaw the school's master's, joint, concurrent, and PhD programs. I also managed staff members in admissions, student financial services/financial aid, the registrar's office, student services, career advancement, and student diversity and inclusion. I chaired both the school-wide Academic Affairs Committee and the Diversity Committee, and was an executive member of the Faculty Steering Committee which includes all of the faculty chairs and determines tenure and promotion for all faculty.

During my tenure at Harvard Kennedy School and my subsequent post at Oxford University's Blavatnik School of Government, I was able to amplify my commitment to global social justice and teach primarily graduate students, senior executives, and global leaders. At Oxford, I worked with an amazing team and launched the Executive Public Leaders Program. Dr. Ngaire Woods, the Dean at the Blavatnik School of Government, one of the most brilliant leaders in global higher education, was extremely supportive of my work, and my transition to my current role as Senior Associate Vice President of Global Faculty Engagement and Innovation Advancement at New York University (NYU). As I reflect on my time at NYU, my greatest pride has been when faculty share with me how my efforts have personally impacted them and their genuine sense of my deep commitment for them to flourish and thrive.

Before accepting any position, whether inside or outside of the academy, ask yourself the following:

- Can I grow here and is there an opportunity for others to grow as well?
- Who are the individuals who will support me? Are there resources available to support others?
- Are there people here who will support Black, Indigenous, and Faculty of Color and women faculty? What is their track record and how have they demonstrated their commitment to faculty advancement and faculty success? If they have not done well as an institution, are they willing to invest the necessary resources to make a change?

These questions have been useful for me and I have shared them with faculty colleagues as they navigate the tenure landscape. Tenure is not just about being promoted, but it is also about creating an ecosystem where you can learn and grow, professionally and personally. It is about having transparency and clarity about the process, as well as understanding who holds the decision-making power. It is important to ask questions and thoroughly research the institution you are interested in to ensure you will have the professional and personal networks of support that will allow you to be successful in your journey toward promotion and advancement.

Commentary on the Scholarly Literature Regarding the Tenure and Promotion Process

In the mid-2000s, few scholars were conducting research that addressed the unique challenges that Black, Indigenous, and Faculty of Color or women faculty faced during the tenure and promotion process. As a Dean at Princeton, I worked with my colleagues on a piece titled "Recruiting the next generation of the professoriate" (Jackson-Weaver et al., 2010) and the question we raised at the end of that piece is as timely now as it was then: Is the higher education community willing to embrace these challenges seriously and labor intensively to resolve them?

In the article, we also highlighted findings from the American Association of Colleges and Universities (AAC&U) symposium where they examined the issue of bias in the academic workplace. During the interactive clicker survey, 45% of the participants ranked race and ethnicity bias as the most important issue for improving the recruitment and retention of Faculty of Color. As an example of racial bias, the symposium report noted that "white males are seen as having instant credibility and meriting attention. As a result, they accrue privilege, solely by virtue of their race and gender" (Viernes Turner, 1998).

In my essay, "Diversity and the future of the professoriate – a call to action" (Jackson-Weaver, 2011), I cited the overrepresentation of white males in the professoriate and the ongoing underrepresentation of Black, Indigenous, and Faculty of Color. Specifically, I highlighted a 2002 study completed by Cathy Trower and Richard Chait at Harvard University which revealed that 94% of full professors in science and engineering were white. Of these, 90% were men. More than 90% of full professors at research universities were white, and more than three-fourths were male (Trower & Chait, 2002).

Although some progress has been made since I published that article, the overall representation of Black, Hispanic/Latino, and Indigenous faculty has changed very little. According to the National Center for Education Statistics, in the fall of 2021, Black faculty comprised less than 5% of tenure and non-tenure track faculty, despite being roughly 13% of the US population (US Census, 2020). Similarly, Hispanic faculty also comprised less than 5% of tenure and non-tenure track faculty s, although Hispanic/Latinos represent approximately 19% of the US population (US Census, 2020). American Indian/ Alaska Native faculty represented less than 1% of tenure and non-tenure track faculty (National Center for Education Statistics, Digest of Education Statistics, 2022). If this rate remains constant, it will take *over 100 years* for the Black faculty percentages to reach parity with the percentage of Black people in the US population, and even longer for Latino faculty (Journal of Blacks in Higher Education, 2009).

Given these statistics, institutions must acknowledge how diversity (or the lack of diversity) impacts scholarly research, pedagogical approaches, departmental climate, institutional priorities, and overall faculty (and student) representation on campus. Much of the literature on Black, Indigenous, and Faculty of Color and women faculty addresses issues related to BIPOC faculty and their experiences with the tenure system, departmental (and school) climate, and institutional barriers to advancement, as well as lack of transparency and support throughout the tenure process (Arnold et al., 2016; DeSante, 2013; Edwards, 2018; Flaherty, 2016; Griffin et al., 2011; Guillaume & Apodaca, 2022; Kelly et al., 2017; Ross & Edwards, 2016; Stanley, 2006; Trower, 2009). Other scholars emphasize the importance of holistic recruitment, retention, and advancement practices, programming, and support systems to combat institutional and systemic racism (and sexism) (e.g., Fries-Britt et al., 2011; Gasman et al., 2011; Harvey Wingfield, 2016; Jackson-Weaver, 2011; Jackson-Weaver et al., 2010; Kelsky, 2017; Rockquemore & Laszloffy, 2008; Turner et al., 2008). In addition, researchers have examined recent shifts in institutional responses to the unique challenges that historically underrepresented faculty encounter, including paying greater attention to experiences of women Faculty of Color and the intersectional challenges they face in the academy (e.g., Domingo, 2022; Ferguson et al., 2021; García Peña, 2022; Perez, 2019; Stripling, 2019; Tugend, 2018; Weinberg, 2008). I am especially grateful to Caroline Viernes Turner for her significant contributions to this field, and the critical research she and her colleagues have conducted in order for institutions to better understand how to groom all faculty for success (e.g., Turner, 1998, 2000, 2002; Turner et al., 2008).

The references at the end of this essay are not meant to be an exhaustive list, but rather a starting point for learning more about the scholarly literature in this area. In addition, they provide a unique opportunity to better understand and proactively address ways to promote women faculty and Black, Indigenous, and Faculty of Color in the tenure, advancement, and promotion process.

Recommendations for the Reader: Seven Keys to Success

As you create a personal success plan for your own journey through the tenure and promotion process, I encourage you to set goals that will position you for success at your institution and beyond. Be strategic about publishing, presenting at conferences, and cultivating relationships in your field. Publish in well-known and well-respected peer-reviewed journals and university presses in your field. Present your papers at conferences that are well attended by leaders in your field. Realize that many will listen to your presentation and possibly consider it an informal job talk. So, prepare your conference papers and any lectures that you present as if they are pseudo job talks. Volunteer to work on committees and task forces within your professional organizations so you are able to establish relationships with colleagues at your home institution as well as peer institutions.

In the midst of all of your rigorous preparation for tenure and promotion, *always prioritize your mental health and well-being*. Furthermore, be clear about your personal values and never compromise on them. Tenure is important, but your values provide a foundation for your identity within the academy and beyond. My hope is that your personal values will be your guide in this process. Take time to examine what is important to you at the various stages of your career and be intentional about identifying a work environment that fulfills your personal and professional needs and values.

As I close, I would like to leave you with seven tips for success in the academy.

1.   Know your value

The meaning of the word *value* is synonymous with the "importance, worth, or usefulness of something" (Oxford English Dictionary). Know *your* worth! During your job search process, work to identify a place where they value you and your research. Look for evidence that you will grow personally and professionally there. Throughout my career, I have been intentional about going to institutions where I felt I could be successful. As I reflect on my personal values of integrity, excellence, respect for myself and others, and knowing my value as a leader, I am relieved that these principles guided me in where I should go, and when it was time to transition.

2. Do an informal assessment of who has tenure at your university

Form a bond with 5 –7 key people at your home institution (within your field and / or closely related fields) who are tenured to gain a greater understanding of how they obtained tenure, and what lessons you can learn from their experiences.

3. Understand the politics of presence

For an institution to invest in you, you must be present. This includes not just showing up for class and office hours, but also attending faculty meetings, and departmental events and gatherings. Overall, the guiding principle to keep in mind is: are you being perceived as a "good citizen" of the department and "are you present?"

4. Have clarity on the decision-making landscape for tenure at your institution

Be intentional about creating an ecosystem of support within and beyond your institution. You should have relationships both within your field of specialty and with decision makers and administrative leaders at your home institution. You will need to have an array of supporters from your department and across your institution, as well as your field or discipline of study (so you will easily secure reviewer letters for your tenure file).

5. Set clear research, publication, and conference presentation goals

Your body of work speaks for you and helps you and others make the case for your tenure and your research contributions to the academy. Take time to be clear and intentional about your publication and presentation goals.

6. Understand the importance of relationships, and how to leverage those relationships when you encounter challenges

Merit has been framed as a central tenet of tenure. However, many of us have witnessed how merit is actually just one part of the tenure process.

In a number of instances, the person under review has established relationships with key decision makers who become important advocates for their case. Understanding how to cultivate these connections while also navigating bias and institutional racism or sexism in the academy is not easy. Because merit alone will not win you tenure, be sure you are purposeful in creating the relationships you need to advance.

7. Create a plan for your success

Make daily, weekly, monthly, and semester plans. The National Center for Faculty Development and Diversity (NCFDD) has a wealth of online resources, workshops, and materials to aid you in creating a plan that positions you for success in achieving tenure and promotion. Prioritize strategic planning at every step of your professional journey and be intentional about carving out the time you need to do the work. Be very clear and specific about what success looks like for you and do so without comparing yourself to others.

I wish you *much* success and invite you to frequently revisit these tips for navigating the tenure process while staying true to your values. Onward!

References

Arnold, N. W., Crawford, E. R., & Khalifa, M. (2016). Psychological heuristics and faculty of color: Racial battle fatigue and tenure/promotion. *The Journal of Higher Education, 87*(6), 890–919. https://doi.org/10.1080/00221546.2016.11780891

DeSante, C. D. (2013). Working twice as hard to get half as far: Race, work ethic, and America's deserving poor. *American Journal of Political Science, 57*(2), 342–356.

Domingo, C. R., Gerber, N. C., Harris, D., Mamo, L., Pasion, S. G., Rebanal, R. D., & Rosser, S. V. (2022). More service or more advancement: Institutional barriers to academic success for women and women of color faculty at a large public comprehensive minority-serving state university. *Journal of Diversity in Higher Education, 15*(3), 365–379. https://doi.org/10.1037/dhe0000292

Editors, *The Journal of Blacks in Higher Education.* (2009). The snail-like progress of blacks in faculty ranks of higher education. www.jbhe.com/news_views/62_black faculty.html

Edwards, W. J., and Ross, H. H. (2018). What are they saying? Black faculty at predominantly white institutions of higher education. *Journal of Human Behavior in the Social Environment, 28*(2), 142–161.

Ferguson, T. L., Berry, R. R., & Collins, J. D. (2021). Where is our space within this ivory tower? The teaching experiences of Black women faculty in education programs. *Journal of Research on Leadership Education, 16*(2), 140–157. https://doi.org/10.1177/19427751211002229

Flaherty, C. (2016). Study finds gains in faculty diversity, but not on the tenure track. *Inside Higher Ed*, August 22.

Fries-Britt, S. L., Rowan-Kenyon, H. T., Perna, L. W., Milem, J. F., & Howard, D. G. (2011). Underrepresentation in the academy and the institutional climate for faculty diversity. *Journal of the Professoriate*, *5*(1), 1–34. https://dx.doi.org/10.1037/dhe0000149

García Peña, L. (2022). *Community as rebellion: Women of color, academia, and the fight for ethnic studies*. Haymarket Books.

Gasman, M., Kim, J., & Nguyen, T. (2011). Effectively recruiting faculty of color at highly selective institutions: A school of education case study. *Journal of Diversity in Higher Education*, *4*(4), 212–222. https://doi.org/10.1037/a0025130

Griffin, K. A., Pifer, M. J., Humphrey, J. R., & Hazelwood, A. M. (2011). (Re)defining departure: Exploring Black professors' experiences with and responses to racism and racial climate. *American Journal of Education*, *117*(4), 495–526. https://doi.org/10.1086/660756

Guillaume, R. O., & Apodaca, E. C. (2022). Early career faculty of color and promotion and tenure: The intersection of advancement in the academy and cultural taxation. *Race Ethnicity and Education*, *25* (4), 546–563. doi:10.1080/13613324.2020.1718084.

Harvey Wingfield, A. (2016). More faculty of color can and should be in the top ranks of universities (essay). *Inside Higher Ed*, September 9. www.insidehighered.com/advice/2016/09/09/more-faculty-color-can-and-should-be-top-ranks-universities-essay

Jackson-Weaver, K. (2011). Diversity and the future of the professoriate: A call to action. *Diverse Issues in Higher Education*, *27*(24), 27.

Jackson-Weaver, K., Baker, E. B., Gillespie, M. C., Ramos Bellido, C. G., & Watts, A. W. (2010). Recruiting the next generation of the professoriate. *Peer Review: Emerging Trends and Key Debates in Undergraduate Education*, *12*(3), 11–15.

Kelly, B. T., Gaston Gayles, J., & Williams, C. D. (2017). Recruitment without retention: A critical case of Black faculty unrest. *Journal of Negro Education*, *86*(3), 305–317. https://doi.org/10.7709/jnegroeducation.86.3.0305

Kelsky, K. (2017). The professor is in: 4 steps to a strong tenure file. *The Chronicle of Higher Education*, October 15.

Perez, P. A. (Ed.). (2019). *The tenure-track process for Chicana and Latina faculty: Experiences of resisting and persisting in the academy* (1st ed.). Routledge.

Rockquemore, K., & Laszloffy, T. A. (2008). *The Black academic's guide to winning tenure – without losing your soul*. Lynne Rienner Publishers.

Ross, H. H., & Edwards, W. J. (2016). African American faculty expressing concerns: Breaking the silence at predominantly white research oriented universities. *Race Ethnicity and Education*, *19* (3), 461–479. doi:10.1080/13613324.2014.969227.

Stanley, C. A. (2006). Coloring the academic landscape: Faculty of color breaking the silence in predominantly white colleges and universities. *American Educational Research Journal*, *43*(4), 701–736. https://doi.org/10.3102/00028312043004701

Stripling, J. (2019). She's a 'star' Latina professor. But not good enough for tenure at Harvard. *The Chronicle of Higher Education*, December 3.

Trower, C. A., & Chait, R. P. (2002). Faculty diversity: Too little for too long. *Harvard Magazine*, *104*(4), 33–38.

Trower, C. A. (2009). Toward a greater understanding of the tenure track for minorities. *Change: The Magazine of Higher Learning*, *41*(5), 38–45.

Tugend, A. (2018). How serious are you about diversity hiring? *The Chronicle of Higher Education*, June 17.

Turner, C. S. V. (2000). New faces, new knowledge: As women and minorities join the faculty, they bring intellectual diversity in pedagogy and in scholarship. *Academe*, 86(5), 34–37.

Turner, C. S. V. (2002). Women of color in the academe: Living with multiple marginality. *Journal of Higher Education*, 73, 74–93. https://doi.org/10.1080/00221546.2002.11777131

Turner, C. S. V., González, J. C., & Wood, J. L. (2008). Faculty of color in academe: What 20 years of literature tells us. *Journal of Diversity in Higher Education*, 1(3), 139–168. https://doi.org/10.1037/a0012837

US Census Bureau. (2020). Population estimates, July 1, 2022. www.census.gov/quick facts/fact/table/US/PST045222

Viernes Turner, C.S. (1998). Keeping our faculties: Addressing the recruitment and retention of faculty of color in higher education. Executive Summary. www.diversityweb.org/diversity_innovations/faculty_staff_development/recruitment_tenure_promotion/keeping_our_faculties.cfm

Weinberg, S. L. (2008). Monitoring faculty diversity: The need for a more granular approach. *The Journal of Higher Education*, 79(4), 365–387.

Getting Your Message Out

20

A Community Conversation

*Robyn L. Gobin[1], Ramani Durvasula, Maryam
Kia-Keating, Terrance Coffie, Doris F. Chang
and Linda Lausell Bryant*

In this conversation, Doris F. Chang and Linda Lausell Bryant speak with Robyn L. Gobin, Ramani Durvasula, Maryam Kia-Keating, and Terrance Coffie, thought leaders and faculty members in psychology and social work who are leveraging the power of the media – in all of its forms – to decolonize psychological science, make mental health education more accessible, and advocate for policies to benefit BIPOC communities. This conversation has been edited and condensed.

Participants

Robyn L. Gobin, PhD, is a licensed clinical psychologist, Associate Professor at University of Illinois, Urbana-Champaign, meditation teacher, DEI trainer, and author of *The Self-Care Prescription* among other books.

Ramani Durvasula, PhD, is a licensed clinical psychologist, Professor Emerita of Psychology at California State University, Los Angeles, podcast host, author of numerous books on narcissism and its impact on relationships, and content creator of the popular YouTube channel, "Doctor Ramani."

---

1 The first four authors are listed in random order, reflecting their equal contributions to this chapter.

DOI: 10.4324/9781003309796-23

Maryam Kia-Keating, PhD, is a licensed clinical psychologist, Professor of Psychology at University of California, Santa Barbara, children's media consultant, and mindfulness and meditation teacher. She is also co-creator of HEROES, a family resilience program, and the founder of Reach and Shine.

Terrance Coffie, MSW, is a social worker, and adjunct faculty at New York University Silver School of Social Work, founder and CEO of The Social Justice Network, podcast host, and activist for criminal justice reform.

Getting Your Message Out: "It's Our Responsibility with What We've Been Given to Get Out There and Raise Our Voice"

Doris: We would like to begin by inviting you to share a story about a moment when you realized, or in some cases decided, that you had something to say – a message that was so important that you had to share it with others. For many of us, that sense of seeing ourselves as worthy of having a platform has not always been present. So we are curious about that moment when you began to see yourself as someone whose experiences, expertise, and point of view *matter*, given that there is so much that keeps us from seeing ourselves in that way.

Linda: In thinking about this prompt, I realize that this is still a question for me. Is there any interest in what I feel like I have to say, outside of my prescribed roles? About a month ago, a former student of mine asked to get together. He wanted to let me know how he was doing, and to share how influential he felt I had been in his life. He suggested that I should write a book and I reminded him that I had done so. He said "No, I mean, a book about you, like your stories. I kept thinking about stories you shared with me when we would meet." And I said, "Well, everybody has stories, there's no need to write a book about that. Everybody's got a story." And he insisted that he would read that book and so would many of my former students. He then said, "I wish it existed." And here I am sitting with all of you and I can't wait to hear about your stories, so I think I'm beginning to realize that yes, there may be a place for my story, not necessarily centered only on my work. I've got a lot of work to do to overcome a lot of imposter syndrome.

Terrance: I'm gonna jump in because I love the prompt that you set for this space, and I don't have to feel all nervous. And even as I sit here with all you doctors, the story that resonates with me was when I was in grad school. I'd had the great fortune of doing my undergrad and graduate studies at New York University. But for those two years, I felt inferior to my classmates, because I come from a very different background, you know what I'm saying? My career actually started in a correctional institution, and me getting a GED, and going to a community college first. And to me, to have an opportunity to attend NYU . . . (pause). So during that time, part of the problem for me is that . . . I wanted to sound like you. There was a gentleman who is now our Dean (Dr. Michael Lindsay) who said to me, "Terrance, don't lose your voice." Because I could talk to him in a way that I hadn't been able to with certain people. There was this apprehension that when I come into certain (academic) spaces like this, there is a questioning of my intellect, a questioning of the depth of what I know. So that was the moment I really began to embrace that part of me, to be able to communicate the issues in a way that these communities could grasp. But I don't think there's just one moment for me. It is a culmination of things that empower our voices on each step of the journey.

Maryam: I agree with Terrance that it's not just one moment. It's a culmination of your life experiences on the personal level, and then professional experiences. When I was young, my family had to escape war, and we ended up going around the world, trying to find a new home. And what it gave to me . . . besides all the challenges, was an opportunity to see the world. I learned from an early age that there was so much wisdom, knowledge and capacity, and innovation and inspiration everywhere, from every kind of community, from every kind of background, from every kind of educational level. The best term I can connect this to is cultural humility.

So the story that stood out for me was starting graduate school and meeting a classmate. I had just started taekwondo classes, I was right at the beginning. She was a student from China, and it turned out she had a black belt, and I was like, "Oh, my goodness, to be you someday." We talked about how there were martial arts classes at the university gym. She had gone to the first class and met the Sensei, and she wore a white belt. And I was like, "What? Why would you wear a white belt?" And she said, "Oh, I would never approach the Sensei that way." It's that sense of humility, you need to start with that connection and relationship. And I just treasured learning that approach. It connected so much to many of my cross-cultural experiences that are quite different from an American approach, which might be about not only wearing the black belt, but doing some moves and showing your skill and being the expert. And I was like, oh, right this is a reminder, there is beauty and strength in starting off with humility.

Ramani: I'm the opposite of Maryam, the moment for me didn't come from a place of humility at all. I had the TV on in the background, and somebody was giving commentary on some mental health issue in the news, and it was a white woman, giving a simplistic and inaccurate analysis of the situation. I live in Los Angeles, and a mother at the school where my children attended worked in the agent management business. I asked her, how do people end up on TV talking about this stuff? This was 2009, before YouTube was as potent a tool for sharing mental health content. You needed an agent to book these gigs. She helped find out who that woman's agent was and I reached out to him. He said, "Send me your info and send me a headshot." I didn't have a headshot. So I sent him a picture someone took of me at a sushi restaurant, along with my CV. And he said, "I like your 'look.' Can you come to New York?" That started an interesting journey into the media, being a commentator on every major news network, being on multiple documentaries, on scripted television. And it really became a class in how colonized this space was. This space was really only telling one story. And sadly, I was participating in the telling of that one story, but there was no way to decolonize that space. If you wouldn't tell that one story, then they were only going to use experts that would.

Then one day in 2017, I said, I can't. I labored for eight years trying to break into that space. I thought – now I'm in Maryam's part of the story – I'm gonna be humble. I'm gonna give back in a different way. Then a young man reaches out to me, "Ma'am, I have a YouTube channel. And I know you talk a lot about narcissism. I'd love to talk to you." He's a kid, like 24 years old, I thought, here's one chance to give back. I sat down and had a really interesting conversation with him. Six weeks later the video went viral. In a very short period of time, it got one and a half million hits. And then around 2018, 2019, two students at Cal State LA reached out and said, "We have read your books, and we love how you teach. It feels you could make a bigger impact on YouTube." I said, That's ridiculous. And they said, Well, give us a chance. They rolled up to my office with an iPhone. And today, we have 1.3 million subscribers, we get 6–8 million hits a month.[2]

In the new media, there's no gatekeeper, no journal editor, no peer reviewer, no producer, no network who's saying nobody wants to hear your story. I told my story. And that story resonated. And I have a podcast now, and the reach has become quite incredible. With people reaching out to us from all over the world saying, "Thank you for giving voice to our story. We're finding ours again." This was a 14-year process of trying to break through a closed media system, spending years writing journal articles that seven people would read. I think every single person who works in psychology and mental health has an extraordinarily important voice, and we have to get the faces of People of Color, queer people, neurodivergent people, different genders . . . we all have to get out there and talk because the space now exists for us to democratize the storytelling. We have to take individual responsibility and go and do that.

Robyn: Everything everyone shared has been so rich, thank you. I've been sitting here thinking what story do I share? I was raised in the South and raised in a Christian household. And it was very much about humility, you know, being seen and not heard, doing well academically, but not necessarily speaking up and using your voice. And so when I got to graduate school, that was something that I took with me. I was the only Black woman in my department (at the University of Oregon). So I thought, I'm going to do well, I'm not going to mess up, I'm not going to speak out unless I have clearly articulated what I want to say. Because a lot of people in Oregon had not engaged with

---

2 Dr. Durvasula's popular YouTube channel, @DoctorRamani, focuses on healing from narcissistic relationships. As of this writing, the channel has 1.49 million subscribers and almost 200 million views.

a Black woman before and I felt this pressure to represent. But I remember that even in trying to show up academically while not speaking, that people always wanted to hear what I had to say. So that was an inkling that okay, maybe I have something to share that can enrich the conversation.

My second year in grad school, I published my first article. I sent it to my family, I was so excited and so happy. I remember so vividly, my uncle texted back saying, "I couldn't get past the first sentence. I could not get past the first sentence. But I'm sure it's amazing. Congratulations." I thought, okay, this cannot be all that I'm doing right? Even though the academy is saying that this is a measure of success, I'm not impacting the people who mean the most to me, which were my family, and the community that I care about. That is when I resolved to share this information broadly, to make sure that the knowledge that I have doesn't just rest in academia where it's not going to reach the people who really need it, and the people who matter most to me.

Doris: One thing that many of you shared, which I really resonate with, is the importance of someone reflecting back to you, "What you have to say is important." The little nudges that each of you got, and the permission that they gave you to take up more space is something that I've experienced as well. Growing up in a Chinese American immigrant household, I was never asked my opinion about anything. My parents decided on stuff, and every now and then they would ask me something. But they never really wanted to know my opinions about anything of substance. So I didn't even realize the extent to which I had assumed that I didn't have anything important to say.

In academia, when you give a talk, you can hide behind your data, your findings. An important turning point for me came when I was invited to give a keynote and decided, screw it, I'm going to weave into this talk a lot of personal details about who I am, my family and my life. At the same time, I realized that I was really scared to do it. That showed me how much of myself I had been hiding in order to fit in. So when I gave that talk, I felt like I was giving myself permission to just be me. I could feel myself relaxing, no longer just performing the role of what I thought a competent academic sounds like. And I saw that what I was saying resonated more with them, they were actually more engaged. And I thought, wow, they actually want to see more of this, more of me. I felt like I shifted into another gear. But it took a long time to get there – this was only about five years ago and shows how long it can take for that moment to happen.

Maryam: We've had to follow a very narrow path in order to succeed in order to obtain our degrees. We're being told by this outside source, what's acceptable and what is of value. So you have to go back to your why and your purpose. So I really appreciate this question, does our whole entire field need transformation, as Ramani suggests? We're not always having the impact that we're saying that we want to have, not making use of the alternative platforms that are increasingly available to us, because the academic gatekeepers are saying, "No, no, don't do that."

Ramani: Who gets to be seen? Those who go through the hierarchy and jump through the hoops that have been laid out. Once you've jumped through enough hoops, then you've "earned" your voice. That kind of transactionality around the earning of voice, not only in an academic system, but in the world at large means that we are having to create a different form of training. Like we were taught, you're a therapist, nobody needs to know about you. Our professors, our supervisors didn't ask us who we were. So if there wasn't even an interest in our stories in the graduate training world, where there was such little representation that looked like us – where would we have ever gotten the idea that our stories were valid? That is the kind of phase shift that the field needs.

Doris: **It sounds like each of you are saying that where we come from and the unique experiences that we've had make us particularly qualified to speak on certain matters of importance to our communities. How do your identities and personal histories inform your work, and your message?**

Terrance: I picked up a mantra that I live by from one of my great mentors, Glenn Martin. He shared that those closest to the problem are also those closest to the solution. And for me, and the work that I do in criminal justice reform as it relates to poverty, intersectionality, and of all these systems . . . it was my life. But when I came into these spaces, I didn't want that life. I wanted to escape it, I didn't know how to embrace it. Even when I was publishing my articles, in USA Today, in Forbes magazine, there was this part of me that was fearful that what I had to say wouldn't matter. That the experiences that I was bringing up, the millions of communities that I represented, the 2.2 million black folks behind them bars, that I represent those struggles, that we would not be heard, because historically that has been the case. But I began to embrace my own lived experience, I began not to be ashamed of it, I began to accept who I was, and who I would be in those spaces. And I know that my life is a representation of a lot of the issues that so many of the men and women that are represented in this space encounter, and are challenged with. So I embrace that and articulate that message to be able to effectuate change.

Linda: **So powerful, Terrance. I feel it in my throat. I feel it welling up and a question for all of us is, how do you go from seeking and working for that external validation to recognizing your intrinsic value? For you Terrance, you started to really focus on the community, rather than on yourself and who was evaluating you in a certain way. You started focusing on your usefulness, and your connection to your community. For the rest of you, what helped you make that shift, from needing external validation to beginning to recognizing your intrinsic value?**

Maryam: To a certain extent, for me, it's been more of a journey of trying to keep going back to the center, back to where you started, and maintain that tie to all this deep ancestral wisdom. But because it's not something we're learning about in school, unless you're lucky enough to be in a family that's like, let's talk about the ancestors . . . you might have to go through your own process of recognizing those ties to the wisdom that came before you, in your own family, in your community, in your culture, and we all come from the same place ultimately, right? For me, it's continuing to return to that. And be centered and grounded with that knowledge to take forward so that the intrinsic becomes what drives me, and that I'm returning to my values and why I'm here in the first place.

Doris: **Thank you, Maryam. Speaking of values, Robyn, I want to bring you in here because we met when you were just an assistant professor and yet you had already published a book about self-care for the general public.[3] I was so impressed that**

---

3 Dr. Gobin wrote the popular and highly rated book, *The Self Care Prescription: Powerful Solutions to Manage Stress, Reduce Anxiety & Increase Wellbeing*, in 2019.

you did that, and also worried for you a little. **Can you share how you decided it was important to you to write this book, even if it took time away from writing those peer-reviewed articles that are so important on one's path to tenure?**

Robyn: It really just came down to, there has to be more than just writing these articles for the academy. Around that time, Jessica Henderson Daniel was the first African American president of the American Psychological Association, and her theme was around "Giving Psychology Away." And so she created this notion of being a "Citizen Psychologist." And it just resonated so much. This is what I want to be about, leveraging the knowledge that I have to improve the communities that I care about. So when the opportunity came up [to write the book], I knew that when I submitted my annual report, this would not be something that [the administration] would be excited about. But it would allow me to get my voice out there, and leverage the knowledge that I have to impact communities who might not ever sit in my therapy chair across from me, who might not ever have the opportunity to sit in a classroom where I teach. So many other people in academia would have told me to wait, you can do it after you get tenure. But I thought, what if I don't live that long? Who will be served by the book versus who am I serving by writing more articles and lecturing more in these classrooms? I have this message in me right now. And connected to what Maryam was saying about values – this was really me saying, it's worth it. This is what truly matters to me.

Linda: It's really bold, right? Because we've all been drinking colonial Kool-aid for years. So it's really bold to go "wait a minute, something's off about this Kool-aid that everyone has said is so awesome."

Robyn: It definitely was not easy. There were a lot of nights of crying and wondering, and definitely after I submitted my paperwork for tenure. I was not confident, because I had done these other things instead of writing more grants and more papers, but I didn't. So it wasn't easy, but I don't regret it.

Linda: **In challenging the status quo, there is often blowback. How did each of you navigate that blowback and pressure as you tried instead to focus on your intrinsic value and what mattered most to you?**

Terrance: The biggest blowback that I get is usually from people, even those on the liberal side, who want to water down the conversation, to make it digestible for the legislators or other policymakers. Even recently, I was part of a conversation about gun violence with key policymakers. So I'm in this room, and we're talking about how we're going to address the spike in gun violence in Black communities. But the different programs and policies that they're setting forth, I see them as temporary, a reactionary response to quell the issue, but not an investment in the ongoing issues that impact those communities. There is this idea that we're supposed to go along with the status quo in these conversations. I've been privileged to be in a place, I hate to say, to be the voice of the voiceless, because I know that they have voices, I just know they're being ignored. And I don't confuse that. They're not voiceless, they're just being ignored. So for me, it is critical that the true issues are represented in the conversations that we are having on behalf of these communities. If that's not happening, then I think we're doing a disservice to the very communities we're talking about trying to empower and uplift. So that's why I'm doing it.

Ramani: I mean, I've had nothing but blowback. Getting old is the best thing ever. Because at 57, there's fewer miles left than miles that I've done. But the thought is not so much, what if I die tomorrow, the visual for me is about my ancestors. I came from a family where my mother had to give up her education for an arranged marriage and move 9,000 miles away to a place where there was no support in a difficult marriage. My great-grandmother had to shear her hair off when her husband died, because she was no longer allowed to be seen because she was a widow. Even though she was very young, she spent the rest of her life with a shorn head, wearing homespun cloth, and did not eat on days when the sun didn't come out. Those are my ancestors, so you better believe I am going to use the voice because too many women suffered. Too many women were silenced to get us to this point, they lived through a colonial regime. So there was a responsibility. Like if I don't use my voice, what am I doing? And then I thought, write the book. If they kick you out of the club, they kick you out of the club. I had to believe that people in academia who saw something good in me would continue to see it. And the people who thought I was a joke, would think I was a joke. The blowback was a lot and in fact, at my university . . . they took little notice when I retired.

It was more of a don't-let-the-door-slam-you-on-the-way-out kind of thing. So, I was like, let's just see where this [a media career] can take you. I internalized that responsibility of having a voice for my own children, for generations and generations of women. I think of the Lao Tzu quote, "Care what other people think, and you will always be their prisoner." I've been a prisoner long enough. So, if people don't like me, I have to learn to be ok with that.

Maryam: The thing that arises for me is this question of the real transformation that's needed, and perhaps a revolution. In psychology, it takes a long time to get prepared to even get into graduate school. And by the time they're out, they're in their late 20s, early 30s, if they started right away. Then they go on to do an internship that pays them poverty level wages, before they get to be called Dr. So-and-So. And I think young people are seeing that it's not necessary to follow that path, that there are other ways to make a difference. There are other ways to get your voice out. There are avenues that don't require all these hoops. I often go back to Audre Lorde, who said "The master's tools will never dismantle the master's house." I think of that quote, all the time, because now I'm at that senior level, and I'm still in the house of the ivory tower. Can we make change from within? I do wonder about a real transformation in education starting from the beginning, in the stories we tell, the voices we hear.

Linda: **Each of your stories describes a revolution in your life. Whereas before, you were asked to be a messenger, but you couldn't own the message. And now you're integrating message and messenger and that is revolutionary. With that integration in mind, you've been getting your message out. What have you learned about how to do that most effectively?**

Doris: **This is now the "how do we do this" part? What's your best advice, your best strategies? That's what we want to hear.**

Ramani: That's what my book chapter was about. Find the way you like sharing your voice that feels most authentic to you. Robyn wrote a book, some of us have podcasts. Some people find power in sharing information via video. It can be blogs, you can write pieces on Instagram, there are many ways to disseminate information. The key piece is for mental health professionals to find what feels most real to them. Find the *way* you want to share your voice, and then figure out *what* you want to talk about. What is it that you feel most connected to? Then figure out *who* you want to be talking to, and what modalities would work in that space. And then you've just got to put yourself out there.

And then either they come or they don't. If they don't, it's not an indictment of you. It just may not be where this group is coming from. So you just keep experimenting, you keep trying things. There are psychologists out there who are making documentaries.[4] Podcasting platforms are free. It's all there for you to go out and experiment with storytelling and content generation and see where it gets you. Terrance is saying how he writes op-eds for newspapers. I've been submitting op-eds for 14 years and no one has ever said yes, so op-eds ain't exactly my friendly space. The key thing is that you believe *this is something important for the world to know*. There are many ways to do this. And it's remarkable how many people can be transformed and affected, because platforms like YouTube are used by everyone all over the world. The platforms are there. People just need to learn to use them.

Terrance: What I do is inform myself on what the community wants, what the community is saying. I like to keep my ears to the streets, and speak a language that the community understands. I change my language to fit the audience I am trying to reach. We have to be able to *code switch*. I can talk to one community and then flip the script and post an article about the exact same thing from a legislative perspective, targeting a different group of people who need to hear that message. As Ramani said, understanding the needs in the messaging and being very authentic. I know what audiences I'm speaking to, and how I'm going to deliver that message to get the greatest response and engagement from that community, on whatever platform that I'm doing it in.

Ramani: This is a marketing game. Marketing is really about getting a message out there. And it goes back to what Terrance is saying. You're not going to sell a car to everyone the same way. You're

---

4 See the work of Matthew Miller, professor of counseling psychologist and documentarian who created SPOKENproject, a video project which centers BIPOC stories about experiences of racism, coping and connection, healing, and resistance: www.youtube.com/@SPOKENproject/about

trying to take this message and meet communities where they're at. And, to Maryam's point, I was chair of the advisory board of the APA Minority Fellowship Program and meeting with trainees and you know what they all said? "We're tired of being broke, we can't pay our rent." When I was in grad school, my professors lived in these multimillion dollar houses in the hills, but they were like, "Go volunteer, take an internship that pays 8000 a year, keep taking those loans, it's noble, you need to care about the people." No, I also need to care about the generations that came behind me because immigrants don't come with cash, not my parents. And we have to communicate to our students that it's okay to want to earn money because at some level, that's going to give them some power in society. And teach them how to market themselves. It's often the first-generation trainees and students of color who do not have access to the resources, family money, connections, or real estate. And they're constantly pedaling faster, paying out loans for a lifetime.

Robyn: The biggest thing that I can share is, "Do it scared." I think a lot of people wait for confidence, and that's a journey that you'll be on for a long time. If you keep waiting, the people who need your voice won't be getting it. So just do it imperfectly, do it scared, and learn as you go. Be open to feedback, be open to pivoting. And I'm actually speaking to myself right now, because this is something that I still work on with myself. I'm speaking to my fellow perfectionists out there. Be okay with not being 100% confident but know that you have something important to share.

And secondly, don't necessarily measure your impact based on likes on social media. I can't tell you how many times I've posted something and people have come to me in private, to tell me how much it meant to them. But I would have never known because it didn't even get any kind of reaction on social media. So have multiple metrics, and trust that your message is having an impact, even if you don't always see it in the number of likes, the amount of reads.

Maryam: My advice is to stay true to your values. That means going back to them over and over again. Connect it to that authenticity, and the passion and your reason for why you're doing it. As Robyn said, it isn't about the likes and the hearts. Don't just be driven by what's popular. We have our pressures in academia, but then it's a popularity contest out there in the world of social media too. And you want to be true, you want to continue to be humble, and cautious with what you're putting out there so that you're putting out things that aren't harmful, but are helpful. We do have a LOT to offer. We have taken the time to learn responsibly, to know and understand some topics in a really deep and meaningful way. And a lot of the loud voices out there haven't necessarily done that. So it's our responsibility with what we've been given to get out there and raise our voice even though we may feel like "Oh, I'm not used to that" or "Will anybody listen?"

Doris: **What are some of the joys and rewards of putting yourself out there? What has your more public-facing work meant to you?**

Terrance: I don't want to sound like I'm about to cry. Because I might. If any of my students from Wallkill see me on the streets, they're gonna think I lost my thug passion. One of the greatest joys that this work has given me is when I became faculty, not only at NYU Silver School of Social Work, but at NYU's Prison Education Program.[5] And I walked into Wallkill Correctional Institution, where I teach a Social Policy program. There are guys there, whom I've taught, who were so empowered, that they have dedicated themselves to becoming social workers, social advocates. I always talk about how our lives come full circle. My greatest joy is seeing the work that I committed myself to . . . these students are being empowered by the message, even behind prison walls. When you go live on the streets, when you walk behind prison walls, and they say your name . . . I have reached, I'm reaching my audience. So that is the joy for me in the work that I'm doing.

Linda: Thank you, Terrance. It must be so powerful.

Terrance: Yeah, it is, I can't even lie.

Maryam: I'll go, since we're all quiet, thinking about joy. I think part of it is perhaps the challenge and struggle of finding the time

5 Founded in 2015, NYU PEP is a college-in-prison program that aims to expand access to higher education within communities impacted by the criminal justice system by offering free college courses to incarcerated and formerly incarcerated students.

to do all the things you want to do, and the things that are most meaningful to you. Part of it is professional, but then on the personal side, having a family and prioritizing them over some of the other things. Because, as you're having impact and making change for the next generation, as a parent, it starts with my own children. Those are the people that I have the most ability to have some impact on, and then hopefully out from there, you know, to communities and beyond. And so for me, that's where the joy is. To be doing the things that I can do in my own home with my own children. And starting with just making a difference for one person's life, so that I don't overwhelm myself or feel like it's never enough, right? Because we've been socialized to feel like whatever we do is never enough. And as soon as you make the next milestone, you're supposed to be on to the next. So really being present with that one person or with a group that you know that you have positively impacted, does truly bring you joy, and continues to revitalize you to keep going.

Linda: Thank you. I'll say what brings me joy is just feeling aligned with my purpose and my calling. And also having those conversations with the people in my family and with the people in my community who I know might not have access, if I didn't open my mouth, if I didn't share, if I didn't write the book. And so having those one-on-one conversations, when people are saying, this changed my life, or this helped me interact in this relationship in a more effective way. Just knowing that what I have to say is actually helping people live more empowered and intentional lives, have better relationships, and a sense of freedom and agency in their lives. That is what brings me joy and keeps me going.

Ramani: What brings me joy is getting to be a storyteller. I think that actually to be a psychologist is to be a healer, and to be a healer is to be a storyteller. I'm getting the opportunity now to hear the stories of many, to respond to their questions and concerns. To see real change, that it actually destigmatizes seeking help for mental health issues. Calling domestic abuse or emotional abuse – abuse. Helping people find the name for what's happening to them, to break through shame and stigma. I've always enjoyed teaching. So there's a way that storytelling is teaching in a very different way, and getting to meet people who are sharing their stories in a way that really is transformative. We underestimate the power of storytelling, that it mobilizes other people, it humanizes their struggles, and helps them recognize they're not alone.

Doris: Thank you all so much. This has been a fantastic conversation, so rich. I feel inspired hearing about your journeys to identify your particular gifts and offer them up to others. And it did feel like there was a revolutionary thread in each of your stories. I hope that readers who want to pursue a similar path can see the importance of challenging what we've been told to value and what is worth sharing. That there is a way through self-doubt, and that you can survive the blowback to have an even more positive and powerful impact in the world. I'm so grateful to each of you for taking the time to be with us today, and for your honesty and vulnerability.

Linda: It has just really been a gift. The themes are resonating with me on a personal level, I can't even tell you. I've got a big birthday coming up, I'll be 60 and I'm thinking, *put that Kool Aid down*. Thank you for the ways in which you've just shared so honestly and so openly. And yes, there is definitely a thread of revolution here. You may not be able to dismantle the master's house with the master's tools. But you are being creative about using the tools to build something else and that feels incredibly revolutionary and powerful to me. I'm really inspired by what you're each doing to decolonize your work. So thank you for the wisdom and the inspiration.

Leading for Change and Impact

Part III

The third section of the book focuses on strategies for transitioning to positions of leadership and influence and leveraging your power – in the media, academia, clinical institutions, government, and social service sector – to address systemic failures that drive racial inequities.

Building on the previous Community Conversation, this section opens with a contribution from Ramani Durvasula, who argues that using the media to educate the public about psychological science and mental health represents a key opportunity for decolonizing knowledge and reaching diverse audiences. A South Asian woman who has built out various successful media platforms, she provides best practice guidelines for using the media in the public interest (**Chapter 21**).

The three chapters that follow offer examples of how BIPOC leaders can drive innovation through inclusive practices that create cultures of belonging and abundance. In **Chapter 22**, Sandra Mattar, a former international Latina trainee now Director of Training at the Immigrant and Refugee Health Clinic at Boston Medical Center, offers suggestions for dismantling colonial and oppressive discourses in clinical training to foster students' personal and professional growth. In **Chapter 23**, Gordon Nagayama Hall, a senior, able-bodied, cisgender, biracial Japanese American psychologist and former editor of *Cultural Diversity and Ethnic Minority Psychology*, demystifies the process of editorial review and illustrates how those involved in the editorial process can make the field of psychological science and related fields more inclusive and rigorous at the same time. In **Chapter 24**, Anneliese Singh, Brean'a

DOI: 10.4324/9781003309796-24

Parker, and Briana Bivens, a racially diverse team of scholars, co-mentors, and antiracist practitioners and organizers, describe how they embodied JEDI (justice, equity, diversity, inclusion) as they co-built the vision and foundations of a college-based JEDI office grounded in compassion, accountability, and truth-telling.

This section ends with two chapters featuring two BIWOC with experiences as organizational leaders and chief executive officers (CEOs) in the non-profit sector. In **Chapter 25**, Jeannette Pai-Espinosa describes her journey as a Korean-American president/CEO of a national non-profit organization that advocates for social and systems change with and for girls, young women, and gender-expansive youth of color. She provides key insights and recommendations for those who are in or aspire to leadership roles in social justice movements. In **Chapter 26**, Linda Lausell Bryant, a Puerto Rican Afro-Latina higher education associate dean, clinical full professor and former non-profit CEO, explores the internalized racist messages and value conflicts she continues to navigate in her various leadership roles in a racialized system of care. She ends with recommendations for leading and managing as a BIPOC, as whole and healthy people, working in community and with purpose.

In our last Community Conversation, we speak with Joseph P. Gone, Helen Neville, and Larke Nahme Huang about Leadership, Impact, and Institutional Change. They discuss their pathways to leadership, the challenges of transforming powerful institutions – higher education, publishing, the federal government, and the mental health care system – and how they navigate barriers and competing demands as BIPOC leaders (**Chapter 27**).

Becoming a Media Contributor
21

Science, Advocacy, and Public Education

Ramani Durvasula

What I had assumed was the end of my career in sharing mental health and psychology in the media, strangely became the beginning. I had been attempting to find my footing in traditional media – as the expert talking head on the news, the commentator on a range of television shows, the therapist on the unscripted show. I had an agent and attended pitch meetings with producers and network decision makers. I also continued in my career as a professor of psychology and maintained a clinical practice. I wrote some public-facing books. None of it was making a big impact. I actually found it frustrating to work with producers who were not culturally or intersectionally informed. I was losing money on the entire pursuit; it appeared that perhaps my age, ethnicity, and gender were all working against me, and I decided to give up. When I finally decided to step away from my attempt at a media career in 2017, I threw myself into other work.

A few months later, a young person with a popular YouTube channel reached out and asked me to speak about narcissism, which was a central focus of my research and clinical practice. I thought, "Wonderful, I can share a little of what I know, and support a younger generation's burgeoning media careers." The interview I did with him performed very well, garnering over a million views, which caught the eye of a producer at a start-up digital mental health platform who then asked if I would do some videos with their team. They came to my home, we shot the videos, and those videos did even better, receiving millions more views.

DOI: 10.4324/9781003309796-25

Two earnest young women who liked my work and had known me through my past work suggested that I share my content on narcissism via YouTube. They believed there was a real opportunity if I were to take what I wrote about in my books (that weren't selling) and present the same content in videos. I had never watched YouTube, but I agreed to try it for a few months.

No gatekeepers, no uninformed producers. Just me, them, and initially an iPhone and a light bulb in an old fixture to light the shot. We started with 500 subscribers. Today, the channel, @DoctorRamani, now has 1.3 million subscribers and counting, and approximately 5 million views per month, making it one of the largest mental health YouTube channels in the world. This was a different media career, of which I was the primary producer and creator and allowed to be responsive to viewers around the world, directly answering questions, and creating content that was congruent with science, lived experience, and clinical practice.

The media landscape has changed (and continues to change). It became clear that in the aftermath of a pandemic that had permanently shifted mental health across the world, a reckoning around ethnicity, race, power, and oppression, and a march toward globalization that was changing how information was shared, but leaving many people unheard and underserved – there was an opportunity to shift how we think about how therapists and scientists could leverage these new tools of communication and disseminate science and clinical knowledge for the greater good.

Psychology in the Public Interest

My media career began 15 years ago when I was watching a TV show. I watched a self-described (but uncredentialed) psychotherapist opining on a newsworthy mental health issue. She was speaking on an issue that required far more cultural awareness and sensitivity than she was bringing. Her conclusions were misleading, and lacked any grounding in empirical, clinical, or psychological theory, leaving me wondering – who gets to be the mouthpiece for the field? If the results and conclusions of empirical research aren't reaching the public in a meaningful way, and the messengers aren't even people trained in our field – then aren't we missing an opportunity to fulfill our responsibility to alleviate suffering and educate the public?

Do we, as psychologists, counselors, academics, and clinicians have a duty or obligation to "give away" what we do to the public? By conducting translational research? Creating ways of increasing access and disseminating mental health and psychological services at low or no cost to large segments of the population? Making education and training in psychology accessible to traditionally under-represented groups? Certainly all of the above, but are there other ways to make our science more accessible, more responsive, and more digestible for the larger public?

Social media and content platforms such as YouTube are increasingly becoming tools by which to share the science, practice, and theories of psychology and mental health and connect them to contemporary life. However, it has not always been that straightforward. Media platforms such as television and radio have traditionally been "gated," requiring access through gatekeepers such as editors, producers, booking agents, and network decision makers. The curators of these media spaces often maintain commercially informed hegemonic representations of racial majority, cis-gender, heteronormative presenters and shepherd content that resonates with similar audiences. Fortunately, the public facing aspect of psychology is evolving. The voices and perspectives that are appearing in public spaces to discuss psychological science and mental health are diversifying, as more BIPOC content creators with backgrounds in all areas of psychology utilize media as a tool to teach, support, and advocate on behalf of their communities.

Drawing on my own experience as a South Asian woman who is a clinical psychologist, professor emerita, media commentator, content creator, consultant, educator, and now executive producer, this chapter attempts to address this gap by providing recommendations on how BIPOC psychologists and other mental health professionals can utilize media to translate and disseminate psychological science and practice to the public.

My Path to Becoming a Media Contributor

In the week before submitting this chapter, multiple paid media opportunities fell through, the representatives repeatedly telling me, "We decided to go with someone else." These moments remind me, especially as a South Asian woman, how important it is for me to manage this space for myself, as myself. Many mentors and colleagues strongly advised me not to pursue this path, with the implication that it was somehow untoward to have strayed away from the regimented world of impact scores, scholarly publications, and extramural funding. The acculturative and assimilative pressures I have always experienced, the implicit assumption that I was "fortunate" to have the opportunity to pursue doctoral work at an R1 institution, and an internalized sense of shame and ingratitude that I was thinking of stepping out of those guardrails stymied my interests in blending media and mental health for a long time.

Despite self-reflection being integral to mental wellness and growth, my training and education experiences more often emphasized keeping your nose to the grindstone and meeting professional milestones. I enjoyed the puzzle of translating science, theory, and practice into something usable, understandable, and engaging, of storytelling and production, and of being in a space that was actually more open to diverse perspectives than traditional strongholds of academic scholarship or clinical practice. While I have been able to grow in this space, retire from academia, and start my own media consulting firm, I continue to do research, provide clinical services, and engage in advocacy work. I have found that media has become an unexpected multiplier that potentiates the reach of my work and elevates its applicability.

My media work has included appearances on major news networks, morning news shows, documentaries, unscripted television, talk shows, digital mental health education platforms, and other people's podcasts and YouTube channels. I have provided consultation to film and television producers. I am also an executive producer of a highly ranked podcast. Participating in a range of media outlets has allowed me to achieve my goal of applying the science and practice of psychology to benefit society and improve lives. Audience comments and feedback have revealed that the content that I have created and collaborated on has helped to demystify therapy, given a name to the painful relational experiences people have endured, fostered global conversations about mental health and treatment, and above all, allowed people to feel heard.

Public Platforms for Mental Health

When I was 19 years old, I attended a university internship and job fair in Rochester, NY, and while I was supposed to be a pre-med major at the time, the idea of journalism and using media to communicate about health and science was already intriguing to me. I even approached the booth of a local news affiliate and asked them about internship and volunteer opportunities. This being the 1980s, I was told "I don't really see a front-of-camera role for you, but perhaps someone 'like you' could be a research assistant or news writer." The entire interaction discouraged me, and sadly reflected the state of media representation at the time.

Listeners and viewers want to hear voices and stories that validate their own experiences. The evolving "democratization" of media represents a still unrealized opportunity for diverse voices to be heard on issues relevant to psychological science, advocacy, and mental health, and to decolonize some of the most accessed spaces in global mental health and public psychology education. Many people may access online resources (Pew Research Center, 2014) before ever being offered psychoeducation by a clinician. Thus, online spaces also represent a key opportunity for BIPOC clinicians and researchers to create culturally responsive and informed content. This content may not only be informational but can meaningfully and accurately address and integrate awareness of culture, race, religion, class, and systemic oppressions in a manner that may destigmatize help seeking, provide resources, and facilitate entry into treatment.

My work addresses narcissistic relationships, relationships often characterized by power imbalances, unhealthy emotional patterns, and significant distress for the relationship partner. The simplistic guidance has often been, "Well if it's so bad, then get out." It isn't that simple, however, and presenting a nuanced framing of the issues of family, culture, and marriage, highlighting that "leaving" is not always an option, and that individuation may feel like hubris, has been a way to validate the experience of people in these relationships around the world and across a range of diverse groups. Through the creation of a library of daily content that is often a touchstone for people struggling in these circumstances, I have been able to provide realistic and empathic guidance to those enduring these circumstances.

There is little guidance for those interested in learning how to utilize media platforms to disseminate information as part of a professional mental health career, nor is media training readily accessible. The current shifts in media represent an opportunity for BIPOC folks to access a variety of platforms such as YouTube, and create their own content, content that traditional news platforms often do not support. Many BIPOC students, interns, fellows, and early career professionals in psychology often grapple with giving themselves "permission" to be seen and heard in these public spaces and may feel unsupported by mentors, faculty, and colleagues, especially in higher education, if they choose to use media as a dissemination tool. At the same time, many are already growing their social media presence on various platforms, but may lack mentorship, guidance, or encouragement to keep building out this presence.

Considerations for Getting Started as a Media Contributor

Despite being discouraged from pursuing this path, curiosity and interest won out, and I started asking questions. There were virtually no mentors to turn to, and the ones whom I approached often did not bring a culturally informed lens or even awareness of the barriers a BIPOC individual would face as they attempted to enter this space. In my case, I had a bit of geographic good fortune, being based in Los Angeles, and a series of conversations with acquaintances fostered a meeting with an agent who was willing to represent me. Even still, it was a frustrating process. For every ten opportunities for which I was considered, I would be retained for one. This early work was expected to conform to what the producers and networks wanted, and while I was showing up as a woman of color, the content was often still not culturally or intersectionally responsive or informed. It was not until I was able to independently generate content that I was able to take the ad hoc "media training" I received from eight years of working on TV and in news media and apply it to what I actually wanted to say.

BIPOC psychologists, researchers, and mental health professionals at any stage of their career can learn to leverage the media as a tool to disseminate research findings, educate the public about important issues related to mental health, and advocate for social change. Below, I offer some practical tips for how you can get started.

1. **Be clear on your goals, values, mission, and vision.** What are you hoping to do by accessing media as a platform? Most commonly people are attempting to provide psychoeducation, but other focus areas include advocacy, sharing lived experience, provision of specific resources, commenting on trends and news in mental health, sharing science in an accessible manner, reviewing content relevant to mental health, and/or providing expert opinion on new programs or documentary style programs. In addition, some people may strive to create linguistically diverse content. Some of you may not want to engage in the public-facing role in media, but rather, act as an advisor to news, film, or television producers to foster more accurate and informed portrayals of a range of issues in psychology.
2. **Adopt a writing style that is accessible and inclusive.** Avoid technical jargon and strive for a more conversational tone, allowing your voice to shine through. Offering to write newsletter submissions for community or professional groups as well as blog or social media posts are simple ways to experiment with this writing style.
3. **Do not solely rely on gatekeepers for access to opportunities to share content in the media space.** Trying to break through via traditional gatekeepers such as production companies, development executives, publishers, news editors, and agents may not only slow a BIPOC person's entry into this space, but also prove to be quite demoralizing. As you

navigate this process, consider open access platforms such as YouTube, podcasting platforms, self-publishing, or blogging platforms. These types of platforms have become a first step toward de-colonizing the media, by increasing access to diverse voices and reaching broader audiences.

4. **Seek ways to interact with your audience to learn how to better customize your content.** Media is now far more interactive, and engagement can be an opportunity to collaborate with communities, shape content to the needs of the communities you are attempting to reach, as well as address any misconceptions.

5. **Remain open to providing your expertise to traditional news, radio, documentaries, and television.** As more content and news channels proliferate, they have a greater need for expert commentary, and mental health practitioners are often in the greatest demand. To make yourself "known" as an expert, colleges and universities may have a media relations office that provides a list of subject matter experts. The American Psychological Association and other professional societies also maintain public affairs offices that connect the media to mental health experts. In smaller markets, consider connecting with local network affiliates who will welcome having a local expert contributor.

6. **Don't assume you need an agent, manager, publicist, or other form of representation.** To generate your own content or serve as a subject matter expert in various news or other content platforms, representation is not needed. Be wary of managers, publicists, or other consultants asking for large amounts of money up front or expensive contracts for services and making unrealistic promises.

7. **Appreciate the value of your training and expertise.** All areas of psychological expertise can provide useful insight to varied audiences. While clinicians are often sought after, areas of psychology outside of the clinical realm are uniquely positioned to provide insights and apply their specific expertise to demystify human behavior.

8. **Seek opportunities for formal media training.** Media training is a useful tool for people to learn how to present themselves clearly and concisely across different media. In-house training is sometimes offered within some employment settings, and larger professional organizations sometimes offer media training as a benefit for members.

9. **Create a video sample of your work.** Producers, news bookers, and others who may be recruiting clinicians and academicians to work on existing media projects may ask for a "reel" or compilation of video clips to ascertain how you sound on tape. You can make your own brief video on a topic that you are knowledgeable about, include clips of videos you

may have shared of yourself on social media, or have someone record a portion of a conference presentation or professional talk.

10. **Be prepared for unkind comments and feedback.** Some of this may even contain aggressive language about ethnicity, gender, or populations you are working with. It is an unfortunate risk of this work. Know your limits and comfort, have safe spaces to turn to for support, and block problematic comments that are unhealthy for you and others who may be participating in your content. Engage in self-care as you do this work, as the unfettered and anonymized world of internet commentary can result in bruising dialogue and attendant discomfort.

Best Practices for Being a Media Contributor

All professionals must remain cognizant about ethical engagement in media, in a way that does no harm, and protects your professional standing. Best practices for working in the media as a psychologist entail multiple standards and considerations:

1. **Be aware of the ethical codes of your profession regarding dissemination of mental health or psychological content.** Remain aware of ethical codes around competency and giving guidance around topics in which you do not possess requisite training (e.g., giving legal advice if you are not also trained as an attorney).
2. **Ensure that you use disclaimers in any content.** This may be done through captions, concluding remarks, or audio disclaimers reminding readers, viewers, or listeners about accessing appropriate emergency services, seeking out consultation, evaluation, and treatment with a licensed mental health practitioner, and that the content is not meant to be a substitute for therapy or other mental health intervention.
3. **Respect client confidentiality at all times.** Do not share any identifiable client information in any public forum, and do not request that clients post or share your content. They may do so on their own, which is their choice. Television and film producers may approach clinicians and inquire about whether you could connect them with clients who are experiencing a particular issue for one of their projects, and that will always be a "no."
4. **Remain aware of your privilege.** Within media spaces, all experts must remain aware of our own privilege in how we use language, interact

with others, and the assumptions we make about others. Remaining aware of differences in access, and making recommendations mindfully is important.

5. **Be aware of your institution's rules and regulations regarding speaking to the media.** If you are employed in any organization or institution – ensure you are familiar with their rules and regulations around your media presence. Be clear on these issues before launching your work in this area.

6. **Keep your professional social media presence separate.** It is strongly recommended that if you are going to use social media platforms to communicate about psychological or mental health content that you create professional sites and keep those separate from any personal social media sites you maintain (APA, 2021). Professional accounts are often public pages; as such, ensure that the content is posted in a manner that is respectful and with the awareness that your clients or students may see it.

Concluding Thoughts

Access to therapy and the latest in scientific discoveries that can benefit diverse communities has traditionally been limited. There are many ways to leverage the media to disseminate science, theory, and practice to a wider audience. The more often this can be done by BIPOC scholars and mental health professionals who work with diverse populations, the greater the likelihood that the content will be presented in a manner that resonates with diverse audiences, fostering greater visibility for issues impacting a range of communities. You may very well find that you and your work are able to shine in these media spaces and reach people in the world on a larger scale compared to traditionally and hierarchically constructed professional spaces.

References

American Psychological Association. (2021). *Guidelines for the optimal use of social media in professional psychological practice.* Committee on Professional Practice and Standards. www.apa.org/about/policy/guidelines-optimal-use-social-media.pdf

Pew Research Center. (2014). *Pew internet and American life project.* www.pewresearch.org/internet

Instituting Anti-Oppressive and Decolonizing Approaches to Supervision and Clinical Training

22

Sandra Mattar

As a young psychologist in training in the United States (US), an international student in the process of obtaining her US residence, a polyglot, born in Venezuela as a daughter of Lebanese immigrants, I had the opportunity of practicing and training in what would be considered highly competitive institutions in Boston, Massachusetts. In fact, some of my supervisors were leaders in the field and their research was the gold standard in clinical work. And yet, many times in supervision and training sessions, I felt misunderstood, mischaracterized, excluded, and stereotyped. I felt similarly about the ways my clients were being perceived and treated. Mainstream narratives of clients tended to be patronizing and even pathologizing in alarming ways.

As a student immersed in a mainly white training environment, I did not have a sounding board to share my thoughts and feelings, nor could I find trusting spaces for having these conversations. I didn't even have the language to have these dialogues, to express what I was experiencing in my life in the US; I was catapulted into an identity crisis. As a white Venezuelan with a Lebanese background, I suddenly became "a foreigner," a "Latina with an accent," and an "immigrant." While used to being "othered"

DOI: 10.4324/9781003309796-26

growing up, I was not familiar with how to navigate being a racialized other in the US, and the target of disparaging stereotypes about Latinx.

Unbeknownst to me at that time, I carried an internalized racism and oppression that is very much prevalent in colonized cultures, in which the white colonizer tends to be the object of aspiration, idealization, and emulation (Freire, 1970) and the local population is dehumanized in order to justify their domination (Fanon, 2001). These implicit dynamics hampered my ability to recognize the insidious ways in which white supremacy and Western European thinking operated in my mental health training and supervision in the US.

My experiences of invalidation were usually centered around feelings of invisibility when sharing my opinions in academic and training settings. I experienced other microaggressions such as minimization of painful experiences by faculty and class peers, dismissal of my intuitive knowledge by supervisors, stereotyping of my cultural background, and an emphasis on evidence-based treatment modalities mainly tested in white populations and inadequate for addressing the most pressing issues experienced by my clients.

Unfortunately, I lacked the power, awareness, and language to name and challenge these pervasive and systemic silencing forces that favor dominant narratives and dominant ways of being. Slowly but surely, stereotype threat and impostor syndrome became a regular part of my training experience. In the process, I lost my voice and sense of self-agency and self-determination, and I doubted myself every step of the way.

Dominant Discourses in the Mental Health Field and Academic Training

Academic discourses and mental health training practices in general are heavily impacted by colonial influences and power structures that perpetuate Eurocentric standards and oppressive dynamics (Galán et al., 2021; Mignolo, 2011). These influences permeate our ideas of what is considered mental health, what treatment approaches are considered optimal for recovery, who defines competencies in supervision and training, and how to be a therapist, among others. The ways we teach and train are deeply embedded in colonial discourses (Carrero Pinedo et al., 2022; Shahjahan et al., 2022).

BIPOC trainees may be especially vulnerable to these oppressive forces in their training and education, and outside of it (Galán et al., 2021). They face significant structural and institutional oppression resulting from the lack of diversity among trainees, faculty, supervisors, and program administrators and faculty, limited social supports and advocacy, implicit biases in academic expectations and evaluation criteria, and white-centered curriculum and training programs (Carrero Pinedo et al., 2022). The result is that BIPOC students report that their cultural, local, and Indigenous knowledge and practices are invalidated and dismissed. Scholarship relevant to their cultural communities, including religion and spirituality, is absent in the curriculum. Instructors fail to acknowledge societal events that have a direct impact on trainees' cultural communities, and a multitude of other slights (APA, 2019). These hegemonic forces are also embedded in the practice of psychological science. For example, as a long-time journal editor, I have had the opportunity to be "behind the scenes" of the publishing process at a major mainstream psychology journal. Publishing becomes a way to legitimize knowledge and amplify ideas and voices. But whose knowledge are we legitimizing and perpetuating when most editorial boards and reviewers are white, male, and based in North America and Europe? (Auelua-Toomey & Roberts, 2022; Buchanan et al., 2021; Mignolo, 2011; Shim et al., 2021).

This same process applies to the development of guidelines in professional practice; while aspirational, they perpetuate an "enforcer gaze" around what is considered "best practices." Do we examine these guidelines regarding representations of diverse voices and experiences? Whose standards of training are we enforcing with these guidelines? When such processes remain unexamined, colonization perpetuates itself (Shahjahan et al., 2022).

The Healing Impact of Culturally Responsive Supervisors

Being exposed to a few supervisors who restored my faith in justice and fairness in the world and validated my own experiences was key to my growth as a person and a clinician. After coming out of a practicum plagued with racist practices, I was lucky to work with a supervisor who never questioned the negative experiences that I had. She never asked me for evidence confirming that they happened. She just listened. She believed me. She also genuinely valued and appreciated my cultural lens when discussing clients, and did not get defensive when I challenged her understanding of the client. Her consistent validation afforded me the space to develop the confidence I needed as a trainee. Most importantly, her validation encouraged my healing process. This process also included the hard work of sorting out what parts of me were privileged, how I used those privileges, and how to dismantle my own racist views about others.

Another key component in my healing process was stumbling upon a multicultural and diverse environment as an early career clinician and academic. I was able to surround myself with a very diverse group of people, including Latinx colleagues. I was exposed to role models and examples of how to handle oppression, power, and privilege. These spaces felt supportive and provided a milieu to have conversations outside of the mainstream narrative, inspiring my activism to create a place where diverse clients, students, and faculty felt represented and included.

Later in my career, I actively sought positions where I could be in the company of a diverse group of colleagues who showed a genuine commitment to improve clients' lives, and empowered the trainees in their charge. While there were certainly challenges along the way – including colleagues who resisted decolonizing approaches to practice, and pressures to adhere to biomedical approaches to treatment and training – these spaces generally afforded me the freedom to use both intuition and cultural knowledge, and to treat my clients using a cultural and intersectional approach. In these spaces, case formulations and assessment procedures acknowledged the complexities of patients' lives and used multiple paradigms to understand their locations and functioning in the world. There were discussions about how systemic injustices impacted our clients and how to address these issues. In these rare spaces, I could be fully and unapologetically myself. I could locate myself along multiple positionalities and feel almost fully seen! Even supervision was a place devoid of a power differential between supervisor and supervisee, while carefully respecting the rules of engagement in training settings.

Promoting Culturally Resonant and Validating Spaces in Training

Training and work spaces like the ones I have described continue to be the exception to the norm up to this day. I made a commitment to create those spaces myself after I became a psychologist and clinical supervisor. I have experienced what Gone (2021) calls "a post-colonial predicament," or the need to "formulate, evaluate, and establish alternative, locally grounded, and culturally resonant professional services" (Gone, 2021, pp. 1518) and training models. As I gained more power and established my professional reputation in the field, I was afforded the freedom to "disrupt oppression" without significant consequences for my career.

My main motivation as a supervisor and trainer is to create spaces where trainees feel seen, validated, and have the space to experience self-compassion, and personal and professional growth. In my current role as faculty and supervisor at the Center for Multicultural Training in Psychology (CMTP) and Director of Training at the Immigrant and Refugee Health Clinic at Boston Medical Center, I have become keenly aware of the ways the Western medical model and the mental health professions continue to favor narratives filled with narrow notions of culture that emphasize demographic variables and discourage explorations of power dynamics, historical legacies of slavery and colonization, immigration, systematized discrimination, and intersectionalities, and spirituality, to name a few. Below, I offer some suggestions for clinical supervisors and training directors seeking to decolonize their approaches to training, and develop more inclusive, culturally appropriate, and anti-oppressive models of education and training.

Decolonizing and Anti-Oppressive Approaches to Supervision and Clinical Training

> For me, decolonizing is a verb. It is an active, intentional, moment to moment process that involves critically undoing colonial ways of knowing, being, and doing, while privileging and embodying Indigenous ways of knowing, being, and doing.
>
> (Fellner, 2018, pp. 284)

It is a challenging proposition to decolonize supervision and training spaces in the mental health professions without considering the multiple and insidious ways that colonial practices permeate every training institution. The ideas I present below have been deeply influenced by exposure to radical scholarship and decolonizing frameworks promoted by scholars and writers such as Frantz Fanon, Paolo Freire, Ignacio Martín-Baró, Edward Said, Lillian Comas-Diaz, Gloria Anzaldúa, Eduardo Duran, and Arthur Kleinman, among others.

According to Millner et al., (2021), in order to decolonize Western mental health practices, it is necessary to deconstruct the European foundation of these practices, to identify power structures that perpetuate these views through discrimination and oppression. Likewise, it is important to recognize the ways the mental health field has traditionally appropriated and erased cultural healing practices and values to support individualism at the expense of community well-being.

Hernández-Wolfe (2011) proposes a decolonization paradigm that decenters the cultural, social, and economic capital of dominant groups, centering the lived experience of the subject, and deliberately providing spaces where people's voices can be heard. She writes, "As people who struggle with using eurocentric ideas about race to represent ourselves and who are habituated to hybridity we have the right to construct, name, author, co-author, and implement healing models and methods that address the worlds we inhabit" (Hernández-Wolfe, p. 298).

The main question becomes, as Hernández-Wolfe suggests, how do we address the "worlds we inhabit" in supervision and training? How do we effectively give voice to and validate diverse cultural experiences, identities, and lived experiences, including oppression and marginalization? What is considered "good quality" supervision? How do we provide freedom in supervision to honor marginalized and neglected discourses, theories, and practices? How do we help supervisees heal from experiences such as imposter syndrome, racial trauma, and minority stress?

To center the needs and experiences of BIPOC students and trainees, I propose a few recommendations for supervisors and clinical training directors that are rooted in decolonizing pedagogies and anti-oppressive approaches:

1. **Create formal opportunities for self-reflection and the development of a decolonized personal and professional identity**

Encouraging self-reflection is a key ingredient in the process of decolonizing training. Self-reflection encourages trainees to center those aspects of their lived experience that can be explored to enrich their clinical work. Exploring paradigms that are familiar to the trainee is a way to validate alternate ways of knowing, being, and doing (Fellner, 2018) and promote self-empowerment. In addition, we advise that the supervisor and supervisee explore and cultivate cultural awareness in the supervision dyad, while engaging separately in self-reflection. Other topics for shared exploration and discussion may include insecurities, strengths, responsibility, and accountability for the care they provide, and how they can each advocate to change oppressive systems of care.

Explicitly discussing the intersection of power and identities in the room between supervisor and supervisee can help create a sense of transparency, safety, and authenticity, and clarify hidden agendas. At CMTP, both interns and supervisors are required to do what we refer to as a "bio" presentation. It is a chance for both groups to make a presentation about their lives and career paths. They locate themselves culturally, speak of major influences in their lives, such as mentors, discuss training and career challenges, as well as sources of healing and support. This is an exercise in cultural humility, cultural affirmation, and an examination of sources of power, privilege, disadvantages, and barriers.

Likewise, we deliberately create a weekly training space called a "mentoring meeting" where a diverse faculty body and the interns engage in dynamic exchanges that center the trainees' experiences, questions, and systemic challenges they experience. We discuss topics such as how to think about power and privilege and to leverage it to advocate for their clients. We also examine issues such as the supervisee's responsibilities, workload, salary, quality of life, and how they express their racial and/or cultural identity in training spaces, including, for example, in their professional attire and the way they wear their hair. Our goal is to provide spaces that allow for both authenticity and full self-expression, in trainees and supervisors. Finally, and perhaps most importantly, trainees have a chance to challenge faculty around their "blind spots" related to issues of diversity. In these weekly conversations, faculty openly acknowledge that cultural awareness and responsiveness is an ongoing process. There is not a final endpoint to learning and growing when it comes to negotiating differences with regards to culture and power differentials.

2. Encourage opportunities for epistemic disobedience in clinical supervision: Theoretical case conceptualization and ethics

Epistemic disobedience refers to the act of decentering colonial discourses and self-serving Western and white supremacist epistemologies with the purpose of transformation, not only reform (Mignolo, 2011). Transformation can occur when supervisor and supervisee engage in an examination of the epistemological constraints of dominant clinical theories, treatments, and case conceptualizations, and "interrogate the privileges of knowledge systems considered universal, delocalized, and applied without question in all contexts" (Shahjahan et al., 2022, p. 76). The goal is to decenter mainstream narratives while creating space for alternative paradigms to explain the supervisor's, supervisee's, and client's behavior and develop culturally relevant clinical interventions tailored to the clients' particular context (APA, 2019). Supervisory conversations also include discussions of the history of discrimination and bias in the field, Indigenous knowledge and practices, as well as the ways that valid epistemologies can also derive from culture, religion, nature, and language, and not just "science."

Strategies to challenge the epistemological status quo include applying interdisciplinary approaches and co-creating knowledge in partnership with communities, placing every co-creator on equal footing. Co-creators also inform clinical practices by sharing their lived experiences and identities (Shahjahan et al., 2022).

3. Integrate body and mind

Mind-body approaches to healing have been used for thousands of years in many cultures yet the mental health field has been very slow to incorporate these practices in teaching and training (Mattar & Frewen, 2020). The practice of decolonizing mental health training in professional practice centers local approaches to healing and wellness, including religious and spiritual practices (APA, 2019), and incorporates these practices into mainstream mental health paradigms (Duran et al., 2008).

4. Address racism, discrimination, and imposter syndrome

Examining the ways that power and privilege, oppressive and colonial discourses, implicit biases, internalized racism, microaggressions, and impostor syndrome have impacted the supervisor and supervisee's life experiences and identity is an integral part of how the CMTP structures supervision and training. The Public Psychology for Liberation Training Model (Neville et al., 2021) is a very helpful resource for this work. This model posits that white supremacist views are generally exempt from scrutiny and rarely questioned, and are deeply embedded in the discipline and training of psychology. It proposes an antiracist and anti-oppressive framework that centers the experience of marginalized individuals from BIPOC communities and the Global Majority, and complements professional psychology training competencies. The model organizes training around five domains that emphasize: a) collectivistic ways of healing; b) ethics that humanize rather than pathologize; c) training that showcases scholarship from the Global Majority, and values the contribution of trainees from those communities; d) reciprocal knowledge between psychologists and communities that values and centers input from those communities; and e) disrupting oppressive practices by offering trainings to address the ways that systemic racism operates within health care systems and beyond. These domains are held together by values such as relationality, respect, responsibility, relevance, cultural humility, care, and compassion, among others (Neville et al., 2021).

Conclusion

Supervision and training in psychology have traditionally emphasized individualistic and decontextualized approaches to mental health, and a separation from community and Indigenous sources of healing. A decolonizing approach to training calls for a radical reconceptualization of healing, one that favors Indigenous and local ways of being, and legitimizes sources of knowledge that are located outside of the confines of traditional Western science. It also forces us to reimagine the supervisor–supervisee relationship as one where there is space for vulnerability and the repair of one's cultural identity fragmentation, development of sense of self-agency, and skills to validate our clients' stories. By decolonizing training spaces, we are not only contributing to the well-being of trainees and supervisors alike, but we are also furthering a social justice agenda while empowering oppressed groups.

References

American Psychological Association. (2019). *APA guidelines on race and ethnicity in psychology: Promoting responsiveness and equity.* www.apa.org/about/policy/guidelines-raceethnicity.pdf

Auelua-Toomey, S. L., & Roberts, S. O. (2022). The effects of editorial-board diversity on race scholars and their scholarship: A field experiment. *Perspectives on Psychological Science, 17(6),* 1766–1777.

Buchanan, N. T., Perez, M., Prinstein, M. J., & Thurston, I. B. (2021). Upending racism in psychological science: Strategies to change how science is conducted, reported, reviewed, and disseminated. *American Psychologist, 76(7),* 1097. https://doi.org/10.1037/amp0000905

Carrero Pinedo, A., Caso, T. J., Rivera, R. M., Carballea, D., & Louis, E. F. (2022). Black, Indigenous, and trainees of color stress and resilience: The role of training and education in decolonizing psychology. *Psychological Trauma: Theory, Research, Practice, and Policy.* https://doi.org/10.1037/tra0001187

Duran, E., Firehammer, J., & Gonzalez, J. (2008). Liberation psychology as the path toward healing cultural soul wounds. *Journal of Counseling & Development, 86,* 288–295. https://doi.org/10.1002/j.1556-6678.2008.tb00511.x

Fanon, F. (2001). *The wretched of the earth* (trans. C. Farrington). Penguin.

Fellner, K. D. (2018). Embodying decoloniality: Indigenizing curriculum and pedagogy. *American Journal of Community Psychology, 62(3–4),* 283–293. https://doi.org/10.1002/ajcp.12286

Freire, P. (1970). *Pedagogy of the oppressed.* Continuum.

Galán, C. A., Bekele, B., Boness, C., Bowdring, M., Call, C., Hails, K., et al. (2021) Editorial: A call to action for an antiracist clinical science, *Journal of Clinical Child & Adolescent Psychology, 50*(1), 12–57. doi:10.1080/15374416.2020.1860066.

Gone, J. P. (2021). The (post) colonial predicament in community mental health services for American Indians: Explorations in alter-Native psy-ence. *American Psychologist, 76*(9), 1514–1525. doi:10.1037/amp0000906.

Hernández-Wolfe, P. (2011). Decolonization and "mental" health: A Mestiza's journey in the borderlands. *Women and Therapy, 34*(3), 293–306. doi:10.1080/02703149.2011. 580687.

Mattar, S., & Frewen, P. A. (2020). Introduction to the special issue: Complementary medicine and integrative health approaches to trauma therapy and recovery. *Psychological Trauma: Theory, Research, Practice, and Policy, 12*(8), 821–824. https://doi. org/10.1037/tra0000994

Mignolo, W. D. (2011). Geopolitics of sensing and knowing: On (de)coloniality, border thinking and epistemic disobedience. *Postcolonial Studies, 14*(3), 273–283. https://doi. org/10.1080/13688790.2011.613105

Millner, U. C., Maru, M., Ismail, A., & Chakrabarti, U. (2021). Decolonizing mental health practice: Reconstructing an Asian-centric framework through a social justice lens. *Asian American Journal of Psychology, 12*(4), 333–345. doi:10.1037/aap0000268.

Neville, H. A., Ruedas-Garcia, N., Lee, B. A., Ogunfemi, N., Maghsoodi, A. H., Mosley, D. V., et al. (2021). The public psychology for liberation training model: A call to transform the discipline. *American Psychologist, 76*(8), 1248–1265. https://doi.org/ 10.1037/amp0000887

Shahjahan, R. A., Estera, A. L., Surla, K. L., & Edwards, K. T. (2022). "Decolonizing" curriculum and pedagogy: A comparative review across disciplines and global higher education contexts. *Review of Educational Research, 92*(1), 73–113. https://doi. org/10.3102/00346543211042423

Shim, R. S., Tully, L. M., Yu, G., Monterozza, E. C., & Blendermann, M. (2021). Race and ethnicity of editorial board members and editors as an indicator of structural racism in psychiatry and neuroscience journals. *JAMA Psychiatry, 78*(10), 1161–1163. https://doi. org/10.1001/jamapsychiatry

Transforming the Research Landscape Through Editorial Leadership Roles

23

Gordon Nagayama Hall

Some may question whether transforming the research landscape and being a journal editor are compatible. Editors may be perceived as gatekeepers whose role is to maintain the status quo. It is probable that many editors function in this way. However, I am part of a community of editors who have created outlets for multicultural research in multicultural and mainstream journals.

I am an able-bodied, cisgender, older man whose father was White. These identities are each sources of privilege. My maternal grandparents immigrated from Japan in the early 1900s to California where my mother was born. She and her family were incarcerated in Poston, Arizona during World War II because of their Japanese ancestry. Being Japanese American has shaped my views on social and racial justice.

My expertise is on cultural contexts of psychopathology with an emphasis on Asian Americans. I have served as Editor of *Cultural Diversity and Ethnic Minority Psychology* (CDEMP) and Associate Editor of the *Journal of Consulting and Clinical Psychology* (JCCP). In addition, I have served on the editorial boards of several other journals. I also served as President of the American Psychological Association (APA) Society for the Psychological Study of Ethnic Minority Issues (Division 45) and the Asian American Psychological Association.

These experiences have taught me that the key to transforming the research landscape is participating in a scholarly community. The African

DOI: 10.4324/9781003309796-27

Ubuntu premise, "I am because we are," characterizes scholarly communities of color that have transformed the research landscape over the past 50 years. Although individual editors can have pivotal roles in shaping the field, lasting change occurs when there is community support.

The overarching framework for becoming a transformative editor is an ethic of citizenship. This means caring about colleagues and mentees in your local setting and beyond, and caring about the health of the profession. Unfortunately, citizenship is not valued by institutions as much as entrepreneurship. A person who can bring in money to an institution is often valued even if they are not a good citizen. So, the service provided by editors is often not rewarded by institutions. But the rewards of good relationships and of advancing science and the profession are much greater and lasting than institutional approval, which can be quite fickle.

The purpose of this chapter is to demystify the process of editorial review and suggest how those involved in the editorial process can change the status quo. The key editorial roles, in increasing order of responsibilities, workload, and power, are: ad hoc reviewer, editorial board member (consulting editor), associate editor, and editor. Ad hoc reviewers are asked to review because of their expertise in a field. This is typically based on existing publications. Those who consistently provide high-quality and timely reviews are often asked to become editorial board members, who are expected to conduct several reviews per year for a particular journal. Associate editors, who have decision-making power on accepting manuscripts and assign manuscripts to be reviewed, are usually chosen from board members. Editors, who guide the journal, assign manuscripts to associate editors, and make decisions on some manuscripts themselves, are usually those with experience as associate editors.

Many researchers will have opportunities to be ad hoc reviewers. A smaller group will be invited to serve on editorial boards. Associate editors and editors are few and far between. However, reviewers in all editorial roles can help transform the field. In this chapter, I will share my personal journey as a recipient of editorial feedback and in different editorial roles.

Early Career: Developing Expertise, Becoming a Reviewer, Networking

"Ironically, this is Pearl Harbor Day." This was the opening sentence of an editor's rejection letter of a manuscript on Asian American personality characteristics that I submitted to a cross-cultural journal in 1980. The letter probably went on to point out limitations of the manuscript, some of which were legitimate (e.g., the sample was from religious institutions) and some of which were less so (e.g., no white control group). I don't remember if these were the actual criticisms. What stuck with me was the opening sentence. I was a graduate student who was stunned and devastated.

The manuscript had nothing to do with Japan bombing Pearl Harbor in World War II. Nor did the editor, a white man, know that my mother and her family were incarcerated in World War II because of their Japanese ancestry. I absorbed this blow alone. My advisor co-author and student colleague co-author were white men. I don't remember any reaction from them.

I don't know the intent of the editor invoking Pearl Harbor Day and I wasn't in a position to ask. But the rejection sure felt as if the editor was somehow seeking revenge. The seemingly adversarial tone set by the opening sentence made the rest of the editor's feedback feel like a personal attack. At that moment, I was not on a trajectory to be in an editorial role myself and I couldn't have imagined myself as such. As you know from my positionality statement, I became a journal editor. Although it is a long, arduous, and labor-intensive road, there is a path for a junior scholar to become an editor.

A harsh editorial rejection is often the end of potential academic careers for graduate students or early career professionals. This could very well have been the end of my publishing career, which began with a previously published article on psychology and theology. And, fortunately, there were journals other than the cross-cultural journal that published work on multicultural psychology.

The path to becoming an editor is publications. There is another chapter in this book with helpful tips on publishing. My own advice is to read and write as much of the time as possible. A conceptual paper based on my dissertation on psychotherapy as a coercive acculturation process, which I termed cultural control, was published in a psychotherapy journal. Unfortunately, this single publication was not enough to land an academic job. Nearly 30 years later at an awards ceremony, I met a faculty member at one of the universities I applied to for a job and was rejected from. He told me he tried to make a case for me and remembered my psychotherapy publication. Had the Asian American personality paper been published, perhaps I would have had a better chance at an academic job and a different career path with a greater emphasis on multicultural issues earlier in my career.

The early 1980s was not a good time for multicultural psychology or for psychology in general. The private view of many that People of Color were undeserving of resources became public and instantiated during the Reagan administration. Affirmative action laws were overturned and community mental health centers were shut down. My only job opportunity was in a state hospital which writer Lawrence Matsuda has compared to the World War II concentration camps that my mother and 120,000 other Japanese Americans were incarcerated in. Although I was there voluntarily, there were constant clinical, administrative, and political stressors at the state hospital, juxtaposed with concerns about physical safety.

There were silver linings to working at the state hospital. Although the state hospital population was about 95% white, I was able to remain part of the Asian American community in my childhood home of Seattle, which shaped my thinking and later research. My job was to do clinical work, but I negotiated 10% time for research. There was a treasure trove of archival assessment data in the sex offender treatment program where I worked. I recruited undergraduate research assistants from local universities. John Moritsugu, who became Co-President of APA Division 45, was the advisor of one of my research assistants. In 1986, Dr. Moritsugu told me about the newly formed APA Society for the Psychological Study of Ethnic Minority Issues (Division 45) and encouraged me to become a member, which I did.

Using a similar methodology to the rejected Asian American personality characteristics paper, I did a study of sex offender personality characteristics based on over 400 MMPI profiles. This was one of the largest MMPI studies of sex offenders and debunked myths about what was considered a typical sex offender MMPI profile. So, I decided with my more senior co-authors to submit the manuscript to *JCCP*, the premier clinical psychology journal.

The manuscript was rejected by the *JCCP* Editor. The feedback was reasonable, suggesting that I had overinterpreted some small effects that were statistically significant primarily as a function of the large sample size. I thought the editor's decision was final, similar to the decision on the graduate school paper on Asian American personality characteristics. I discussed the rejection with a friend and colleague, Maria Root, who I had met during my postdoctoral fellowship at the University of Washington medical school. She suggested that I appeal the rejection. I didn't know this was possible. However, I successfully appealed and the *JCCP* Editor reassigned the manuscript to Associate Editor Larry Beutler. Dr. Beutler subsequently accepted the manuscript for publication in *JCCP* and also published other studies on sex offenders I conducted.

Because I had publications in *JCCP*, Dr. Beutler invited me to be an ad hoc reviewer for *JCCP*. I was conscientious about completing reviews well before deadlines out of respect for the editors and the authors waiting on editorial decisions that in some cases could make or break their careers. Given my traumatic graduate school journal rejection, I tried to be constructive in my criticism and not to include anything that might be interpreted as a personal attack. Learning to offer constructive criticism proved valuable later in my career as I assumed greater responsibility in the editing process.

Reviewing manuscripts submitted to *JCCP* exposed me to good (and not so good) research, which improved my own skills and helped me develop publishable manuscripts of my own. In 1987, I was surprised to be invited by Dr. Beutler to be a Consulting Editor for *JCCP*. I was the only person on the editorial board working at a state hospital.

My publications from my five years of work at the state hospital and my status as a consulting editor allowed me to land an academic job that I had coveted when I completed my PhD. Dr. Beutler wrote a letter of recommendation for me, which was highly influential. Kent State University was a respite from the constant stress of the state hospital. But there were major costs to moving from Seattle to Ohio. My wife and I were isolated from our families and Asian American communities on the West Coast.

Despite the isolation from my communities, Kent State provided an opportunity to mentor graduate students of color. Juanita Martin was my first PhD student and did her dissertation on Black and feminist identity among African American women. The *Journal of Counseling Psychology (JCP)* had published research on similar topics and Dr. Martin's dissertation was published there. Again, my experiences as a reviewer were beneficial as a co-author in getting Dr. Martin's dissertation published in *JCP*. Throughout my career, my editor experiences helped me mentor BIPOC students and colleagues in publishing their work, which helped transform the research landscape.

Mid-Career: Leadership and Editorships

A benefit of an academic job was the flexibility to become involved in national psychological associations. This national visibility opened editorial opportunities, as well. In 1993, my Seattle friend Dr. Root persuaded me to run for President of Division 45. Although I had been a member of Division, I had not been active, but was elected.

One of the responsibilities of the Division 45 President is a presidential address at the APA Convention. The work of the seven Division 45 presidents who preceded me involved multicultural psychology, so their addresses flowed from their work. Apart from my multicultural work in graduate school and my co-authored Black/feminist identity article with Dr. Martin, my work was on sexual aggression. Richard Suinn, who was the first Asian American President of APA in 1999, had the solution for my presidential address and research career direction. Dr. Suinn was on the Division 45 Executive Committee when I was President and I became his APA presidential campaign manager. He suggested I integrate my interests in sexual aggression in contexts of communities of color. This was the topic of my Division 45 presidential address and I developed it into an article that was published in the *American Psychologist* with graduate student Christy Barongan as co-author.

As Division 45 President, I became friends with Division 45 founder, Lillian Comas-Diaz, who in 1995 founded the journal *Cultural Diversity and Mental Health (CDMH)*, which later became *CDEMP*. Involvement in national professional organizations offers exposure to broader perspectives than is available in one's local institution. Such national involvement is important for those in editorial work.

One of Division 45's initiatives in its 1992 strategic plan was to establish a Division journal focusing on multicultural psychology. In 1998, Dr. Comas-Diaz's journal, *CDMH*, was acquired by Division 45 and expanded to become *CDEMP* to include multicultural psychology beyond mental health. Because of my visibility as past president of Division 45, as well as my publication and reviewing record, Dr. Comas-Diaz selected me to be an Associate Editor of *CDEMP*.

Our goal as the *CDEMP* editorial board was to establish a top-tier outlet for multicultural research and to mentor our colleagues in publishing. I learned much from Dr. Comas-Diaz about seeing potential in all work that was submitted and providing feedback that was as kind and encouraging as possible. Even when we rejected manuscripts, we offered feedback on how to improve them. Our goal was to balance rigorous journal standards with inclusivity. This approach succeeded over the years, as *CDEMP* is now the flagship multicultural psychology journal and has the highest impact factor (4.035) of the 18 top ethnic studies journals.

Associate editors have the daunting task of identifying reviewers to evaluate manuscripts submitted to the journal. I was fortunate to know many potential reviewers via my networks in Division 45 and the Asian American Psychological Association. Several other reviewers who I knew only by reputation also immensely helped in the reviewing process. Conscientious reviewers often are selected to be journal editorial board members and board members may be selected to be journal editors. William Liu was one of my most conscientious reviewers with a breadth of expertise. Dr. Liu is now Editor of *JCP*, the flagship journal in counseling psychology. So, being responsible and timely with reviews can position a person for greater influence over the publication process.

A rewarding aspect of being an associate editor was mentoring graduate students in journal reviewing. New journal reviewers tend to be overly critical in an effort to prove themselves. I'm sure I erred in this direction to some degree when I started reviewing but this tendency was tempered by my own experiences of rejection. Student reviewers benefit by contributing to the review process and by learning firsthand about the elements of quality manuscripts. These elements include a strong conceptual framework, quality data, rigorous methodology, and accurate data interpretation. In turn, the students I recruited as reviewers benefitted the field by making the reviewer pool more diverse.

Having served for several years as a Consulting Editor for *JCCP* and Associate Editor for *CDEMP*, in 2005 I was invited by Annette La Greca to become an Associate Editor for *JCCP*. This would mean simultaneous associate editor responsibilities for two major journals, *CDEMP* and *JCCP*. Associate editors were given no compensation at the time and my university did not allow course releases for editorial responsibilities. However, being an action editor for *JCCP* would allow me to influence the flagship clinical journal, so I accepted the invitation.

I helped diversify the *JCCP* reviewer pool by inviting reviewers from my previous *CDEMP* work. One of my major accomplishments as a *JCCP* associate editor was publishing Joseph Gone's qualitative study, "A community-based treatment for Native American historical trauma: Prospects for evidence-based practice" in 2009. Qualitative publications are rare in *JCCP*, as are publications on Indigenous communities. Thanks to my *CDEMP* network, I was able to identify reviewers having expertise on qualitative research with Indigenous populations. Dr. Gone's article has had a major impact on the field and has been cited more than 500 times. I am honored to have had a role in getting *JCCP* to think "outside the box."

A career highlight was being selected as Editor of *CDEMP* in 2005. One of my goals for the journal was to reduce editorial lag time, which is the time from when a manuscript is submitted to the editorial decision. As indicated previously, scholars' careers often hinge on timely editorial decisions. At this point in my career, I had a strong cadre of conscientious colleagues who served as associate editors and editorial board members. Our average editorial lag time was approximately eight weeks.

The purpose of *CDEMP* was to be a journal that encompassed all areas of multicultural psychology. In the 2000s, Americans of Middle Eastern and North African (AMENA) heritage were not represented in Division 45 nor were there many *CDEMP* publications on this community. One of my proudest accomplishments as *CDEMP* Editor was publishing Germine Awad's article, "The impact of acculturation and religious identification on perceived discrimination for Arab/Middle Eastern Americans," which appeared in 2010. This article has been cited nearly 400 times. Dr. Awad has been an effective advocate for AMENA, becoming the first AMENA member-at-large of the Division 45 Executive Committee in 2015, co-founding the AMENA Psychological Association (AMENA Psy) in 2017, and being elected AMENA Psy President in 2022.

I also engaged in advocacy in the editorial process with my mentees. In 2007, one of my graduate students conducted a study of Asian American personality characteristics, similar to but much more sophisticated than the one I had conducted as a graduate student. Because I was Editor of *CDEMP*, I did not want the study submitted there to avoid the appearance of conflict of interest. So, my student submitted the study to the same journal that I had submitted my 1980 study to. The initial result was the same – rejection. However, some of the criticisms of my student's study seemed unreasonable. Unlike my advisor in 1980, I wrote to the action editor (a different one from the 1980 editor) and expressed my concerns about the review. Unlike 1980 when I was a graduate student, I was a full professor and I was in a position to ask the action editor about their decision. I also mentioned my experience as a student in 1980 and contended that the journal's lack of receptiveness to multicultural work was a deterrent to me and other scholars from submitting their work to this journal. The action editor relented and the article was eventually accepted for publication. Nevertheless, without my advocacy, my student's important work might not have seen the light of day.

Late Career: Creating Special Publishing Opportunities

My most recent editorial board assignment was as Consulting Editor for the *American Psychologist*, the flagship journal of the field. In this capacity, I got to co-edit three special issues of the journal. The first special issue, published in 2019, on "Racial trauma: Theory, research, and healing" was co-edited with my longtime friend Dr. Comas-Díaz, who was an Associate Editor of the *American Psychologist*. We co-edited the special issue with Division 45 Past President Helen Neville. The special issue allowed us to bring mainstream attention to racial trauma and healing among African Americans, Indigenous populations, Japanese Americans, Latinx immigrants, and AMENA.

In 2021, only 7 of over 8,700 articles published in the *American Psychologist* over the past 40 years focused on Asian Americans. The 2021 special issue of the *American Psychologist*, "Rendered invisible: Are Asian Americans a model or marginalized minority?" co-edited by Tiffany Yip, Charissa Cheah, Lisa Kiang, Dr. Comas-Diaz, and I addressed this vacuum. Central themes were intersectional identities and de-bunking the model minority stereotype.

APA formed the Task Force on Strategies to Eradicate Racism, Discrimination, and Hate in 2021. Task Force Co-Chairs were Drs. Awad and Gone, whose groundbreaking work was discussed previously. The Task Force advised APA on developing a historic Apology to People of Color for APA's Role in Promoting, Perpetuating, and Failing to Challenge Racism, Racial Discrimination, and Human Hierarchy in the US. Drs. Awad and Gone, and Task Force members Kevin Cokley, Dr. Comas-Diaz, and I, are in the process of co-editing a forthcoming special issue of the *American Psychologist* on "Dismantling racism in the field of psychology and beyond."

Take Home Messages

I leave you with the following take home messages on editorial leadership as a mechanism for transforming the field of psychology and related disciplines to be more inclusive and rigorous.

- Don't give up! My career started on the margins of the field, and with the support of others, I moved into positions of influence.
- Read and write as much of the time as possible.
- Develop your expertise via publications.
- Create a professional network beyond your local one.
- Be a good citizen, accepting service and leadership roles. Get involved with professional organizations, such as the American Psychological Association or Society for Social Work Research. But be selective and be sure that the roles you accept are ones that will have an impact vs. cleaning up someone else's mess.
- As a reviewer, balance rigorous journal standards with inclusivity. Be conscientious, kind, and constructive. We are socialized to be critical and our default needs to be to see the potential in all work rather than finding reasons to exclude it.

- In editorial roles, mentor and advocate for students and junior colleagues, especially those from underrepresented groups.
- Take risks as an editor, getting your journal to "think outside the box." With great power comes great responsibility. You may have an opportunity to help your colleagues reach a wide audience with a publication in a flagship journal, extending their influence and impact on the field.

References and Resources

APA Journals (2021). *Equity, diversity, and inclusion toolkit for journal editors.* www.apa.org/pubs/authors/equity-diversity-inclusin-toolkit-journal-editors.pdf

Awad, G. H. (2010). The impact of acculturation and religious identification on perceived discrimination for Arab/Middle Eastern Americans. *Cultural Diversity and Ethnic Minority Psychology, 16*(1), 59–67. https://doi/10.1037/a0016675

Comas-Díaz, L., Hall, G. N., & Neville, H. A. (2019). Racial trauma: Theory, research, and healing: Introduction to the special issue. *American Psychologist, 74*(1), 1–5. https://doi/10.1037/amp0000442

Gone, J. P. (2009). A community-based treatment for Native American historical trauma: Prospects for evidence-based practice. *Journal of Consulting and Clinical Psychology, 77*(4), 751–762. https://doi/10.1037/a0015390

Syed, M. (2017). Why traditional metrics may not adequately represent ethnic minority psychology. *Perspectives on Psychological Science, 12*(6), 1162–1165. https://doi/10.1177/1745691617709590

Yip, T., Cheah, C. S. L., Kiang, L., & Hall, G. C. N. (2021). Rendered invisible: Are Asian Americans a model or a marginalized minority? *American Psychologist, 76*(4), 575–581. https://doi/10.1037/amp0000857

Zárate, M. A., Hall, G. N., & Plaut, V. C. (2017). Researchers of color, fame, and impact. *Perspectives on Psychological Science, 12*(6), 1176–1178. https://doi/10.1177/1745691617710511

Living Our Equity, Diversity, Inclusion, and Antiracism Values in the Academy

24

Engaging in Social Change Across Generations

Anneliese Singh[1], Brean'a Parker and Briana Bivens

We are writing this chapter as a collective of early-career (Brean'a and Briana) and mid-career, tenured (Anneliese) scholars, co-mentors, and higher education EDI (equity, diversity, inclusion) and antiracist practitioners – situated across different disciplines in education and social service professions – who worked together between 2016 and 2020 to shape DEI[2] (diversity, equity, inclusion), racial healing, and antiracist change in the Mary Frances Early College of Education (COE) at the University of Georgia. We are each positioned differently in relation to structural power, and we each hold a diverse range of social identities, knowledge, and experiences that shape how we engage in critical liberation work in the academy and in our communities (which we discuss in a moment). Now, after all our years working and dreaming together, we are finally writing together, reflecting on our shared leadership in a DEI Office and the qualities that made our collaboration so special, authentic, and transformative. Our hope is that our stories will inspire

---

1 Denotes shared first authorship.
2 Please note that we alternate use of "DEI," "EDI," "JEDI," "IDEA," and other important acronyms in the work.

DOI: 10.4324/9781003309796-28

you as a reader to not only own your own expertise in DEI work, but to also trust your lived experience as a guiding North Star for how you may (or may not) choose to contribute to DEI work in your personal and professional lives. Throughout this chapter, you will see us leaning into the freedom and joy that comes with using, alternating, problematizing, and uplifting different acronyms and terms in JEDI (justice, equity, diversity, inclusion) work.

The Roots of Our DEI Stories

When we think of our collective IDEA (inclusion, diversity, equity, access) journeys, we know that these journeys are rooted in our individual and family stories. We share our positionalities to help set the context for how and why the collective DEI work we engaged in unfolded, as well as to invite you as the reader to consider that DEI work is additive in many ways for Black, Indigenous, and People of Color (BIPOC). We should not have to engage in the work, and yet our personal lived experiences and our chosen paths of study often lead us down the metaphorical DEI road. In addition, we all have a DEI "origin" story. What is yours? Why is the work important to you? As we will share throughout this chapter, we have come to believe that BIPOC people should not have to lead the work to "undo" racism and other intersectional oppressions. Yet we have done so for multiple generations before and after abolitionist movements in the country we now call the United States of America. We have done this work because we have ancestors who have passed on to us clear visions of what liberation and freedom look and feel like. EDI work at its best follows this vision, seeks to manifest freedom, and helps people understand liberation for all as an attainable experience, process, and aim. Embodiment of the work is such a crucial part of JEDI strategy and change efforts. Just like your dissertation or that last article you published – and just like how many of us analyzed every lyric of Beyonce's *Renaissance* – doing IDEA work involves a series of goals, a systemic-change mindset, an understanding of the inevitable challenges and opportunities along the road of change, and embracing the joy and pleasure that come with the work of undoing intergenerational societal oppressions for humanity.

Anneliese's Story

The core of my journey to becoming a community organizer was seeded early on by my parents. As an interracial couple (South Asian immigrant father and white Southern multigenerational "American" mother), my parents raised me in the Sikh religion – teaching me that this spiritual tradition came with expectations of "seva" (community service) and that truthful living came in the form of compassion, love, and determination to ensure that all people were treated "equally." As a mixed-race child, I noticed the harsh realities of racism and xeno-prejudice that my family experienced. Amidst this racist content, I discovered my queer and genderqueer femme self in New Orleans, a city famed for its gender and sexual freedom. However the city's reputation was not a lived reality for everyday queer and trans BIPOC communities. I joined environmental activists fighting for clean water and air in poor and working-class Black and white communities and marched with the NO AIDS Project – eventually making and delivering meals to homebound people when people were dying from AIDS rather than living with HIV. I was fortunate to receive mentorship from countless queer and trans BIPOC community organizers, many of whom engaged in survival sex work and were the backbone of the New Orleans queer and trans community. As I pursued my graduate studies in counseling and counseling psychology respectively, I immediately noticed my activist communities were missing in the textbooks I was reading. When a peer passed along a job announcement for a tenure-track assistant professor at the University of Georgia that entailed building a social justice counseling doctoral program, the rampway into the professoriate appeared – as did my increased access to educational privilege and social class power. As I was becoming a full professor, I was asked by my Dean to serve as the inaugural Associate Dean of DEI in the college, and a dream-come-true began to unfold in the work with Brean'a and Briana as we built the DEI Office and embedded EDI values into the COE.

Breana's Story

I came into justice work through reading and learning about Black womxn, trans, non-binary, elders, and youth, whose ancestors experienced forced displacement during *Maafa*, a Swahili word depicting the genocide, terrorism, and forced enslavement of African ascendent people. As a Black womxn taught by my familial and cultural ancestors, family members, and mentors to use my voice, knowledge, and culturally grounded praxis to resist the hyper invisible forms of prejudice, erasure, and degradation of Black community members, I fell in love with storytelling and building community with people who were passionate, courageous, and unapologetic about resisting the multilayered forces of racism, sexism, homophobia, transphobia, and ableism among other forms of interlocking oppressions. Moreover, I fell in love with the knowledge of ancestors like bell hooks, Audre Lorde, Fannie Lou Hammer, and Ida B. Wells who fought tirelessly through creativity, community building, dream work, education, and active resistance to dismantle the dehumanization and violence toward Black communities. Moreover, I fell in love with how Black feminist, and radical queer feminism and womanism gave me not only words to document my experiences and those of others, but that it also introduced me to the human privilege of joy, pleasure, love, and building in and through relationships to counter the impact of oppression. This led me to become a counselor and later get my doctoral degree in counselor education and supervision. It was during this time that I committed myself to do intentional work in the same college I was training in and experienced institutional and programmatic forms of inequity – where I was also able to meet amazing accomplices in the fight for justice, equity, diversity, and inclusion. I joined Dr. Anneliese Singh to begin building the foundations of the DEI office and was able to create a large current of change when another co-conspirator, Briana Bivens, came into the office.

Briana's Story

I came to justice work through community organizing in the US South during my master's program, when I felt compelled to translate the feminist and anti-oppressive theory I was learning in the academy into concrete material change. Outside of my graduate studies and restaurant serving job, I spent several hours each week working on electoral campaigns, in non-profit organizations (*Athens for Everyone* and the *Economic Justice Coalition*), and with grassroots collectives to lead political education and capacity-building workshops, coordinate volunteer recruitment, and shape organizational process and strategy – all with the aim of advancing racial, social, and economic justice through local and state policy change. I embraced this work with an open-minded curiosity and a deep desire to hone my capacity to contribute ethically to justice work as a white woman who benefited from educational privilege and family wealth. I grew up in a politically conservative family, and neither my parents nor my older sibling graduated from college, so my critical educational studies and political advocacy generated familial suspicion, if not backlash. This background served as a constant reminder for me of all the (un)learning I had to do, an undeniably lifelong process made more possible and enjoyable in community. To join Anneliese and Brean'a in the Office of DEI, then, seemed like a fantastic next step! I strived to not only engage with the transformative work taking root within the academy, but also to grow the circle of accountability and care I had begun crafting in community spaces. My collaboration and friendship with Anneliese and Brean'a has been nothing short of life-changing for me. I experienced the true joy and magic of what it looks like to be part of truly caring, just, and accountable relationships modeled off the same JEDI values motivating our shared scholarly and advocacy work.

Living Our JEDI Values: Putting Diversity, Equity, and Inclusion into Action with Antiracism as a Foundation

The Office of DEI, as we built it to be, was not just some bureaucratic arm, a space for the university to perform lukewarm DEI values. Those of us who had a hand in crafting the office saw it as a transformative changemaking space. Embedded in a historically white state flagship institution, we knew we couldn't take this aspiration for granted. Ahmed (2017) reminded us of the tendency for universities to claim the existence of the diversity, equity, and inclusion office as itself the enactment of diversity, equity, and inclusion – a sort of mechanical box-checking. So to do something different – something bolder, more transformative – took intention, trust, and deep collaboration. To realize our aspirational DEI space, we saw it as our charge to create programming and advocate for policy change that advanced equity and justice in our college, but also to be "in right relationship" (Brown, 2017, p. 24) with each other in the ethical and sociopolitical frameworks shaping our office programming and our personal commitments to the work.

As a BIPOC scholar, once you have explored your own positionality, assessed why DEI efforts are important to you, and reflected on aligning your practice with DEI values, it is helpful to have an organizing framework and to establish a common vocabulary in the work. There were important moments where we as a team and COE community slowed down and got clear about a common vocabulary. For our community, "diversity" was an important hallmark term that reflected the intergenerational resistance work of Black and other BIPOC scholars in education and counseling that called for access, justice, and belonging for BIPOC communities within higher education. Our community defined "inclusion" as a term that recognized that all people with historically marginalized identities had a "voice" and a way to communicate their needs, and inclusion denoted a collective commitment to uplifting these voices and ensuring a metaphorical seat at the decision-making table. Snuggled between "diversity" and "inclusion" was the term of accountability –

"equity," which our community defined as the central organizing work of all our justice and liberation work and meant that we sought to build a community in our COE where equity was normative and an expected process and outcome. As we paused to develop this common vocabulary, we were able to articulate that we all embraced intersectionality as a guiding theoretical framework (Crenshaw, 1989). This meant that the aim to dismantle systemic racism wherever we could – in the policies, procedures, and practices within our DEI Office and within our college – required naming and addressing the multiple systems of oppression that complexify, intensify, and work alongside racism.

Building JEDI Infrastructure Within the College of Education

Once we immersed ourselves in the current scholarship of IDEA change efforts within higher education and examined existing qualitative and quantitative data within our college, we were ready to design, develop, and implement DEI interventions and activities. We cannot emphasize enough how important it was to continue building our relationships with one another and our support of one another which served as a foundation of trust and embodiment that we could rely on when resistance and pushback arose in the college and university. Our relationships served as a liberatory template for how we interacted with others in JEDI change with compassion, accountability, and truth-telling in some of our interventions below. They include the following:

1. **Staff DEI retreats.** Annual staff retreats were in alignment with our praxis of slowing down and reflecting on the work we have done within and set out to do within our college. This was also an opportunity to celebrate, connect, and become re-grounded with the work we collectively committed ourselves to doing. The retreats were essential to checking in on our well-being while also getting away to engage in play, joy, and dream work necessary to continue to make change.
2. **Educational DEI workshops and webinars.** A major foundational principle was the role of education, training, and opportunities for COE faculty, staff, and students to learn about what JEDI encompassed and their responsibility in creating a learning, training, and physical environment that was both inclusive and affirming to people who held intersectional identities and lived experiences. Our educational workshops were

focused on moving attendees from awareness, knowledge, and skills in IDEA work to JEDI action to uplift BIPOC, queer and trans, international, women, disabled, and other historically marginalized communities.

3. **Annual DEI conference.** While we did not invent the concept of an annual DEI conference, we opened up these conferences to community members, students, and staff, when traditionally it was only open to faculty. We invited faculty, staff, and students across the five department areas to participate as a conference committee to mobilize around a social justice theme – such as intergroup dialogue, radical self-love and disability justice, racism and classism – and discuss how we can get folx involved in presenting sessions, trainings, and workshops at the conference.

4. **Exploring White Privilege Group.** Our office also coordinated the "Exploring White Privilege Group," conceptualized as a space for well-meaning white folx to come together to dialogue about how to contribute to antiracist action without taking over or re-centering whiteness. Students, faculty, and staff met monthly to participate in the dialogue, and we often structured our conversation around a particular resource or concept, such as Singh's (2019) racial healing prompts from *The Racial Healing Handbook*.

5. **Graduate Students of Color Research Mentoring (GSOCRM) program.** As an office situated within the academy, we were acutely aware of how inequity, underrepresentation, and lack of access existed within our college specifically for BIPOC graduate students. This led to the creation of the Graduate Students of Color Research Mentoring Program, which offered graduate students access to Faculty of Color and transformative intellectuals to learn about topics such as grant writing, navigating tenure and promotion, engaging in transformative and radical scholarship, and academic writing. This cohort-based group utilized horizontal mentorship, which encompasses mentorship and the sharing of knowledge and experience by everyone, in contrast to the traditional top-down intellectual–learner model.

6. **Faculty of Color Thriving program.** We were aware of the differential experiences of Faculty of Color and the impact of navigating predominantly white institutions on the persistence and sustainability of BIPOC faculty. Thus, imperative to our mission and value of JEDI was having monthly spaces for Faculty of Color to discuss challenges and barriers, provide support and mentorship networks, and learn how students can pour back into faculty to support their thriving.

7. **Build community and capacity.** Oftentimes what can make this work feel laborious and impossible to sustain is that we are often working in silos or alone. Thus, we need a network of helpers with various resources, talents, connections, and natural abilities to create a system of justice, resistance, and transformation. You cannot do this on your own, so begin building your community and resource capacity not only for the work, but also for the community of support and healing.

8. **Center the margins.** In alignment with the work of bell hooks (1984), centering the margins requires that our goals and ethics are aligned with those of community members and organizations that are currently engaging in this work. This step requires that we work in collaboration with advocates and co-conspirators across campus and across our community. We recognize that while we have diverse perspectives, knowledge, and information, our advocacy, training, and supportive spaces are enriched when we center members at the margins of our hierarchical society, both in the creation and execution of our work. Centering the margins within our topics and makeup of our committees, facilitators, and consultants both held us accountable, while also helping to ensure that our work was in alignment with justice and liberative action.

9. **Bring in "outside" voices.** In higher education we sometimes have the habit of *preaching to the choir*, e.g., engaging in conversations with people who are like-minded and occupy the same space as we do. The greatest thinkers, creators, and radical agitators are both within and outside the ivory tower. When we connect and bring in the work, voices, and bodies of community members who are already intimately engaging in justice-based and equity-grounded work we begin to expand how we can engage in systemic change and transformation.

10. **Embrace the intergenerational, abolitionist, and liberatory work of JEDI.** Reading abolitionist and liberatory works and connecting with community organizers who embodied DEI change work held us accountable to a larger vision of where DEI work "fit" in the larger intergenerational movements of social justice change. For example, our relationships with students (e.g., Marques Dexter, Bekah Estevez, Elizabeth Cardenas Bautista) across multiple disciplines provided us with the opportunity to "live" the social justice texts they were reading in their courses alongside them. Our relationships with faculty across rank and power (e.g., Drs. Cynthia Dillard, Bettina Love, Darris Means, Chris Linder, Chris Mojock, Ed Delgado-Romero) helped us mobilize faculty to move out of their micro-expertise worlds to engage in collective

social justice action and mutual accountability. Our staff, alumni, and community-based relationships (e.g., with Broderick Flanigan, Julia Butler-Mayes, Umesh Patel, Chris Risse, Andy Garber, Meg Evans, Rashad Small) kept our work viable in the "real world" in terms of accessibility and accountability for our change efforts.

11. **Understand resistance and "good trouble."** Situated as we were in the public flagship institution in a state that has long been hostile to justice work, we knew our antiracist, anti-oppressive efforts would meet resistance. Yet, because we built a community around our work, we felt more equipped to confront institutional resistance and justify our office programs and activities as the collective brainchildren of a diverse coalition of students, faculty, and staff that they were. We also remembered that resistance is an inevitable feature of authentic JEDI work, because the work entails rearranging power relations, challenging the status quo, and interrogating how the communities and institutions where we live, learn, and work have been complicit in systemic oppression.

12. **Capture the work.** Taking pictures, keeping a narrative journal of what we have accomplished, assessing how people feel they have changed because of us and our work, and celebrating our achievements are ways that we are able to capture (think photograph) and genuinely reflect on our work. Moreover, this is how most movements are known to us today because their legacy is kept alive by someone recording what they did and the impact the work had on liberation.

Conclusion

As we end this chapter, we hope that you are reminded to trust yourself as a BIPOC scholar and the wisdom and blueprint of your ancestors. We certainly did as we came together as a collective DEI Office to engage in JEDI change in a way we never expected to do. By reflecting on our own relationships, practices, and activities we facilitated in a DEI Office, we hope to offer a reimagining of what JEDI work can "look like" within and outside of higher education.

References

Ahmed, S. (2017). *Living a feminist life*. Duke University Press. https://doi.org/10.1215/9780822373377

Brown, a. m. (2017). *Emergent strategy: Shaping change, changing worlds*. AK Press.

Crenshaw, K. (1989). Demarginalizing the intersection of race and sex: A black feminist critique of antidiscrimination doctrine, feminist theory and antiracist politics. *University of Chicago Legal Forum*, 1(8), 139–167.

hooks, b. (1984). *Feminist theory: From margin to center.* South End Press.

Singh, A. A. (2019). *The racial healing handbook: Practical activities to help you challenge privilege, confront systemic racism & engage in collective healing.* New Harbinger Publications.

Rooted in Justice and Joy

25

Collaborative Organizational Development

Jeannette Pai-Espinosa

Why Write This?

My goal in writing this chapter is to share honestly, candidly, and clearly – as a woman of color – about my process of being and becoming in a white supremacist, patriarchal world. From my heart to yours, I share wisdom gleaned from decades of struggle, challenges, lessons learned – **and joy**. Data and facts, like everything else, can be manipulated to make invisible, judge, dismiss, and oppress those of us who don't fit neatly into socially constructed boxes. Less quantifiable are the bonds that women of color build with one another – the support after a difficult company meeting, the laughter over lunch, the happy hours where we decompress in solidarity. The veracity and wisdom that comes from our own experience can only be questioned if we allow it. I stand behind every word on these pages, and hope you will see your reflection in them – as validation for what you, too, have experienced, as insights regarding what you might be experiencing now, or what may be coming down the road. My hope is that the **nine insights** I share with you in this chapter will resonate in your heart and mind to remind you that you are not alone; that you're not imagining the microaggressions; that you are, in any given moment, so much more than enough; and that you, and we, are powerful beyond our wildest imagination – otherwise why would they work so hard to keep us down?

DOI: 10.4324/9781003309796-29

The Backdrop

In 2006, I stepped into the role of leading a team of two (including me) in the reinvention of The National Florence Crittenton Mission, founded in 1883 to support the needs and potential of "wayward and fallen" girls, young women, and women across the country. Seventeen years into this adventure and several name and brand modifications later, we changed our name in 2023 to align with the heart and soul of who we are today. Today, I am the President of the (renamed) Justice and Joy National Collaborative and our tagline is ". . . unapologetic advocacy." It has been a long and interesting adventure wrapped in unpredictable challenges and successes – more on this later.

Up until the point that I accepted the position, I had been fortunate to have had an amazing set of professional experiences and opportunities, journeying through different positions in public and private higher education, local government, and consulting, and enjoying the scenic route of a not-so-traditional, not-so-linear path. There was no blueprint that guided me, but rather a set of choices made to accept, stay, and move on from jobs, guided by my core values and my deep commitment to advancing justice on all fronts.

Staffing the watchdog work of local human and social service commissions, and being a senior staff member for a Governor of Oregon and responsible for overseeing affirmative action in all 119 state agencies made me a target and scapegoat. This confirmed for me the need to build and nurture strong alliances and trust with the communities most impacted by the issues being addressed because we are so much stronger and authentic together. As Audre Lorde (1979) said, "Without community, there is no liberation." My career has been grounded by my commitment to lead from the center and guided by the mantra of "nothing about us without us,"[1] not only because it is the right thing to do, but because it was and is, for women of color, a matter of survival. I recall, as many of you may, many sleepless nights calculating whether it was time to leave a job before I was kicked out, because for change agents who work from within systems and organizations to change them, that is our reality. The clock is always ticking, and feeling safe is a mirage. As challenging as this sounds, our truth is the awakening, passion and strength experienced when people step into their own power. The resulting collective power is well worth the time we spend looking over our shoulders.

---

1 A phrase invoked by South African disability rights activists in the 1990s.

My Herstory (in Brief)

I am the child of activists. My ancestors fought for Korean independence. My mother worked at Planned Parenthood, and my father was a college professor. I was the first to be born in the United States on both sides of my Korean family, and grew up in New Jersey, Missouri, and Kansas in predominantly white, conservative communities. Most of my friends were white but I gravitated to anyone of color with whom I could establish a relationship. In grade school, I played and ate with the few kids of color in the school who were Black and Native American. Although it was segregation that placed us together, our solidarity in shared experiences – even if we couldn't articulate our "otherness" at the time – was a joyful and an enriching part of my childhood.

The everyday indignities, casual and outright racism, and xenophobia we experienced served as constant reminders that we didn't fit in, much less matter. It was clear that it wasn't safe to be me. My friends and parents taught me that community can also be built through resistance, and activism was often where we found it. Truly, the need and search for belonging and acceptance is a life-long journey. If we are fortunate, our families provide a foundation. But the road is long and we travel much of it alone, until we feel in our hearts that we belong and can accept ourselves, no longer dependent on the expectations of others and the social norms and practices that attempt to define and confine us.

My husband is from Mexico, and over more than 36 years together with our four children, we have built a life, careers, an extended family, and a diverse community that resonates with the kind of belonging and acceptance that comes from the hearts of those who have lived many moments of "otherness." We have cultivated our otherness into joy, and steered our children to do the same. It has not been a straight or easy path and there have been plenty of unfortunate side trips, but guided by love and the core shared values of compassion, justice, humility, authenticity, inclusion, and responsibility, the way forward reveals itself – sometimes just in time.

The Challenge

With my professional and personal backdrop, I stepped into the job with Crittenton believing that it was possible, together with others, to create an intergenerational, collaborative, powerful organization free from the vestiges of oppression and patriarchy. A place where women of color across generations can safely bring their whole selves. Where we can be all that we are and aren't with transparency, vulnerability, bravery, humor, brilliance, and more, in order to exert our power to change the world. The challenge before me was to lead an organization's reinvention aligned with a vision and set of values informed by my own experiences, positive and negative, and by the collective experience of the myriad women of color that I have had the honor of working with over the more than six decades of life and work.

Interestingly, the values of Mr. Charles Crittenton and Dr. Kate Waller Barrett, National Crittenton's founders, were in many ways similar to mine, though seen and experienced through a very different lens and time. I could not shake my disbelief and my rage at the depths of the invisibility of girls, specifically those who were system impacted and of color. In 2004, there was no national advocacy presence, and this has changed very little since then, though across the country the movement for girls and gender-expansive young people has grown. Systems do what they were designed to do: distracting us from our own needs, ignoring our deepest truth and power, and preventing collaboration. Yet once we shake free, we change the game.

On January 1, 2007 I woke up in a panic. Despite my professional successes and lived experience, insecurities and doubts stemming from internalized oppression flooded my head and heart. My ideas on shared power and collective action had always been threatening to people, organizations, and institutions entrenched in rugged American individualism. We are stronger together, and gatekeepers know that. I was reminded again that our socialization to white patriarchal norms is so ingrained, effective, and insidious that often we are **complicit in our own oppression**, and that of our allies. There have been countless times in my life when persistent internalized oppression popped up in the form of self-doubt, imposter syndrome, and fear of inadequacy, even today at age 66. It passes more quickly now, but it still arises. I wonder what my younger self might have done differently had I understood that it was almost never about my inadequacies. I can see now that in my younger years, my internalized oppression often made me part of the problem – part of what propped up the system by justifying inequity in the name of equality, largely by holding myself and others back. When we hold ourselves back, we prop up the status quo and risk becoming part of the problem and creating barriers to change. Healthy self-reflection is important, but self-sabotage is often disguised as excessive self-doubt. By sharing our truths across generations and addressing our internalized oppression, we sustain and support each other, ensure that we are not part of the problems we are working to solve, and step into our unmitigated power.

The reinvention of National Crittenton was intentionally built on a set of core values – compassion, justice, humility, authenticity, inclusion, and responsibility – intended to transform the oppressive systems that shaped us. Today, as the Justice and Joy National Collaborative, we are an intergenerational, multiracial, multiethnic organizing and advocacy team of 25 women of color ranging in age from 23 to 66. We collaboratively work as a team and with external partners to advance social, economic, and political equity to ensure that young People of Color can live unapologetic lives without fear of violence or injustice. We are silo busters using a root cause approach in our advocacy. We are intentionally intergenerational because the experiences, wisdom, and leadership of girls and gender-expansive young People of Color must be at the forefront of social change, but we also know and hear from them that they want and need support from allies with different perspectives and decades of lessons learned. It is the give and take that is critical to constructing an enduring ecosystem for gender and racial justice that encompasses many organizations, leaders, and movements that together can withstand the test of time and stop decisions like the Supreme Court ruling on *Dobbs v Jackson*.[2]

The Way Forward

Leadership that is adaptive, conversations that are vulnerable and courageous, and an iterative practice of unlearning the cis heteronormative white supremacist patriarchy sustains the advocacy ecosystem. This has never been clearer than in recent years as we have witnessed the fragility of our democracy. Young People of Color in particular are demonstrating that merely surviving isn't enough; we deserve dignity, joy, rest, and safety. Our liberation is intertwined, and when historically oppressed, excluded, and marginalized communities show up for one another, we heal together, strengthen movements, and disrupt the status quo.

---

2 *Dobbs v. Jackson Women's Health Organization* is a US Supreme Court Ruling, decided in June 2022, that the Constitution does not confer a right to abortion, overturning *Roe v. Wade* and *Planned Parenthood of Southeastern Pa v. Casey* and paving the way for states to ban abortion.

The insights shared below emerge from my experiences, observations, and lessons garnered over nearly 50 years of activism, starting in the seventies as a college student. I share them (in no particular order) with the hope that they will support you in some way during your own journey of being and becoming.

- **Live your life and do your work guided by a set of unwavering core values.** Women of color at all phases in our lives are pressured to produce, nurture, fight, succeed, persevere, thrive, compromise, and, above all, feel "grateful" for the opportunity. As a result, I believe that for women of color across the span of our lives, our core values are a super power and an essential survival skill that we often do not recognize in ourselves. Each day, we face choices that require us to weigh what or who is worth making a sacrifice or fighting for, because we are always aware that we live life "at risk of." This is not martyrdom; it is the reality that society and systems were never built with us in mind and we were never expected to survive, much less thrive. These values ground us and fuel our passion, dedication, courage, and brilliance. Values are the bedrock of our bottom line. Moreover, we instinctively know that shared values can be used to reframe disagreement or conflict, to get people pulling in the same direction rather than being locked into opposing positions. Living a values-driven life is a superpower, so let's seize it.

- **Shift your thinking to one of radical abundance.** Internalized oppression and inadequacy coupled with the fear of letting each other down propels us toward scarcity rather than abundance. We know that scarcity is a myth created by those who hoard power and control, but that myth has disastrous impacts if we allow it to go unchecked. Operating from a center grounded in abundance opens the door to collective power, impact, and liberation, creating unlimited opportunities for leveraging shared knowledge, resources, connections, and more. Growing power as we share it.

- **Recognize and dismantle white patriarchal capitalist competition in your work and life.** There is no doubt that white patriarchal capitalism pits people and groups against one another. Community agreements and recurring practices of self-reflection and evaluation can help mitigate misunderstandings, assumptions, and biases that affect the collective work. But we must never forget that society and systems of oppression function as they were intended – to separate, police, and polarize those deemed to be "the other." We must be vigilant in supporting each other to avoid playing into the oppressor's hands. We must see the success of others in the movement as ours, too. Perhaps most importantly, we must recognize how deeply internalized oppression lives in all of us, whether we are 12 or 92. We must support each other in identifying it and supporting each other as we actively refuse to be a tool of oppression by silencing ourselves and others.

- **Don't become a gatekeeper.** As a consultant working on a wide array of strategic communication and public awareness campaigns, I saw, time and again, passionate advocates who, intentionally or not, became barriers in the narrative shifting and courageous conversation efforts in which they were deeply involved. As advocates, we need to engage in ongoing introspection to ensure that we don't become the gatekeepers trying to control and "own" the conversation, determining the tactics and solutions without input. In a world where power exists in the hands of the few, we must always check our individual need for power and control, and interrogate ourselves about the biases that we hold about the groups we are trying to reach and engage.

- **Create courageous spaces.** Our ability to trust is profoundly entwined with the events that have caused us to experience trauma as individuals, families, cultural groups, and as a society. At National Crittenton, we have grappled with how to create a safe space for our very diverse team of women of color across the age range of 23 to 66, with vastly different life experiences, to be able to have tough conversations. In the end, we have shifted our focus to creating *courageous* spaces because there is always the possibility that we will unintentionally hurt each other. We cannot guarantee anyone's safety and it seems disingenuous to claim that we can. While we are still crafting our courageous space, we know it must make room for vulnerability, mistakes, restorative practices, mutual support, and commitment to continuing the dialogue.

- **Engage the leadership of those most impacted.** "Nothing about us without us" is a commonly articulated principle these days. Clearly, raising issues and creating solutions for pressing issues must always be led and informed by those most impacted. Their voices and experiences help guide us to identifying and eradicating root causes, while also addressing specific problems rather than simply solving problems in isolation. Bandages don't heal blood clots; the same logic applies here too. But often we fall short by asking them to share their wisdom and then advocating on their behalf, or scripting them like a commercial for our work. When we advocate for those who can do so for themselves, we embody the colonizer mindset. When we put words in their mouths, we have added ourselves to the list of people and organizations who have exploited them.

- **Context does matter.** In all that we do, we partner with girls, young women, and gender expansive young People of Color with lived experience as leaders and advocates. They bring the sum total of their past and present life experiences into every room and situation. But once in the room, they are viewed within a different context, whether it is a hearing room in Washington, DC, a conference, or a workplace. We often forget that when we invite them to share the context of their lives in these spaces, they are received and often judged against the values and standards of everyone in that room, suddenly shifting the context of their lives forever. We must meet them where they are, and we must apply equitable empathy rather than equal standards for performance and participation. We must provide support and time for reflection, utilize liberatory feedback and asset framing strategies.

- **Cultivate a culture where mistakes are welcome.** We live in a world where perfect lives and people portrayed in social media collide with our very real imperfection, our complex journey to self-acceptance, internalized oppression and the drive to prove that we are the best. Somewhere along the path, we have forgotten that we learn by making mistakes – that they are a sign of our courage and growth. We cannot be afraid of making mistakes and should welcome and embrace them by building cultures of work and relationships that support us in doing so.

- **Create and embrace your joy.** In the early days of the COVID-19 pandemic, I decided to order flowers to be delivered to myself on the first Friday of every month. I love flowers and harbor a dream of being a florist when I retire. The joy I felt when they arrived was special and still makes me smile today – a stark contrast to the bleakness of social isolation and uncertainty of that time. I was 63 when I placed that monthly order and remembered how simple it is to create my own moments of joy, even during a pandemic. I knew this before, but in the pressures of life, work, travel, and world events, I lost sight of it. Today, creating those moments of joy for myself with family and friends is a priority, as it should be for all of us.

Closing

I am and have been honored to be surrounded by an intergenerational community of women of color, along with some trusted white allies, who mutually nurture, support, and challenge each other to work toward our collective liberation. Through mistakes and successes, betrayals and loyalties, laughter and tears, I hope the insights I have shared here will resonate with your past experiences or illuminate a situation with which you are currently struggling. To the mental health professionals of color reading this, I thank you for stepping into this work with your head and hearts. Be fearless as advocates for healing, health, and justice. How different the lives of girls and gender expansive young People of Color will be because you will bring your perspective and experiences into the work.

References and Resources

Brafman, O., & Beckstrom, R. A. (2006). The starfish and the spider: *The unstoppable power of leaderless organizations*. Penguin Group.

Collins, J. (2005). *Good to great and the social sectors: Why business thinking is not the answer.* Harper Business.

Kennedy, F. R. (1976). *Color me Flo: My hard life and good times*. Prentice Hall.

Lorde, A. (1979). The personal or the political – II/Conference on feminist theory, 1979 (Tape 1), Lesbian Herstory Archives AudioVisual Collections. http://herstories. prattinfoschool.nyc/omeka/items/show/50

Lorde, A. (1984). *The master's tools will never dismantle the master's house* (Comments at the "The personal and the political panel," Second Sex Conference, New York, September 29, 1979). In *Sister outsider*. Sister Visions Press. (Original work published 1979)

Schaef, A. W. (1981). Women's reality: An emerging female system in the White male society. Winston Press.

Leading and Managing While BIPOC

26

Emphasis on Goal Not Role

Linda Lausell Bryant

I begin writing with this question for myself, and also for you: Looking back at your career so far, or looking forward to the career you desire, what would make it transformative? After 37 years in social work, spanning middle, senior, and executive leadership roles in non-profit and governmental agencies, and now in the academy, I reflect on my career as a Puerto Rican Afro-Latina woman and first-generation college graduate. I have served in a range of roles, including division director, associate commissioner, and executive director, which was a dream come true for me and my entire family. While I am deeply grateful for every career opportunity I have had, my standards for what constitutes a transformative career are evolving.

Workplaces in the mental health field, whether psychiatry, psychology, social work, marriage and family therapy, or academia, can be centers of race-based stress, despite the elegantly articulated codes of conduct that guide these professions. Neither classrooms, board rooms, therapy rooms, nor conference rooms are exempt from racism, prejudice, and biased beliefs, attitudes, and perspectives. These beliefs and attitudes can, and often do, become codified in the policies, protocols, practices, and cultures of organizations and institutions. Think of the case of an organization that celebrates its colorblind hiring of clinicians for a largely Black and Brown clientele, in pursuit of only the "most highly qualified" clinicians, which turns

DOI: 10.4324/9781003309796-30

out to be those with psychoanalytic institute training. There are likely good intentions, assumptions, and blind spots underlying this approach and these will all impact the services that BIPOC people receive. For all who are in, or pursuing leadership roles, there are many such dilemmas of conflicting values and perspectives. How can you avoid replicating racially biased perspectives and practices in a managerial role? It is helpful to contemplate these questions, in the context of your own history as a Person of Color. Cultivating a practice of self-reflection can be an important tool for those who are in these positions and those who aspire to be.

The Leadership Lens

Like so many people in the helping professions, I received no training in leadership throughout my post-secondary education. What I gleaned through observation was that leadership meant being in charge, responsible, and making sure that work got done by people, which to me meant working hard and taking care of people, being a "good" boss. I was well into my tenure as the CEO of the youth-serving non-profit organization when I was introduced to the adaptive leadership framework, developed at the Harvard Kennedy School by Ron Heifetz and Marty Linsky. I appreciated the conceptualization of leadership as separate and distinct from position or role, with the implication that anyone could take up leadership. According to Heifetz et al. (2009), leadership is not centered on a single person identified as the leader. Leadership however, is action, activity, a practice for bringing about change. Authority, on the other hand, is related to role and position and is often conflated with leadership.

Consistent with this framework, in this chapter, I refer to management as connected to your role of authority (director, supervisor, etc.) where you are distributing, organizing, and directing behaviors in order to accomplish a work-related goal or task. Leadership or leading is about activity that focuses on mobilizing people to do the hard work of change, not relying on authority. I found this framework to mesh well with social work, with its focus on changing systems, and engaging multiple perspectives. It anchors my leadership practice in inclusion, welcoming different perspectives, and engaging multiple shareholders within the system. If I am leaning mostly on my own ideas, it is my cue to pursue other perspectives. Good ideas can come from many sources and I want to create a climate where people feel that their ideas are welcomed, listened to, and explored. When I joined New York University in 2015, I brought adaptive leadership into our social work curriculum to address the dearth of leadership development training for social workers. While a full description of adaptive leadership is beyond the scope of this chapter, I have included recommended resources in the references. The next sections of this chapter will discuss aspects of my own history and lessons learned.

The Endless Audition

My sense of what I needed for professional success had been conditioned as far back as my childhood growing up in Brooklyn, New York and Carolina, Puerto Rico. Success looked like American (white) culture and white people seemed to own success in a way that other groups did not, especially immigrants and Black and Brown people, like me. I consumed a steady diet of messages at school and at home that encouraged assimilation to American white culture (Liu et al., 2019). Although Puerto Ricans have been US citizens since 1917, the lived experience is overwhelmingly one of an outsider, even as we board airplanes to and from Puerto Rico without a passport. I learned that the real "passport" to success is tied to speaking English without a Spanish accent and keeping other tell-tale signs of our culture hidden, willingly assimilating. This is a perverse trade-off even if the intention was to help me succeed in a context that was not friendly to Puerto Ricans. Sadly, what I learned was that I could succeed as long as I relinquished my own culture and pledged allegiance to the dominant culture. I learned that this is the price of success. The table was set for the emergence of the imposter phenomenon.

Imposter phenomenon has been described by Clance and Imes (1978) as a debilitating mental state marked by feelings of incompetence and of being a professional fraud. I had already internalized the need to prove that I had the "goods." Behaviorally, this manifested as strong gratitude for every opportunity, which I saw as a blessing, rather than something that I had earned or deserved. It also showed up as a willingness to work harder, longer, and beyond my scope, to establish that I was not just good enough, but exceptional. Regardless of my titles and rank, I have consistently been the worker with the largest caseload, the largest portfolio, and the least amount of tangible support. Psychologically, I have experienced my career as an endless audition. It doesn't matter how many times I get the "role." Every day is an audition to prove that choosing me was a sound decision. Accompanying my imposter phenomenon is a cluster of personal work survival traits that I have coined my *"Pendejita* Syndrome." The term *pendeja* or its diminutive form, *pendejita* (little pendeja) is a Spanish profanity that is roughly translated to mean *idiot, dummy, gullible, fool.* If I were describing Pendejita Syndrome for the DSM-5, it would consist of a cluster of behaviors such as people pleasing, extreme self-sacrificing, self-deprecation, prioritizing the needs of others over my own. I am a recovering *pendejita*, resisting this self-deprecating description, with compassion for "Little Linda" who did not know better.

Social Work, Management and Leadership: Home Training

A range of strengths developed because of, or in spite of, my upbringing. These strengths have played a key role throughout my career. The pressure of growing up female, and the oldest child in a Puerto Rican household in the 1960s and 70s, helped me to develop a strong sense of responsibility. I learned to spring into action before being asked. My mother's sharp tone stating, "Can't you see that the floor needs sweeping? I should not have to tell you," taught me to observe my environment, to identify work that was needed, and to act without being asked. I learned to listen to the adults speaking, to read between the lines, sense tensions, and solve problems, mediate and keep peace. My brother, who is two years younger than me, was babied and indulged by my mother. In contrast, I was expected to be a little adult. This double standard and emphasis on my housekeeping skills infuriated me. Nonetheless, I was a "good girl" and delivered what was expected of me. I was often angry on the inside at this perceived injustice. I channeled these emotions into excelling in school, where I received validation for my academic strengths and even my athletic skills. In school sports I could be as tough as I wanted, without penalty for not conforming to girly gender expectations. I learned how to project strength, even if I felt scared. This is consistent with characteristics of the "Superwoman Schema" which include the obligation to show strength and help others (Woods-Giscombé, 2010). I was "Supergirl" growing into a "Superwoman."

I learned the value of hard work, and graduated high school, as valedictorian, at 16. At 20, I became my family's first college graduate. A few years later, I pursued my MSW and later my PhD in social work, another first in our family. I embodied and embraced being that exception, that model student, daughter, and worker.

Dilemmas in Leading and Managing While BIPOC

In the range of leadership roles that I have held, I have faced dilemmas, gained wisdom (and weight), while losing sleep due to stress. On one hand, I felt fortunate to be in these roles, where I was often breaking gender or racial-ethnic barriers and was inspired by the possibility of working for change. On the other hand, I felt the tension of being a representative of and co-conspirator with some values that I did not share. As I got more experience in more organizations, I began to see a pattern of conflicting values permeating the entire human services apparatus that serves BIPOC youth, adults, and families as clients. I was vexed by the "soft bigotry" of low expectations for the BIPOC young people and their families that I was working with. I observed the never-ending dance for funding, which I describe crudely as an exercise in "packaging" BIPOC people to be sufficiently appealing to, and worthy of, a donor's interest and dollars. In practice, this looked like telling the story of a client's most grueling traumas, and pairing it with evidence of their amazing resilience and potential to become a triumphant success, indeed, one of the "exceptions." Even though this would be carried out with a level of compassion, it would trigger a tightness in the pit of my stomach because I felt complicit in showcasing their pain in order to get resources to help alleviate their pain. I also felt identified with them because their stories could have been the story of any of my family members or me.

The emotions that surfaced were a mix of shame, rage, and helplessness. Despite effort and skill to fundraise with compassion, consent, finesse, and sophistication, this isn't uncommon in human services for poorer BIPOC people. This unresolved tension is rooted in the history of charities and social services in the US with its embedded racially biased perspectives (Salomon, 2012; Miller & Garran, 2017).

When I was CEO of a non-profit agency for pregnant and parenting teens in foster care, our annual fundraising gala would celebrate youth honorees along with corporate honorees. I experienced a conflict between helping our attendees experience the humanity of the young people and the question of whether we were prostituting our clients to help us raise funds. That was neither our goal nor intention, but I found myself interrogating the ethics of this. As a BIPOC CEO, in a ballroom of over 500 current and prospective donors, I also felt like I was on display, as the embodiment of what our young clients could be and that our donors could support. Even writing this, I feel the familiar knot in my stomach. Despite many good intentions, the whole non-profit system based on charitable help has an air of superior benevolence that fails to address fundamental structural inequities. Why should we have to package and sell the stories or anyone's pain for charitable donations? What impact does it have on BIPOC people to be the consistent "face" of need for charitable social services? (Schaffer, 2016; Wake, 2021).

In the early 2000s, many funders were focused on the concept of ROI (return on investment). Service provider agencies were expected to articulate a broad algorithm describing the ROI for their funding dollars, for example, every teen pregnancy prevented saves a certain amount of dollars in future public assistance costs. So many young people are in circumstances through no fault of their own, and the case for caring should be based on more than reducing our tax burden. Why not make the case that supporting young people to have every chance to succeed is a wise investment for all of us? As parents, do we invest in our children to help them fulfill their potential? Or to prevent them from draining our resources later in life? Why then should we think about funding services for youth in this way? I think the lens matters. These are some of the ways in which I experienced the seeds and fruits of racism showing up in managing and leading social services agencies.

Lessons Not Learned and Trophies Earned

What I did not learn in my early career was that being an exception is not enough. We won't achieve equity or inclusion by including a few exceptions in demographically and culturally white organizations, like decorative chocolate sprinkles on a vanilla-frosted cake. I did *not* learn that working hard could also include boundaries and respect for other dimensions of my life, like rest, exercise, joy, and time for loved ones. I didn't learn how to ask for help. My orientation was one of sacrifice, striving to succeed at all costs because I felt a responsibility, as one of so few in these spaces, to represent my whole ethnic group. I felt that my success was success for every Puerto Rican person and that my failure would reinforce the belief that we all are failures. That's quite a load to carry and this is not a unique experience. Many of my BIPOC colleagues attest to taking on the burden of representing their groups.

In my 37-year career, I have received awards, recognitions and other "trophies" which have come with a concomitant cluster of what I like to call "sad" trophies, testaments to both the lessons I learned so well, and the ones I didn't. These sad trophies include exhaustion, anxiety, depression, obesity, hypertension, breast cancer, knee replacements, and all of their aftermaths. Fortunately, I have been blessed with teachers, colleagues, sister-friends, a loving husband and children, and a great therapist, all who support me in revising those early lessons and forming new insights and wisdom.

Reflections on Managing and Leading While BIPOC

My subjective experience of leading and managing while BIPOC has been one of having multiple jobs within one job title. Being BIPOC is not just my identity, but on the job, this identity is leveraged to meet the quest for diversity across the organization. You may (and likely will) be called upon to serve on committees, workgroups, or in meetings that are focused on diversity, equity, and inclusion issues, whether to develop training, improve organizational climate, or represent the organization externally. Rarely do these additional tasks come with additional compensation. You will be a support for other BIPOC colleagues, (formally or informally) listening, supporting, mentoring. This is both the extra labor of being BIPOC in systems where you are a minority, as well as a way in which we uplift each other and stay in solidarity, striving to co-create a more equitable workplace and stay strong while we get there.

Leading and managing while BIPOC means working hard to stay "on your game" and produce high-quality, excellent work, ever aware that you are in a role that few other BIPOC have had the opportunity to be in. Whether you are the first or the third, you don't want to be the last, so your margin for error is slim, because you are a representative of BIPOC excellence and worthiness. It also means using the privilege of your role to highlight the skills, talents, and gifts of other BIPOC and to advocate for all of us.

Working in overtly or benignly hostile environments means speaking truth to power with diplomacy. There will be moments where diplomacy is not the first language you want to use. However, I prefer to stay connected to my humanity and decorum, even when provoked. Surviving, let alone thriving, requires grounding in a meta-framework, which I find in my faith. It grounds me in a set of values and the love of a just God. Grounding yourself in something bigger can consist of other spiritual practices and take many forms, like meditation, yoga, and other practices. Grounding myself in my faith helps me feel less vulnerable to the forces of racial bias and reminds me that I am part of a larger purpose.

Recommendations

I offer three key recommendations for leading and managing as a BIPOC and holding on to yourself, holding steady against the damaging impacts of racial bias and staying focused on progress.

1. Know your value and values

If we are destroying ourselves at work, we are keeping oppression alive and well by signaling our availability for exploitation. Let's commit to engaging in the process of discovering and embracing our value. Show yourself some compassion. It is hard to know your value amidst a torrent of messages that devalue People of Color. Make a conscious inventory of your strengths and intentionally curate relationships in your life that affirm your value and reduce the power and positioning of those that don't. Identify supportive peers or mentors that can see strengths that you may not appreciate in yourself. Practice articulating your unique strengths, to trusted people, or in the mirror. To this day, I struggle to introduce myself in a way that feels authentic. Aim to inhabit the role you are in, defining it with your unique self in it. The audition is over. You got the role!

Social work and other mental health professional practices are grounded in values. In addition to the explicit values (in social work these include social justice, respecting the dignity and worth of each person), there are also implicit values that may conflict with the explicit ones. Interrogate yourself often, and reaffirm why you've chosen to work in this profession. Consider joining or launching a support group for BIPOC managers. Leadership is not a solitary activity. Draw strength in community with other BIPOC managers.

2. Ground your leadership and management in purpose

Anchor yourself in your purpose, your "why" for doing this work. Our purpose sustains us to persevere during the challenging times, and serves as a North Star to guide, sustain, and mobilize you. Separate your job tasks and responsibilities from your purpose so as not to conflate them. My purpose in work is to build the leadership capacities of BIPOC to engage in the change work needed for us to leverage our collective strengths to thrive. Now that you have the authority of your role, consider how you can use your voice to advocate for BIPOC, being mindful of identifying the risks within the system you're in.

3. Seek the strength of different perspectives

The exercise of leadership requires acting out of self-awareness, rather than by default. Get comfortable with different perspectives because in managing teams, you are managing differences. You are also helping to build collective capacity to appreciate differences and still be able to work together. Lean into the discomfort of difference with genuine curiosity. Name different perspectives in your group, team, or staff as normal, a strength, and essential to the work.

Conclusion

I began this chapter with a question: What would make your career a transformative one? For me, a transformative career is characterized by wholeness, community, and alignment. This translates into health and well-being for us and for the people we work with. Our destinies are linked. I have written this statement of affirmation to remind myself, and now you, to put away the superhero cape and bring yourself, whole and healthy, to the work, *with* communities and *in* community.

> My skills, talents and passion are devoted to honoring, preserving, protecting and restoring the wholeness of people and communities whose humanity has been dishonored and attacked. I am a whole, integrated vessel. I need not check my identities at the door, as the price for doing this work. I need not forfeit my Blackness, my Latinidad, my life experiences, my lips, hips or hair, for my career. I need not sacrifice my health while investing in the health of others. I work in a context of aligned values and deep commitment to providing restorative care. I work in community. I am not a lone hero or a sacrificial lamb. I am uplifted as I uplift.

It is my hope that this chapter will provoke you to consider your own aspirations for your work and our professions. You may not find employers who provide support for you as a whole human, yet you can work to request it, demand it, create it, and mobilize others to co-create it with you. May we be the force for change that we are capable of being, as whole and healthy people, working in community and with purpose.

References and Resources

Clance, P. R., & Imes, S. A. (1978). The imposter phenomenon in high achieving women: Dynamics and therapeutic intervention. *Psychotherapy: Theory, Research & Practice, 15*(3), 241–247. https://doi.org/10.1037/h0086006

Heifetz, R., Grashow, A., & Linsky, M. (2009). *The practice of adaptive leadership: Tools and tactics for changing your organization and the world.* Harvard Business Press.

Lausell Bryant, L., & Coltoff, P. (2021). *Social work: A call to action – A time for reflection and reckoning.* NYU Silver School of Social Work.

Liu, W. M., Liu, R. Z., Garrison, Y. L., Kim, J. Y. C., Chan, L., Ho, Y. C. S., & Yeung, C. W. (2019). Racial trauma, microaggressions, and becoming racially innocuous: The role of acculturation and White supremacist ideology. *American Psychologist, 74*(1), 143–155. https://doi.org/10.1037/amp0000368

Miller, J. L., & Garran, A. M. (2017). *Racism in the United States: Implications for human services.* Springer.

Salomon, L. M. (2012). *America's nonprofit sector: A primer* (3rd ed.). Foundation Center.

Samimi, J. C. (2019). Funding America's nonprofits: The nonprofit industrial complex's hold on social justice. *Columbia Social Work Review, 8*(1), 17–25. https://doi.org/10.7916/cswr.v8i1.1967

Schaffer, J. (2016). Poverty porn: Does the end justify the means? Nonprofit Quarterly, June 10. https://nonprofitquarterly.org/poverty-porn-do-the-means-justify-the-ends/

Thomas-Breitfeld, S., & Kunreuther, F. (2017). *Race to lead: Confronting the nonprofit racial leadership gap.* Building Movement Project Report, June.

Tran, N. (2023). From imposter phenomenon to infiltrator experience: Decolonizing the mind to claim space and reclaim self. *Peace and Conflict: Journal of Peace Psychology, 29*(2), 184–193. https://doi.org/10.1037/pac0000674

Wake, E. R. (2021). *Are you paying to perpetuate poverty?* | Elizabeth Ross Wake | *TEDxUofISpringfield.*www.youtube.com/watch?v=IzlaFaxZ9iA

Woods-Giscombé, C. L. (2010). Superwoman schema: African American women's views on stress, strength, and health. *Qualitative Health Research, 20*(5), 668–683. https://doi.org/10.1177/1049732310361892

Leadership, Impact, and Institutional Change **27**

A Community Conversation

Joseph P. Gone[1], Helen Neville,
Larke Nahme Huang, Doris F. Chang and
Linda Lausell Bryant

In this conversation, psychologists Helen Neville, Larke Huang, and Joseph Gone speak with editors Doris F. Chang and Linda Lausell Bryant about their pathways to leadership, the challenges of transforming institutions – higher education, the federal government, and the mental health professions – and how they navigate barriers and competing demands as BIPOC leaders. This conversation has been edited and condensed.

Participants

Joseph P. Gone, PhD, is an international expert in the psychology and mental health of American Indians and other Indigenous peoples. A professor at Harvard University, Gone has collaborated with tribal communities for nearly 30 years to re-envision conventional mental health services for advancing Indigenous well-being. As a clinical-community psychologist

---

1 The first three authors are listed in random order, reflecting their equal contributions to this chapter.

DOI: 10.4324/9781003309796-31

and action researcher, he has published over 100 scientific articles. He is an enrolled member of the *Aaniiih*-Gros Ventre Tribal Nation of Montana.

Helen Neville, PhD, is a counseling psychologist and Professor of Educational Psychology and African American Studies at the University of Illinois at Urbana-Champaign. She has held numerous national leadership positions and has co-edited eight books and (co)-authored more than 90 journal articles and book chapters on race, racism, and diversity issues related to well-being, with a focus on the lived experiences of Black Americans.

Larke Nahme Huang, PhD, is a Senior Advisor in the Office of the Assistant Secretary for Mental Health and Substance Use and Director of the Office of Behavioral Health Equity (OBHE) at SAMHSA (Substance Abuse and Mental Health Services Administration). As a licensed clinical-community psychologist, she has worked at the interface of policy, research, and practice in behavioral health for nearly 35 years.

Leadership, Impact, and Institutional Change: "Believe in Yourself and the Power That You Have to Make a Difference"

Doris: **There are so many connections between each of us in this room and we are hoping that our gathering today can prompt some reflection and sharing of stories about your respective journeys into positions of influence. We want to begin by asking you to introduce yourself with a story about when you first began to see yourself as a leader.**

Larke: That's a hard question obviously.

Joe: Well, I went to three different colleges over five years, and I did a stint in the United States Army in between as an enlisted person and ended up going to West Point as a cadet. As a West Point cadet, you're being trained in leadership, military leadership in particular. Obviously, military leadership is quite different from leadership in lots of other contexts. I think the time when it became most apparent to me was in graduate school, at the University of Illinois in Urbana-Champaign, in the clinical-community psychology program. My faculty mentors were really supportive of thinking outside of the box and doing unusual things. And one thing they let me do was to leave campus to go to my home reservation in Montana for an entire semester, giving me practicum credit just to do stuff on my reservation. So I went there to teach at our tribal college. And we were trying to launch a grassroots cultural society for our tribal community. We called it the White Clay society because our name for ourselves, *A'aniiih'nin*, can be translated as "White Clay People." It was a small group, like half a dozen or maybe eight people, and there were some tribal leaders involved. And part of it was getting organized as a cultural society to handle things like repatriation of human remains back to our community and things like that. Well, all I did was listen and write things up and try to keep things a little structured and document what people were doing. And because of that, some of those tribal leaders came to me and said, "Look, we have a vacancy for the person who's running our tribe, what we call a Tribal Administrator. We want you to do it." And I thought, me? I had done stuff for my tribe after college, little things, but nothing like that.

So I spent the next six months or so serving in that role before going back to graduate school. I inherited 200 staff and 50 tribal programs, and there wasn't really one person who could tell me how it was all organized, and what was going on. Millions of dollars were flowing through. So that's sort of where it dawned on me that I had to learn how to be a leader in a really distinctive context, where there are competing leadership paradigms at work. There's the old traditional Indian way of leadership in which a lot of what makes you a leader is having resources to be generous with. And so your followers are people that you share with, things that they wouldn't otherwise get. That is very different from federal bureaucracies, funding agencies, in which every dollar has to be accounted for and has to be shown to be going for programmatic purposes. People would come through the tribal agency, into my office and say, I need help with this and that, and of course there's no program that's meant to help everyone just in the way they wanted. So, trying to navigate my way through those very different leadership paradigms, I also had to manage the tribal politics that so heavily influenced my bosses on the Tribal Council.

Helen: I'll just share a little bit. Growing up as an African American girl, and then a woman, in multiracial, diverse Los Angeles, but going through public schools that were racially diverse but with no Black people in them, I experienced intense anti-Black racism, as well as this sense of solidarity. I did not grow up thinking that I could be or was a leader, even though I showed leadership. As a Black girl growing up in that environment, I was not told, "You are a leader." A lot of my career has been mostly other people asking me, would you serve in this capacity, will you do this, and not as much self-initiated. So I have stumbled in terms of having formal leadership (training), even though I was engaged in more informal leadership. So if I were to think about one critical moment in my development as a leader, it would have to be after I was asked to co-chair our university's strategic planning around diversity and create a ten-year strategic plan. After that, I was asked to apply for this Provost Fellow Program,[2] which was affiliated with what was then known as the CIC [Committee on Institutional Cooperation]. They would identify Provost Fellows for each of the institutions that were part of the Big 10. So it was then that I began to see myself as a potential leader. It was this external validation, and then, engaging in a year of activities where you really reflect on what it means to be a leader? How do you impact change? What kinds of things do you need and then getting mentorship about how to create structural change. So it was later in my career that I began to see myself as a formal leader but I think that experience empowered me to say, how can I use those skills to make a difference in other kinds of settings. One of the most impactful things that the Provost fellowship provided was the chance to travel to other institutions to meet other fellows and attend various programs. And as part of that, the President of the university would have this quiet chat with you behind closed doors about what it was like to be a leader. People were very real and honest and authentic and it humanized the experience of being a leader. It allowed me to say, "Yes, I can be a leader." Not necessarily the leader the university wants me to be, but a leader in other capacities.

Larke: So I don't think I have the answer to this question yet. I've never strived to be a leader. But I am . . . drawn to problem solving, and trying to figure out how to solve problems, whether it's a big societal problem, or how to teach my kids to tie their shoes. In terms of seeing myself as a leader . . . I suppose it was when there was external

---

2 The Provost Fellows Program provides academic leadership experience in key campus administrative roles for distinguished faculty at the University of Illinois Urbana-Champaign. Fellows also participate in the Council of Independent Colleges' Academic Leadership Program.

recognition that I could actually influence people that I highly admired or who were much more senior to me. I realized that they might have incredible depth of expertise, but they don't really know how to solve problems. I see that a lot in the federal government, where we have tremendous thinkers, but as Joe alluded to, the federal bureaucracy is extremely complex, and you have to know how to navigate the rules, regulations, turf issues, and people and personalities in order to solve problems to get things done. I realized that I'm not going to be of the stature and prominence of some of the people I most admire. But while they define the problems and the drivers most eloquently, they often fall short of testing solutions, even incrementally. And I think that's something that is at the heart of everything that I do, that there's a problem that needs to be solved and there's a strategy that needs to be crafted.

That flexibility of thinking and being drawn to problems that don't have easy solutions are probably what helped me to get into leadership roles that I didn't volunteer for. I will often say to my teams, "I'm the accidental fed." I didn't go into the federal government with intention, I kind of slipped into it, and then I realized that your reach is great, for better or worse (laughing) in the federal government. So once I was there, it was hard to think about a different kind of position. Growing up, I had to assume leadership in my family in ways that young children typically don't have to. I was fiercely protective of my family, and I think that probably instilled the ferociousness I sometimes still have today. So [my pathway to leadership] was a culmination of different kinds of experiences and nobody anointed me as a leader of anything and I didn't run to be a leader of anything, but I have had opportunities to shape different things and build strategies that I feel are important.

Linda: **I love this thread that ran through the three of your responses. Each of you ended up being thrust into leadership or told, this is something you can, should do, we need you to do – or as Larke characterized it, you became an** *accidental* **leader. Was there a point that you began to own the sense that, "I bring some unique things to this work." How do your identities and your personal history connect you to the kind of change work you're involved in today?**

Helen: I know a lot of people don't believe this, but I am introverted. So doing leadership takes a different kind of energy from me. When I think about a leader, I think of somebody who has an extroverted leadership style who says, this is my vision, this is what we're working for. At a diversity conference years ago, Patricia Arredondo impressed upon me that counseling psychologists have a lot of transferable skills – good listening skills, being able to have people come together, as well as the values of social justice, freedom, etc. And through my Provost fellowship position, we learned that there are multiple ways of being a leader. I've come to realize that my leadership style is more of a collaborative collective leadership style, the understanding that things don't fall on one person, the importance of working within a team in order to create a collective vision to move forward on and have the impact. So those are some things that have been really important insights along my journey.

Early on in my career, I knew I was passionate about antiracism work. But the work I want to talk about is my newer work. I did this Fulbright at the University of Dar es Salaam in Tanzania. And being there for so many months, I experienced a level of liberation and freedom that I had never experienced in the US. While there were some issues that I experienced there, I did not experience racism. And because Tanzania did not have a history of settler colonialism, it didn't have white people living there, they also don't have the internalized whiteness that goes with it. So it was incredibly liberating. Around that time, somebody asked me to run for president for Division 45, the Society for the Psychological Study of Culture, Ethnicity, and Race (a division of the American Psychological Association). And at that time, I'm like, okay, maybe I could do this because I want to focus my whole energy on People of Color. When you do antiracism work, some of the work is directed toward white folks to get them to understand certain things. I really wanted to center People of Color and our experiences, and how we are able to heal and thrive in the face of incredible adversity. I was fortunate enough to work with some really good people to develop a Radical Healing paradigm[3] that builds on ideas that others have been working on, a framework to understand what is our lived

---

3 The Psychology of Radical Healing Collective is a group of BIPOC scholars and healers who produce scholarship and frameworks that elevate community resources, ideas, and actions that are strength-based. The Collective aims to encourage social justice action and commitments among psychologists and other healers to foster individual and collective healing for BIPOC and people of the Global Majority. For more information, see: https://psychologyofradicalhealing.com/

condition, what gifts can we give to people that are hurting now. And doing it in a way that is not, "This is my singular vision," but as a collective vision and a collective effort. And now I am President of Division 17 (Society for Counseling Psychology) and want to build on work that we did in Division 45. So my initiative will center personal and collective healing, which includes justice and joy, transforming healing practices, and counseling psychology and beyond.

Larke: Justice and joy, that is a really interesting combination of concepts. I'd love to learn more about how you put those together.

Helen: Wole Soyinka (the Nigerian novelist) says, the first condition of humanity is justice. And community psychologists say, you have to have justice in order to have both individual and collective well-being. But often when we focus on justice, the focus is on how we've been oppressed, how we've been downtrodden. But we are more than the oppression that we experience. No matter what else is going on, there is joy through our cultural celebrations. We know through the science and psychology of joy that it adds to well-being. Personal individual joy, as well as communal and collective joy, as resistance and as cultural strengths.

Larke: I really like that because especially in the time we're in now, we don't really find the joy in our day, we just find the division, the hate, the anger, and the oppression. So I like that combination. And, it connects to my own leadership style, which is often about bringing contrasting concepts together. The way I try to organize my life – how I live at home with my family and what I take to work and vice versa – is not as divided as some people think it is. And the team piece that you're talking about, Helen, is really a critical part of how I think about leading, too. This sounds really trite, but I feel that being a leader is also about being a lifelong learner. I'm always surprised when people say, you really spend time learning from your children. But it's important for me, because many of the

---

4 In July 2023, the White House Initiative on Asian American Native Hawaiian and Pacific Islander (WHIAAPI), the Substance Abuse and Mental Health Services Administration (SAMHSA), and the US Department of Health and Human Services (HHS) convened a summit focused on improving equity and access to behavioral health care for AA and NHPI communities. For more information, see: www.hhs.gov/about/whiaanhpi/index.html

people I'm leading are in their generation as well. And I thought it was striking when you said you're an introvert because I never really thought about that until one of my fellows said to me, "I watch you as an introverted person leading these meetings and I realize, there's hope for me." So I think again, it's putting together contradictory concepts. That creates new leadership paths too, because not they're not necessarily traditional modes of leadership.

Doris, you were at the summit that we had last week, the White House summit.[4] And what brought me tremendous joy about that Summit was when I sat back in the audience and saw the people who are leading the Summit now. The facilitator there, the subject matter experts, the people who we invited to be panelists, the people who were moderating panels, many of them were my interns, or people I hired early on in their careers. And I sat back there just looking at that stage full of people that in some ways I had been connected to their lives, and felt, *Okay, I can RIP, I can "retire in peace" now*, because it feels like there's a transition to a new generation of emerging and confident leaders. And it was actually just thrilling to me. Although I had provided leadership in the design of the program, and who was going to be in attendance, to observe this generation of new leadership was deeply satisfying. And I thought, for me, I guess it's a kind of quiet leadership. I push, I feel like I try to shape, I try to mold even when confronted with resistance. I see growth and development and change. And, it's very exciting to see.

Joe: Yeah, you know, I think pretty early in my career in graduate school, it became very apparent that my desire to train in clinical psychology and mental health services would have certain strong limitations with a swath of people in my home community. I think of more traditionally oriented Indigenous people in particular. And that led me then to want to start thinking through, well, what are the disconnects between conventional counseling and psychotherapy, the kinds of things that I'm being trained in and the things that traditionally oriented relatives, or others at home, might not find very helpful. And so that led really to a series of linked project-based inquiries. One question is, how would we characterize what we might call the cultural psychology of my own people, and other Indigenous peoples. I wanted to learn more from Indigenous people themselves: what are the distinctive facets or aspects of our own cultural psychologies? The second parallel effort was to try to unpack the cultural orientations and assumptions of the mental health professions and how those map onto the distinctive facets of Indigenous cultural psychology (or not). And the third endeavor explored what therapeutic treatments or services are needed to better reconcile those disconnects. That's what my career has been about. I've aspired to take the knowledge of my ancestors, my people and other Indigenous peoples, and to bring it into psychology, particularly into applied psychology and to health service psychology or mental health work. I hoped to better open up what we consider to be "true" (or authorized) knowledge about psychology, as well as to try to harness it to be more practically beneficial for my own people.

I've drawn inspiration from certain of my ancestors. My great-great-grandfather was called The Boy. He was often referred to as the last chief of the Gros Ventres, of our people. And one thing he had was a treasury of Indigenous ceremonial knowledge, especially from the old days, that was really no longer viable in the reservation era with Christian missionaries and government agents suppressing Indigeneity as savagery. He made sure that all that knowledge was written down because he wanted it preserved for the future. And I look back to that knowledge as one way to help influence psychology today. And so my goal in keeping with an anthropological approach to culture, if you will, is to keep it quite specific, tied to particular communities and particular traditions.

Doris: **Thanks, Joe. It sounds like you're mapping out a more expansive and inclusive vision for what you're hoping the field can be. And I'm struck by how each of you are working within these so-called traditional institutions, some of the oldest institutions we have. I'm curious about your decision to invest in trying to change those institutions, whether it's APA, or your universities, the federal government, your scholarly discipline. We're seeing a trend toward lots of younger folks deciding to opt out of these existing institutional structures, deciding instead to build their own thing. That is exciting and important. And yet these institutions are still really powerful. Can you talk about first, your decision to invest in these institutional spaces. And second, what are some of the key approaches you've taken to try to shift and change those institutions for the better?**

Larke: I don't think about changing the federal government. But I think about the federal government's reach and its power to influence service delivery at the state and local levels by deciding who gets research funding, who gets grants, what kinds of services are available. So the way I try to influence things is to embed social justice and equity issues deeply into the mechanisms and the operations of government. I've served under four different presidential administrations and have seen expansion and shrinking of civil rights. I think societally, now we are in a period where rights are being taken away, so I think it's imperative that we expand opportunities. In my office, the Office of Behavioral Health Equity, we are really trying to expand the reach of our funding apparatus to those populations that are not traditionally receiving significant federal grants. We started an initiative about ten years ago, called the Disparity Impact Strategy,[5] where we changed the language and set the expectation in our grants, that funding was going to be linked to the populations served, and requiring greater inclusion of populations who are more disparity vulnerable or traditionally underserved in the catchment area of the grant.

We were able to get people to think differently about the distribution of their resources, because we tied it to funding decisions and also required them to report who they serve, what services they get, and what the outcomes are, disaggregated by race and ethnicity and sexual gender minority status. And so it has been very transformative for our agency, because it affected every operation in the agency, those who were writing the grants, those who were administering them, those who were reviewing them, those who were deciding whether they would get a continuation of award, etc. So it really penetrated deeply into the operations of our agency. And now it's part of how we do our funding. And it goes back to what you were saying, Joe, that leaders are those people who have the resources. We're trying to send a message through our agency, because they are making decisions that really affect people's lives in sometimes life and death ways by who is getting resources and who is not. But it's also very data driven. We expect the grantee, the applicant, to really examine their data – who is and who is not being included. I just wanted to share this initiative because when

5 The US Department of Health and Human Services Office of Minority Health's (OMH) Disparity Impact Strategy is a comprehensive data-driven approach for identifying and addressing health disparities to promote health equity for racial and ethnic minority populations. For more information, see: www.minorityhealth.hhs.gov/omh/Content.aspx?ID=22540&lvl=2&lvlid=12

you think about change in the federal government, it can be slow and tedious. But every now and then you get a "win." And not surprisingly, fundamental to this change is building on relationships and allies.

Helen: I'll share what I'm thinking. At this point, you know, I spend a lot of my career invested in institutions, trying to make them change, but it's realizing at what level of the investment so I realized early on, it's not at the administrator level, I can't think like an administrator, because I've got the heart of faculty, staff, and students in mind more than taking up the perspective of the administrator. And I was told repeatedly that don't think like an administrator, I'm like, well, thank you. I realized over time that I would rather use my energy in other ways. There is a point where you feel like, let me invest in the institution and create change. There was probably a decade and a half where I was that. Now, I'm in this season of life of *divesting* from this institution. Do what is asked of me, but conserve my energy for things that I can change outside or make a difference in students' lives on a very real level. Students are hurting now, and I'd much rather invest in students than institutions that are reticent.

Doris: **Helen, I do think of you as an institutional leader, within APA and within the field of counseling psychology. Especially with regard to your work developing your Psychology of Radical Healing collective and framework, and building teams of people who are co-creating new ways of thinking about mental health research and services for BIPOC communities. I think of those as also falling into the category of institutional change processes. I wonder if you see it that way or not?**

Helen: Okay, so that institutional change, again, a lot of my things are by invitation, not by like," Oh, let me go ahead and get up, get up in here and do this . . ." I feel like the past few years have been tough. Maybe it's the case for everybody, but Black women have been asked to stand up, step up, step in, lean in, as most People of Color. And I guess I'm in the season of being exhausted, to be honest.

Linda: **I'm appreciating your honesty because we don't say that part out loud. You know, and it can literally hurt us from a career perspective to say it. So, I'm applauding that. Totally.**

Joe: For me, I'd say the first thing that happened in terms of institutional change was also not voluntary in any way. I arrived at Michigan as a faculty member in Clinical Science. And our chair said, form a mentoring committee of senior faculty, get their advice on how to get tenure here. So I called together some folks who I knew would be supportive of me getting tenure, and went through a presentation: here's who I am, here's what I study, here's why it matters, here's the kind of research I want to do. When I was done, there was silence for a minute. And then one of the faculty said, "Well, that's well and good. But if you want to get tenure in this department, shelf all of that until ten years from now, because it's too risky for a bunch of reasons." I talked to my mentor, Julian Rappaport at the University of Illinois, who said, "Why would you want tenure in a department that doesn't actually value what you care about?" So I decided that I would have to do enough work, publications that I'm proud of, and if they don't want to tenure me on that basis, that's okay. I can live with that. So I proceeded in the way that I had in mind with this vision I've told you about. So there were some things that have happened in my career by virtue of the right support, the right luck, whatever I can bring to it in terms of diligence and whatever talent I have.

In terms of thinking about institutional change now, I told you about my philosophy of psychology and wanting to contribute Indigenous knowledge to our field. The way I tend to do that predominantly is through published scholarship. I really try to actively circulate, to go out to the margins of our discipline, where there's more humanistic and interpretive kinds of inquiry going on. I have tried to take what I have learned, the ideas, the exchanges, which I think are really rich and interesting, and then carry them back to a more central place in our discipline, which I'm able to do because of the applied focus and the mental health focus. I feel like I'm constantly circulating, I cross over disciplinary boundaries, and go into anthropology, to Indigenous Studies, etc. So that's a kind of effort to transform an institution or a discipline.

More concretely, I've been at Harvard for five years. Harvard changed my life as an undergraduate. I would not be who I am and doing what I do if I hadn't gone to Harvard. And I want to make that possible for a broader swath of people. Harvard has been around since 1636, and there's baggage. So part of what we're also needing to do is to say to Harvard, look, for example, at the way you've treated Indigenous people in the New England area. There are bad things in that history, which need to be remedied. Since I've been Faculty Director of the Harvard University Native American

Program, we now have over 300 Indigenous-identifying students at Harvard, which is higher than we've had before.

Helen: I'd like just to add that predominantly white institutions aren't the only institutions that we've been involved with to make change. I have consistently made a commitment to being involved with other institutions, whether it's through ABPsi (Association for Black Psychologists), or other [BIPOC-centered] community organizations that are pushing for institutional change. I don't want to say that my gaze has always been toward white folks, because that's not my orientation at all.

Doris: **Great point, Helen, I'm so glad you clarified that. As each of you describe ways that you have and continue to push for institutional change in your various contexts, I'm wondering, how do you deal with blowback or challenges to your work?**

Helen: It depends on where you are in your career. Where I'm at now, maybe I'm tired. I just can't be bothered. It's people both within my circle and outside my circle, and people you think should be allies that aren't allies. And of course, it hurts when people undermine the issues. But I think my best approach is first, to gain a little bit of distance, and not take it personally when there are attacks, then to name what is really at play here. Is it that my energy is pulling out the worst possible energy in that person? Is it that we have different agendas? So really trying to name what's critical here to not make it personal. And then to find some solutions. So for example, I do this when I have leaders who do things that I disagree with. I try to put things into perspective by acknowledging that we have different interests in mind. My interests are related to faculty and students, their interests are related to the institution or something else. And so it's not about who this person is, but what is it that we need to do to protect or advance something and how can I build alliances to get to that? I try not to personalize it and get some distance from it. It doesn't mean things don't hurt, but I have to pull up a forcefield, personally.

Joe: I'll just give you a recent example of instances in which I decided that certain kinds of responses are not acceptable and tried to do something about them. A student and I submitted a manuscript to the leading journal in our subfield, an APA journal. The editor wrote back and said, thanks, but sorry, we don't publish qualitatively analyzed studies. And I wrote back and I said, well, actually, I published a qualitative study in this journal 12 years ago, so I'm surprised to hear that. And she wrote back and said, well, it's the policy now. I said, okay, and we ended up publishing it somewhere else. A few months later, I got an invitation from that same journal to review a qualitatively analyzed study, for a special issue on race and ethnicity. So then I got mad. I said to the editor, okay, so you're upholding certain methodological standards, as you would define them, in regular submissions. But when it comes to race and ethnicity, you're open to supposedly "lowering" those standards in a way. And her response did not really make sense to me.

So I took it all the way to the APA Publications Board. I had a meeting with them and said, this is unacceptable. It's actually structural racism to have a policy like that, when we know that so many research psychologists are trying to represent our communities, and our communities themselves have said that qualitative analysis better represents our voice and our perspectives and adds things in ways that variable analysis doesn't. But there's a lot of autonomy for journal editors. I didn't really know this editor that well, but this is a Person of Color. And so this is an example of what can happen when you adopt narrow procedural norms. One thing we have to be on the lookout for is being open and committed and dedicated politically to advancing certain causes, but then when it comes time for review and tenure, reviewing an article, or reviewing a grant, somehow we shift back into those myopic views in which we've been trained to operate in a procedural fashion, and that can exclude opening up things. And I think that's something we all need to be on the lookout for, whether we're folk of color or not.

Larke: I look at "blowback or challenges" as part of the work. I've always engaged in initiatives that are calling for some form of redistribution of power and privilege. This by its very nature will challenge the status quo and make people feel uncomfortable. So, I think it is important to anticipate it and think about steps that could be taken to minimize its undermining of an initiative. Identifying and making the right "allies" is critical. For example, when I was serving on a school board, I asked questions about how issues – whether academic, financial, or psycho-social – were handled with students from culturally diverse backgrounds. Soon, I was asked to Chair the subcommittee on Diversity and Inclusion. Recognizing that if I led this as a new Board member and the only woman of color on the Board, that it could easily be tokenized and would be totally powerless. So I only agreed to do this if the Chairperson of the Board would be my Co-Chair on the subcommittee on Diversity and Inclusion. Over the course of my time on the Board and Co-Chairing the subcommittee, there were many contentious issues under discussion, but having the "power" of the Board Chair enabled our committee to make some important system changes. In other situations, the end-users of the system or program are often the "undeniable" voices. Partnering with people or youth with lived experience of the issue at hand . . . although they are often at the "bottom of the power hierarchy" they often present irrefutable perspectives. So combining their stories with relevant data often serves to slightly quiet detractors. But I think it's important to expect "blowback" and recognize that it's an important part of the "work."

Doris: **I appreciate how each of you adopt different approaches to dealing with naysayers – including those internal shifts you make to cultivate empathy and not take things personally, to speaking up and saying "that's unacceptable" when lines are crossed, and identifying, cultivating, and strategically using "allies" to be more effective, especially when dealing with contentious issues. And I appreciate that these different approaches highlight that there are a million ways to be effective, depending on your specific position, context, and as Helen said, where you are in your career.**

Linda: **Well said. For our last question, what is one piece of advice that you would give to your younger self or someone who is like your younger self.**

Helen: "Be yourself." One thing I've always done is lived by my principles, I have never done anything in terms of my career that compromised my values or my principles. Believe in yourself and the power that you have to make a difference. I think that many times, for Black women in particular, and maybe other people as well, there are many ways in which people try to undermine our intelligence, our leadership. So believe in yourself. Believe in your potential and dream big. Because one of the things that I have realized that the younger generations have, is they have big bold dreams and they go for it. When I was socialized, we were socialized to keep our dreams down to a minimum. So yep, believe in yourself and dream big. Go for it.

Larke: For me, two things come to mind. First, I learned from my children: Get 1% better each day, always try to improve, but you don't need to move mountains every day! Second, invest in relationships – vertical and horizontal – this is a rich resource of learning, of understanding trust and respect, and how to navigate and influence complex situations. While it's important to be humble and giving, it's equally important to be forthright and demanding and to communicate expectations.

Joe: In terms of what to tell my younger self, I would say that, in a career path, planning matters, but serendipity is huge. I would suggest keeping a balance between preparing and planning the best that you can for the decisions that are in front of you, like where to go to graduate school, who is a good mentor, those kinds of questions. But at the same time, all that planning can go away as soon as a path appears that you never imagined, as you're walking your trail. And I think being attentive to and cognizant of when those paths appear and not having ever considered that but trying to see what value there might be. Because I could never have predicted my career journey. As I said, I went to three colleges over five years. I was in the Army in between. No one would plan that. But it's created a valuable set of experiences that I can draw on to this day.

Doris: **Great way to end. Joe, thank you so much. Thank you all so much for sharing your experiences and wisdom with us all.**

Linda: **Appreciate it. Thank you.**

Concluding Chapters

Part IV

We close this volume with two concluding chapters in which we summarize emergent themes with specific messages for BIPOC and for white racial justice allies. In **Chapter 28**, we reflect on core themes from the book, including race-related stress, healing, and resistance, calling on readers to strategize and mobilize for transformative change in their careers and communities.

We are joined by Lisa B. Spanierman to offer a final bonus chapter (**Chapter 29**) specifically for white peers, supervisors, faculty, and administrators who seek to support their BIPOC colleagues as allies and accomplices in the fight for racial healing and structural change. Drawing from the experiences and lessons shared by the BIPOC contributors in this volume, we highlight key themes and insights that we hope will support white readers to advance racial equity and justice in your spheres of influence.

DOI: 10.4324/9781003309796-32

Conclusion   **28**

Find Strength in This Community

Linda Lausell Bryant and Doris F. Chang

Dear Colleague,

Thank you for picking up this book. In its opening chapter, Linda Juang (Chapter 1) wrote, "You chose this book because you are on your way to a career in mental health (or are already in one) and may be seeking some inspiration for this path. Know that there are people out there who care about you, who share similar experiences, who know what it is like to question ourselves along this pathway. Find strength in this community" (p. 21).

It is our hope that you have found value in this community of BIPOC mental health clinicians, educators, researchers, administrators, and activists who shared their stories and advice. Perhaps you felt a pang of recognition in their stories of alienation, or felt inspired by their bold, original, and courageous responses. While each story is unique, their plots feature common themes, including that of *awakening* to the lies that we have been told about our inferiority, *reclaiming* one's cultural and communal resources, and *creating liberatory spaces* through naming and resisting norms and practices that maintain white supremacy and other systems of oppression. For BIPOC, these shared experiences mirror the affective, cognitive, and behavioral processes of ethnic-racial identity development (Marks et al., 2020), as over time and with guidance and support, we may grieve what we have suffered, recognize our innate worth, and begin to share our gifts with the world.

DOI: 10.4324/9781003309796-33

The Three Pillars of a Transformative Career in Mental Health for BIPOC: Healing, Social Change, and Community

Illustrated through first-person narrative accounts, this book argues that for BIPOC, a transformative career in mental health requires maintaining a delicate balance between inner and outer work, that is, the twin pillars of *healing* and *social change*. Naming our pain, identifying its intrapersonal, interpersonal, institutional, and structural causes, and prioritizing our own healing are transformative acts because they challenge the myth of the neutral scientist, the therapist-as-Zen-master, the BIPOC leader who is the exception to the rule. Speaking honestly about our struggles can create opportunities for more authentic relating to our students and trainees, peers, and leaders and can begin to create more compassionate and inclusive spaces for training, education, and practice.

Of course, not everyone is prepared to receive the fullness of our experience (see Chapter 29 for aspiring white racial justice allies), which is why a third pillar of transformation is needed, that of *community*. As Hector Adames and Nayeli Chavez-Dueñas (Chapter 4) note, "Surviving and thriving in systems not built by us and for us is difficult, and we cannot do it alone . . . you will need a community to support you as you navigate systems anchored in white supremacist capitalist heterosexual cisgender patriarchal values . . . Having a squad that understands what it is like to be you, supports you, and helps you navigate challenging times is the fuel to get you through when you feel like giving up" (p. 56). In discussing the tenure process, Karen Jackson-Weaver (Chapter 19), advises that before taking a new position, BIPOC faculty should carefully assess whether the environment offers the "professional and personal networks of support that will allow you to be successful in your journey towards promotion and advancement" (p. 213).

And where there is no community, we can create our own. Helen Neville et al. (Chapter 16) show us how we can cultivate a healing and social justice community for students of color that can promote transformative change in academic and institutional settings, as mentees go on to become mentors and leaders themselves. Their approach integrates Black feminist and intersectional theories with their model of radical healing (French et al., 2020), which situates healing in the "dialectical space between resisting interlocking systems of oppression and envisioning possibilities for a socially just future" (p. 182). Building on these theoretical insights and the personal stories of hardship and resistance in this volume, we see how the third pillar of community supports the other two pillars of healing and social change, to create the conditions for

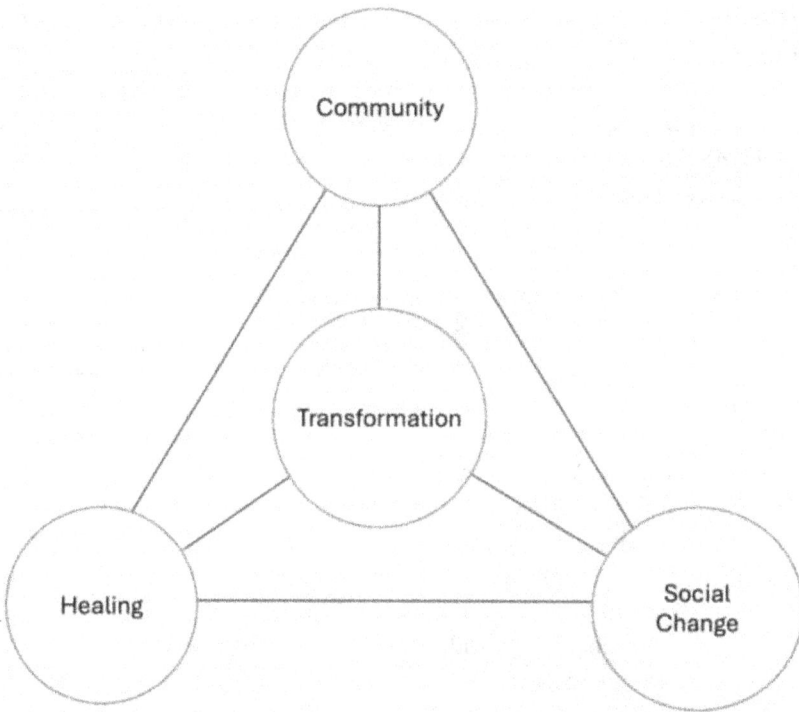

Figure 28.1 Tripartite Model for a Transformative Career in Mental Health for BIPOC

a balanced, sustainable, and transformative career for BIPOC in the mental health professions (see Figure 28.1).

Tending to our inner wounds and relying on community support gives us a solid foundation from which to engage in social change work in a healthier and more sustainable way. Research points to the disproportionate service contributions of BIPOC and high rates of burnout among BIPOC professionals in higher education (Domingo et al., 2022; Jackson et al., 2023). We are often spread too thin, trying to occupy too many seats at too many tables (how many of us have permanent seats on diversity committees?). Reflecting on their complex lived experiences, the chapter contributors illustrate diverse ways of engaging in multi-level social change work, whether through teaching and mentoring, program development and direct service delivery, research or policy – relying on self-care practices and relational supports to restore equilibrium. We invite you to reflect on where you stand in the balance between prioritizing your own health, safety, and wellbeing and engaging in the critical work of institutional and social change, and what community supports you have in place to sustain yourself. Below, we revisit some of the key nuggets of wisdom that the chapter contributors share about their efforts to find the balance in their own careers, and explore implications for training, education, and practice.

Chronic Stress, Resistance, and Healing

Managing race-related stress and cultivating sustainable approaches for resistance has been the hidden curriculum for survival and professional advancement as BIPOC. These are professional development issues that should be brought to light and formalized in our training, education, mentoring, and evaluation processes. In their work and personal lives, the authors in this volume describe surviving and navigating imposter phenomenon, microaggressions, stereotyping and othering, epistemic injustice, police violence, incarceration, and the psychological and material legacies of colonization, genocide, and slavery. The energy expenditures required to maintain balance and equilibrium in the face of oppression are significant, affecting their work, health, relationships, and overall quality of life. This too should be systematically acknowledged and addressed as a training and development issue. This means extending beyond abstract, academic discussions about racism and white supremacy, cis-sexism, heterosexism, classism, ableism, nativism, and other forms of oppression, and creating space for reflection, healing, and relational repair in training and workplace settings.

Many of the authors in this volume describe how active, daily practices of resistance allow them to carve out spaces of refuge. These resistance strategies include, for example, focusing on something (a community, a set of beliefs) that grounds them in belonging and purpose, a guiding "North Star." In the first Community Conversation (Chapter 9), E. J. R. David shared that his family and community are his purpose: "I just work *at* the university, I don't work *for* the University. I work *for* my people" (p. 115). Facing police brutality and institutional racism, Derek Suite turned inward and drew on his spiritual center: "I needed to create something that would help heal me. I kept looking outwardly for it and wanting somebody to validate me and then I realized that nobody is going to do that . . . you have to go inward first because the answers are not outside" (p. 111). As he and others remind us, our biggest sources of power and magic are often those parts of ourselves that we have been taught to hide away. Reclaiming our identities and our values is central to the process of decolonization and liberation. As you read the book, what other examples of reclamation did you identify? What do you want to reclaim?

In the ongoing battle for our lives, we are also reminded of the importance of rest and celebration of the beauty of life. During the dark early days of the pandemic, Jeanette Pai-Espinosa (Chapter 25) began ordering flowers to be delivered to herself each month: "The joy I felt when they arrived was special and still makes me smile today – a stark contrast to the bleakness of social isolation and uncertainty of that time. I remembered how simple it is to create my own moments of joy." Robyn L. Gobin (Chapter 13) reminds us, "being joyful amid oppression is an act of resistance (Lu & Stelle, 2019). Our ancestors sacrificed so we can live a good life – one where we can intentionally access joy while still in pursuit of liberation for ourselves and our communities" (p. 158).

Challenging and Transforming Institutions

Personal experiences of marginalization, invisibility, violence, and injustice drive many of us to engage in social justice work. While painful, our experiences also allow us to see things from a unique vantage point and can drive innovation. Encountering the work of Clance and Imes (1978) on the imposter phenomenon (IP), which focused on women's feelings of inferiority in male-dominated environments, Kevin Cokley had a flash of recognition: "I began to reflect on my experiences as a Black undergraduate student, and how gratified I was to know that there was an actual term to describe my feelings and experience in college . . . I wondered how IP impacted African American and other minoritized students" (p. 83). This breakthrough moment eventually led to a productive and high-impact program of scholarship that has documented the harmful effects of IP among minoritized students and inspired advocacy efforts and initiatives to address it in higher education.

As we progress in our careers, we can draw on our diverse experiences – of trauma and strength – to begin to transform our institutions into more inclusive spaces of learning and growth. Sandra Mattar reflected on the healing impact of culturally responsive supervisors and being in a multicultural environment during her training years. She wrote, "These spaces felt supportive and provided a milieu to have conversations outside of the mainstream narrative, inspiring my activism to create a place where diverse clients, students, and faculty felt represented and included" (p. 251). Now a faculty member, supervisor, and director of training, she has the power and position to establish policy and develop more inclusive, culturally appropriate, and anti-oppressive models of education and training.

Finally, for those of you who hesitate to see yourself as a leader, know that the field needs you and your unique set of insights, talents, and passions. Lest you think that leaders are born, not made, many of the authors in this volume never actively pursued leadership positions. In our final Community Conversation on Leadership, Impact, and Institutional Change (Chapter 27), Joseph Gone, Helen Neville, and Larke Nahme Huang each described being recruited into leadership roles, and only later coming to appreciate what they uniquely had to offer. Their backgrounds, knowledge, and experiences became a cluster of character strengths that they could harness for good. In Huang's case, she "had to assume leadership in my family in ways that young children typically don't have to. I was fiercely protective of my family, and I think that probably instilled the ferociousness I sometimes still have today" (p. 301), an asset in her policy, research, and advocacy roles within the federal government. Learning to persist in the face of institutional resistance to change is a skill that minoritized groups unfortunately have had to hone for survival. It is made easier when we work together and use our power to expand opportunities for others. Writing about transforming the psychology discipline through editorial leadership (Chapter 23), Gordon Nagayama Hall invoked the African Ubuntu premise, "I am because we are" in describing the "scholarly communities of color that have transformed the research landscape over the past 50 years. Although individual editors can have pivotal roles in shaping the field, lasting change occurs when there is community support" (p. 259).

Our Hopes for You

We hope that this book will support you in your own transformative change process, beginning with owning your distinctive and powerful voice (Part I), and using it as a force for change. We hope this book inspires you to take a courageous leap (Part II), whether embarking on an established path or a road less traveled, and trust that you will find your way. Finally, as your own career develops, we hope you will seize the opportunity to lead for change and impact (Part III). Our impact grows when we work together with our BIPOC colleagues and white allies toward transformative, systemic change. Not only will our shared burden feel lighter, but with our combined brilliance and ingenuity, we can address the most intractable problems of our time.

Our work honors the efforts of those who came before us, those actively engaged in the struggle, and those who are preparing to join us. Our healing and liberation are as much for them as they are for us. This book details change strategies at various levels and in a wide range of settings, whether you are starting your career, winding it down or any phase in between. We hope that these stories of challenge, healing, social change, and community will help you feel supported and prepared to take action with clarity, conviction, and most of all, hope.

In closing, we leave you with the words of former President Barack Obama, "Change will not come if we wait for some other person, or if we wait for some other time. We are the ones we've been waiting for. We are the change that we seek."

Pa'lante! 加油！

Yours in solidarity,
Linda and Doris

References

Clance, P. R., & Imes, S. A. (1978). The imposter phenomenon in high achieving women: Dynamics and therapeutic intervention. *Psychotherapy: Theory, Research & Practice*, *15*(3), 241–247. https://doi.org/10.1037/h0086006

Domingo, C. R., Gerber, N. C., Harris, D., Mamo, L., Pasion, S. G., Rebanal, R. D., & Rosser, S. V. (2022). More service or more advancement: Institutional barriers to academic success for women and women of color faculty at a large public comprehensive minority-serving state university. *Journal of Diversity in Higher Education*, *15*(3), 365–379. https://doi.org/10.1037/dhe0000292

French, B. H., Lewis, J. A., Mosley, D. V., Adames, H. Y., Chavez-Dueñas, N. Y., Chen, G. A., & Neville, H. A. (2020). Toward a psychological framework of radical healing in communities of color. *The Counseling Psychologist*, *48*(1), 14–46. https://doi.org/10.1177/0011000019843506

Jackson Preston, P., Brown, G. C., Garnett, T., Sanchez, D., Fagbamila, E., & Graham, N. (2023). "I am never enough": Factors contributing to secondary traumatic stress and burnout among Black student services professionals in higher education. *Trauma Care*, *3*(2), 93–107. https://doi.org/10.3390/traumacare3020010

Marks, A. K., Calzada, E., Kiang, L., Pabón Gautier, M. C., Martinez-Fuentes, S., Tuitt, N. R., Ejesi, K., Rogers, L., Williams, C. D., & Umaña-Taylor, A. (2020). Applying the lifespan model of ethnic-racial identity: Exploring affect, behavior, and cognition to promote well-being. *Research in Human Development*, *17*(2–3), 154–176. doi: 10.1080/15427609.2020.1854607

Relational Approaches to Transforming Institutions

29

Guideposts for Aspiring White Racial Justice Allies

Doris F. Chang, Linda Lausell Bryant and Lisa B. Spanierman

Jan Michaels is a social worker and clinical supervisor at a multiservice agency that provides wraparound services to families who are predominantly Black and Latinx. Although Jan is a cisgender white woman, many practicum students of color seek her supervision because of her specialization in trauma-informed care. She is privy to many of her white colleagues' disparaging and racist comments about some of those very students. One student in particular, a queer Cambodian American student named Phuong, has drawn the attention of other supervisors who describe them as "difficult," "resistant," and "defensive." At their most recent supervision meeting, Phuong shared that they are feeling isolated and frustrated by the training they are receiving at the agency, and are considering trying to find a different placement. While Jan had an inkling of Phuong's struggles, she was surprised that they may want to leave. Jan thought that she had a good relationship with Phuong, but now begins to wonder if her colleagues are right, that Phuong really is too difficult to work with and a liability to the agency.

Dr. Zayas is an Afro-Latina professor of counseling at a predominantly white university. Waiting for the monthly faculty meeting to start, she

DOI: 10.4324/9781003309796-34

notes that on the agenda is a faculty vote regarding a DEI (diversity, equity, and inclusion)-focused faculty search. The search committee presents several candidates, emphasizing their publications and grants. Dr. Z wonders if they will discuss what the department needs with respect to DEI. Her thoughts are interrupted by the insistent vibration of her phone. Her colleague, a Mexican-American non-tenured faculty member, is venting about feeling "freakin' triggered" in this meeting. Dr. Buckman, a white colleague, texts, "Are you angry? You look irritated." Dr. Z feels a wave of panic as she wonders if her great poker face is betraying her. Ignoring the sweat pooling in her armpits, Dr. Z blurts out, "What are we hoping these candidates will actually do for this school in terms of DEI?" The department chair, a white woman, responds that all of the candidates have already met that threshold and now we just need to select the most qualified ones. Dr. Z feels shut down and mentally checks out for the rest of the meeting. Afterwards, Dr. Z's phone is convulsing with texts. No fewer than four white faculty colleagues are "checking" on her and apologizing for not having supported her with their own voices during the meeting. She considers, yet again, whether it's time to leave the academy. She's not interested in their self-flagellation nor in soothing it.

Despite the documented benefits of diversity in a range of educational and workplace settings (Stevens et al., 2008), recent challenges to diversity initiatives – including the June 2023 Supreme Court decision to effectively eliminate affirmative action programs in higher education – are making it increasingly difficult to cultivate mental health training and practice environments that are inclusive, diverse, and equitable. As a result, efforts to promote social justice within mental health organizations and training sites may increasingly depend upon white insiders and gatekeepers whose overrepresentation in positions of power will persist without significant systemic efforts (Matias et al., 2022). In this chapter, we explore how white individuals in the mental health professions can use their power and privilege to help shift institutions toward racial justice and more effectively collaborate with and support their BIPOC students, colleagues, and leaders. Drawing on the experiences and lessons offered by the BIPOC contributors in this volume, we highlight key themes and insights from their contributions that we hope will support you, our white readers, in your efforts to advance racial equity and justice in your institutions. Whether you are a school dean or department chair, faculty or clinical supervisor, classmate or colleague, practitioner or trainee, each of you has the opportunity to make a difference in the lives of the BIPOC individuals that populate your schools and workplaces, and to shape the values and practices of the organizations and systems that you are a part of, in ways big and small.

The ideas in this chapter are informed by the diverse backgrounds and professional experiences of the three authors. Doris is a cisgender, straight Chinese American woman and clinical psychologist who was previously faculty and Director of Clinical Training in a psychology program before joining the faculty of a school of social work. Linda is a straight, Puerto Rican Afro Latina clinical professor of social work and associate dean for academic affairs who previously served as CEO of a child welfare agency. Lisa is a white cisgender heterosexual Jewish American woman, professor of counseling psychology, and associate dean for academic personnel. All three of us have been actively involved in racial equity work for our entire careers, through our research and writing, teaching and mentoring, clinical and social service practice, as well as our involvement in numerous DEI-related service roles in the academy and the profession at large.

The Context and Culture of White Supremacy in Mental Health Training, Education, and Practice

Because white people are socialized into the dominant position in a racialized social system (Bonilla-Silva, 1997), they have the privilege to be oblivious, to engage in willful ignorance, and to inadvertently cause harm to BIPOC despite good intentions. Feagin's (2020) concept of the white racial frame provides a framework for explaining the societal justification of racial oppression and white privilege and at the same time serves as a lens through which to understand everyday experiences. For example, the white racial frame positions white people as superior, virtuous, and hard-working, whereas BIPOC are deemed inferior, lazy, depraved, and/ or dangerous; these ideas are transmitted through stereotypes, images, prejudicial attitudes, and emotions. Because white healthcare professionals are socialized within the same cultural practices and institutions as everyone else, the white racial frame consciously and unconsciously shapes the way they experience and understand race and racism. A recent review found that healthcare providers, including those in mental healthcare, held significant pro-white/anti-Black, -Hispanic, -American Indian and dark-skinned implicit bias (Maina et al., 2018).

White people, including mental health professionals, often operate from a racially color-blind perspective that denies or minimizes the influence of race and racism (Neville et al., 2013). They may be socialized to believe that discussing race itself is a racist act, which prevents open and honest dialogue and instead perpetuates subtle forms of racism. In some cases, racially color-blind white people experience awareness-inducing events (e.g., training on racial health disparities or witnessing racial discrimination directed toward a BIPOC friend), which may shatter their obliviousness about societal racism. According to Helms's (1995) white racial identity development model, these events may propel white people into the status of "disintegration" (i.e., cognitive dissonance about loyalty to their own group versus moral and humanistic values). Disintegration involves painful emotions, such as guilt and shame, for not knowing (or doing) better sooner. Consequently, white people may return to their racially color-blind perspective, justify their earlier position of white dominance, or seek to learn more about structural racism and white privilege.

Although institutions of higher education often are considered bastions of liberal and progressive ideals, their histories may be connected to white supremacy. In the book *Ebony and Ivy: Race, Slavery, and the Troubled History of America's Universities* for example, Wilder (2013) shows how US Ivy League institutions received economic support from slave owners and in turn provided scholarly justification for slavery. Scholars also have documented ties between predominantly white universities and white supremacist organizations, such as the Ku Klux Klan (Jaschik, 2017). Given this historical backdrop, it is not surprising that even as colleges and universities seek to diversify their students and faculty, white faculty continue to be overrepresented at the highest ranks (American Psychological Association, 2019) and BIPOC continue to face daily racial microaggressions and other attempts to exploit and/or subjugate them (Anthym & Tuitt, 2019; Louis et al., 2016; Zambrana et al., 2017).

Germane to the contemporary context of higher education, Gusa (2010) identified *white institutional presence* – referring to a culture of whiteness embedded in the norms, traditions, practices, and ways of knowing in the academy. Although BIPOC students, staff, and faculty may be keenly aware of white institutional presence, its markers are often invisible to their white counterparts. White institutional presence is also inscribed in mental health and social service agencies, as evidenced by documented disparities in access to and utilization of mental health services. In addition to stigma and distrust in such services, members of BIPOC communities often receive lower quality care due to a lack of culturally sensitive providers (Mongelli et al., 2020; Wells-Wilbon et al., 2021). Even when BIPOC clients seek and obtain access to mental health services, a culture of whiteness embedded in the norms and practices of these organizations may reinforce subtle messages of white superiority. For example in this volume, Hardy (Chapter 10) reflected on the color-blind racial ideology embedded in his early training as a marriage and family therapist: "Like many of my white counterparts, I had been trained to view the slow or minimal treatment progress of a client of color as evidence of their resistance to the process or an indication that they were probably not working hard enough. Not once did I consider, or was I ever trained to even hypothesize, that maybe what I was generously offering was grossly misaligned with what they needed" (p. 121).

Understanding BIPOC Experiences of Mental Health Training, Education, Practice, and Leadership

The vignettes that open this chapter highlight common challenges and coping responses of BIPOC mental health trainees and professionals that are explored further throughout this volume. These challenges include a) chronic exposure to race-related and other minority stressors at each stage of one's career, b) the need to invest significant time and energy to navigate those stressors on top of other professional responsibilities, and c) intentional efforts to strengthen the discipline and promote institutional equity by leveraging personal and cultural assets. Many of us eagerly discuss these issues in BIPOC-oriented spaces where we gather to provide validation and support, laugh and cry, and share practical survival tips and strategies. Yet, these issues and experiences are often difficult to talk about with white colleagues due to fears and direct experiences of othering, dismissal, and/ or retaliation. We invite you to review the chapters referenced below, to be a "fly on the wall" in these conversations to deepen your understanding of the lived experiences of your BIPOC colleagues and students, cultivate greater empathy and compassion, and ready yourselves to engage in critical action in your spheres of influence.

Chronic Exposure to Race-Related and Other Minority Stress

A common theme in this book is that BIPOC individuals experience significant race-related stress in mental health training and educational institutions, even those that explicitly frame social justice as central to their mission. Like Jan Michaels and Dr. Zayas's white colleagues in the opening vignettes, white faculty and supervisors may be surprised to learn that many of their BIPOC students, supervisees, and colleagues – even the most "successful" by conventional standards – are struggling to cope with everyday stressors such as discrimination and microaggressions (Lee et al., this volume), racial violence (Suite, this volume), imposter syndrome (Cokley, this volume), internalized oppression and shame (David, this volume), and the loneliness and pressure of being "one of the only ones" (Adames & Chavez-Duenas, this volume). Fear – of failure, of racial harm, of squandering opportunity that others were not given – often hovers just beneath the surface. As Gobin (this volume) noted, "Deeply rooted ancestral trauma caused me to fear the consequences of not constantly jumping through hoops to prove my value to others." (p. 150).

These stressors and challenges have been documented at each step of the educational and professional journey, although the power and skills available to meet them may shift over time (see Mattar, this volume). For example, Suyemoto (Kim & Suyemoto, this volume) described graduate school as "an actively oppressive experience for me, an experience that pathologized my experience as a queer Person of Color, while also enacting passive oppression in its almost complete inattention to race, culture, or ethnicity in the curriculum" (p. 192). This experience sparked a desire for her own students to have a radically different kind of educational experience, leading to a professional interest in transformative education and critical pedagogy.

Hidden Labor: Expending Time and Energy to Survive and Thrive

Because BIPOC students and professionals frequently face race-related and other minority stressors, it is important to recognize the additional energy expenditures needed in order to maintain one's equilibrium while performing basic work functions. As highlighted in the reference to Dr. Z's "great poker face," many BIPOC work mightily to put on a brave front, to project competence, serenity, and confidence in white dominated spaces to avoid being seen as "a problem" or activating negative stereotypes such as the "angry Black woman" (see Lee et al., this volume). It is notable that much of this effort is directed toward proving one's value, seeking belonging, and ensuring one's survival in oppressive systems (Woods-Giscombé, 2010). For example, Cokley (this volume) wrote about managing imposter syndrome, "The thing about impostorism is that it makes people work incredibly hard in the constant pursuit of proving themselves as smart enough, as good enough, and as truly belonging" (p. 88).

As the vignette about Phuong illustrates, those who are more vocal about their experiences of race-related stress and discrimination, or who dare to challenge white supremacist cultural norms (Liu et al., 2019), are frequently marginalized or suffer reputational damage or other punishments. To maintain balance and a positive self-concept, many BIPOC invest significant time and energy filling in the gaps of an ethnocentric training curriculum (see Juang, this volume), seeking and creating community in BIPOC-affirming spaces (see Neville et al. and Pai-Espinosa, both this volume), engaging in activism and radical self-care (see James and Gobin, both this volume). For example, Miao and Zhou (this volume) described how international student trainees expend significant time researching legal restrictions pertaining to clinical training and employment because many programs fail to properly advise their students about these critical issues. To mitigate these stressors, James (this volume) emphasized the importance of restorative practices, including finding joy, to buffer the impact of trauma: "It is how my ancestors and other oppressed people have survived the horrors of this world" (p. 175).

Leveraging Personal and Cultural Assets to Strengthen the Discipline and Transform Institutional Practice

In spite of these structural, historical, and institutional challenges, all of the chapter authors have had a significant impact on their respective fields and have worked to shift institutional practices toward greater justice and equity. Nearly all describe a point at which they began to move out of survival mode and align themselves with a greater purpose. For many, this marked a *return* to core values, forged out of early experiences that affirmed their value and connection to family, culture, home – a psychological and communal place of safety and belonging. Jackson-Weaver (this volume) recalled her delight as a child in "playing school," a love that connects her diverse experiences in educational leadership. In a community conversation, Coffie (Gobin et al., this volume) described how he began to embrace his own lived experience of incarceration as a source of insight and inspiration for his work in criminal justice reform: "I began not to be ashamed of it. . . my life is a representation of a lot of the issues that so many of the men and women that are represented in this space encounter, and are challenged with. So I embrace that and articulate that message to be able to effectuate change" (p. 228).

Given pressing challenges to the nation's health and well-being, institutions would do well to recognize and leverage the cultural wealth and strengths of BIPOC students and faculty, mental health practitioners, and leaders. Yosso's (2005) cultural wealth model describes six types of cultural capital that marginalized groups bring into educational spaces: aspirational, linguistic, familial, social, navigational, and resistance capital. Applicable to more than educational settings, this model highlights the strengths and resilience of BIPOC – their hopes and dreams, communication skills, connections to family and community, resourcefulness, and historical legacy of working to advance social justice. Proulx (this volume) reflected on the relationality that shaped his upbringing in the Mohawk matrilineal tradition and where his "bond with the natural world was deepened by the interconnectedness between humans and nature in Indigenous culture" (p. 92). His decision to focus his research on Indigenous well-being and health was born out of a recognition that "these were strengths that society did not promote or investigate as strengths and my goal was to leverage those strengths towards a better planet" (p. 93). Centering the values, experiences, and ways of knowing of historically oppressed individuals can offer new perspectives and healing wisdom to benefit all living beings (see David, this volume).

How White People Can Stand with BIPOC as Racial Justice Allies

Having deepened your awareness of the experiences and cultural resources of BIPOC, how can you help? Many of our white colleagues want to support their BIPOC students and colleagues but may not know how to do so, or they may succumb to inaction for fear of making a mistake. In the vignette about Dr. Zayas's experience at the faculty meeting, colleagues reached out privately to provide support, rather than showing their public support during the meeting. As is often the case, Dr. Zayas felt pressure to assuage her white colleagues' remorse for not having spoken up earlier. Although there is no one-size-fits-all approach to intervening effectively, there are guideposts that white people should consider.

In this section, we discuss five key ways that white individuals can support their BIPOC colleagues and students as racial justice allies by disrupting the cultural and structural norms of white supremacy in mental health training, education, and practice. We acknowledge criticisms of the term *ally*, which suggest that white people work only to support their BIPOC counterparts rather than work to create a more just and equitable system for people from all racial backgrounds. Some have used the terms *accomplice, comrade*, or *co-conspirator* to signal shared interests in the struggle against racism. Regardless of the terminology, our position is clear. Namely, white people's primary responsibility is to work in their own communities to dismantle the structures that maintain individual and institutional racism (Carmichael, 1966). At the same time, when white people work in solidarity with members of BIPOC communities, they must be informed by the insights of those communities. Informed by critical consciousness theory, we emphasize the importance of critical reflection – i.e., engaging in an analysis of how individual and interpersonal behaviors are shaped by systems of oppression – in guiding our social justice actions (Jemal, 2017). This analysis should encompass how each of us, unintentionally, upholds institutionalizing practices of white supremacy that perpetuate racial harm and inequity in our clinics, agencies, colleges, and universities.

While institutional change work takes time, and critical consciousness involves a continuous process of development, we call on you to consider how you can meaningfully support the BIPOC individuals in your places of work *now*. We focus on relational encounters, whether in a dyad or a group, formal or informal, that provide an opportunity for white colleagues and leaders to respond in meaningful ways to mitigate race-related stress, and proactively work to advance equity and justice at an organizational level.

1 Self-assessment: Examine your motivations, intentions, and knowledge gaps

In a synthesis of the interdisciplinary literature, Spanierman and Smith (2017) outlined potential hazards and aspirational characteristics for white racial justice allies. For example, white helping professionals might behave paternalistically, inadvertently positioning themselves as "saviors" of members of BIPOC communities. Additionally, white allies might over-identify with some BIPOC clients or colleagues and express false or misguided empathy (e.g., "As a white woman who has experienced sexism, I feel your pain as a Black woman"). They may focus their efforts on individuals and ignore more subtle institutional and structural manifestations of racism. Finally, because racial justice work is hard, and mistakes are inevitable, white ally efforts oftentimes are superficial or transitory.

In contrast, Spanierman and Smith (2017) offered a set of aspirational characteristics of white racial justice allies. For instance, white allies demonstrate a nuanced understanding of structural racism and white privilege. They enact a continual process of self-reflection about their positionality and feel a sense of responsibility to use their privilege to disrupt racism and promote racial justice. Rather than centering themselves, they work in collaboration and solidarity with People of Color; at the same time, they work actively in their own communities to educate other white people. Antiracist educators (Goodman, 2011; Kivel, 2017) and white racial justice organizations (e.g., Showing Up for Racial Justice, n.d.) emphasize the importance of understanding how white supremacy harms *everyone* in the system and elucidate our mutual interests in the fight against racial injustice.

Ask yourself: What biases and assumptions am I making about my BIPOC students, colleagues, and leaders? What knowledge gaps do I have and how can I address them? How does my positionality inform my experiences and understanding of the world, insulate or expose me to diverse perspectives, and affect my impact and influence in working with my BIPOC colleagues to advance racial justice? What are the larger structural deficits or assets of my institution? Where can I have the most positive impact in my specific setting?

> For example, before expecting Dr. Z to open the discussion about how the job candidates might contribute to the DEI efforts of the department, her white colleagues might have paused to reflect on their expectation that DEI work is the primary responsibility of BIPOC faculty. Interrogating that assumption may yield insights into the associated costs to Dr. Z (i.e., political capital and emotional labor) and the effects on the system as a whole (e.g., who benefits when BIPOC individuals are distressed, overworked, burned out, and marginalized?), as well as how their silence perpetuates the idea that DEI issues are irrelevant to white faculty.

2 Mindful presence: Take the time to listen and observe

As described above, many BIPOC are reluctant to talk with their white counterparts about their experiences of race-related stress and often feel the need to hide the labor they invest in managing it. If a BIPOC student or colleague does confide in you, demonstrate that you are worthy of their trust by taking the time to truly listen. Rather than jumping to conclusions, moving to problem-solving, or getting lost in your own thoughts and feelings, bring your mindful attention to what is being shared with you. Listen without judgment, interpretation, or criticism. Convey a stance of openness, curiosity, and compassion. Ask questions to deepen your understanding. If you are in a situation where you are observing an interaction in real time (as in the faculty meeting with Dr. Z), notice how BIPOC individuals in the space are being affected by what is unfolding.

> Upon hearing that her student Phuong was contemplating leaving the agency, Jan initially felt surprised, then guilty, that she had not known about the stress her student was experiencing. She felt defensive and anxious, worried about what her colleagues would think. After pausing to reflect, she realized that she had not taken the time to really ask Phuong about their experience of the practicum or as one of the few BIPOC students in their program. In their next meeting, Jan checked in with Phuong, apologized for cutting their discussion short the previous week, and asked if Phuong would feel comfortable sharing more about their experience of the practicum and their concerns. As Phuong spoke, Jan focused on her goal of listening with curiosity, openness, and care. When she noticed her own insecurities and judgments cropping up, she reminded herself of her desire to learn about Phuong's experiences and to invest in their growth by providing support and helping to address their concerns.

3   Critical reflection: Conduct a critical analysis of the situation

After mindfully listening to or observing your colleagues/students during moments of race-related tension, take some time to critically reflect on what you have learned and what this brings up for you (Spanierman & Smith, 2017). This includes examining taken-for-granted assumptions, beliefs, and thoughts (e.g., those shaped by the white racial frame) and identifying how so-called normative practices have evolved to maintain and perpetuate systems of inequity (Diemer & Blustein, 2006; Watts et al., 2003). What role are you playing in the system? How might internalized, interpersonal, and structural oppression be affecting your individual experiences and interpersonal/group dynamic? What feelings are present for you? Are you feeling anxious, angry, sad? Surprised, curious, hopeful?

This process of critical reflection is challenging and often emotionally charged. Do you feel an urge to dismiss your colleague's/student's perspectives or avoid the situation altogether? Try to embody the perspective of your BIPOC colleague or student. Does your view of the situation change? Acknowledging that allyship is difficult, ask yourself: How do I want to show up at this moment? What would it look like to align my actions with my values and ethical principles? What potential actions, even small ones, might you take to promote equity within your own practice setting? Is there anything getting in the way?

> Dr. Z's colleagues (or at least those who were paying attention) witnessed her distress after the Chair shut down her idea to discuss the candidates in the context of the department's DEI priorities. Although four colleagues cared enough to text her later to apologize for their inaction, none of them paused to ask themselves what it meant to really show up for Dr. Z., one of the few BIPOC faculty in the department. What did they fear would happen if they had spoken up? Beyond the minimal investment of a texted apology, what might genuine allyship look like? What is getting in the way?

4 Private actions: Provide emotional and instrumental support

For many white mental health professionals, providing emotional and instrumental support to persons who are suffering comes naturally. We are socialized to turn toward pain and try to alleviate it where we can. Yet research shows that neural, physiological, and affective empathic responses are greater when observing pain experienced by individuals of the same race compared with those of other races (e.g., Cikara et al., 2011). By making intentional efforts to listen to and get to know your BIPOC colleagues and students in a more authentic way – including directly asking them how you can support them – your circle of concern expands, your sense of interconnectedness grows, and prejudice decreases (e.g., Davies et al., 2011). Be proactive and enter those conversations with humility and some awareness of the potential stressors and challenges that your BIPOC faculty and students may be managing. Neville, Lewis, and French (this volume) offer additional guidance for social justice mentoring with students of color to facilitate their personal and professional growth.

> In her conversation with Phuong, Jan was able to listen empathically, validate Phuong's concerns, and help them brainstorm strategies to improve their experience at the agency in both the short and long term. Jan expressed support for Phuong's idea of reaching out to the training director to ask for staff training on creating antiracist and queer- and transgender-affirming spaces. While Jan felt good about her ability to be more emotionally present and supportive of Phuong in their private supervision meetings, she felt anxious about advocating for Phuong

with the senior administrators in the agency, including those who had described her as "difficult," "resistant," and "defensive" in prior team meetings.

5   Public actions: Be bold in visibly leveraging your power and privilege

While private actions are important, public actions – especially by senior leaders – are critical for transforming institutions. Jan's efforts to repair her relationship with Phuong helped them to feel supported in the moment. Yet to address the root causes of Phuong's marginalization in the agency and to prevent other trainees from experiencing the same, Jan needs to use her power and position for institutional change. Examples include proactively advocating for policies and practices to promote diversity, equity, inclusion, and belonging, challenging bias and discrimination at all levels, and expressing public support for your BIPOC colleagues and students. In classrooms and in meetings, elevate their contributions and expertise, as BIPOC voices and achievements are often overlooked and minimized. Invite them to collaborate on research projects and grants. Sponsor, mentor, and nominate them for roles that will help them develop as leaders. Your public actions will likely be experienced as a challenge to the power structure and you may experience blowback. Seek support and community with other colleagues who share your values and commitments. As you engage in a continuous cycle of reflection and action, it is important to examine your motivations and fears, analyze and boldly leverage your power and privilege, and work in solidarity with BIPOC.

> After the faculty meeting, Dr. Z felt very alone, depleted, and angry. She found herself thinking, "I'm so tired. Will this ever change? It's just an academic issue to them, but for me, it impacts how I feel here." Frustrated, Dr. Z decided to reach out to Dr. Buckman, a senior white professor with whom she had a warm, collegial relationship. Dr. Buckman listened carefully and came to understand how her silence during the meeting had hurt Dr. Z. She realized that she was afraid that people would think that she was trying to look "woke," and she feared being marginalized by some faculty for that. Yet, she realized that by remaining silent, she was undermining Dr. Z's efforts, while also failing to personally invest in the DEI mission of the school. She decided to have informal individual conversations with a few other white faculty about the candidates and the school's challenges regarding DEI. After speaking with Dr. Z, they all decided

to approach the Chair about putting the topic back on the agenda for the next faculty meeting. This time, they all came prepared to share ideas for policy and program changes, including advocating for a cluster hire, more financial aid for students, and training to improve faculty mentoring of BIPOC students. This helped to frame a more substantive discussion about each candidate's potential contributions to this broader vision of institutional change, which is what Dr. Z had originally proposed. This time, she wasn't alone, and with the support of the colleagues, the Chair was more receptive to their ideas.

Final Thoughts

Like Dr. Z., we have had moments where we have been so disheartened and hurt by an institutional culture working to maintain white dominance that we have contemplated leaving our positions. Our work is devoted to a future in which institutional racism is no longer a threat, and that BIPOC can apply their creative energy and talents to other problems and concerns. In the meantime, we call on you to seek ways to mitigate your BIPOC colleagues' race-related stress by holding yourself accountable for actions that may be perpetuating harm, and by supporting your colleagues both publicly and privately. We ask that you work in your own communities to disrupt the normalization of racial color-blindness and other forms of racism that maintain white supremacy. We emphasize the importance of critical reflection, mindful listening, and intentional efforts to deepen your empathy and understanding, in order to partner effectively with BIPOC to advance racial justice in your institutions. The two vignettes illustrate that even when you struggle to respond in the moment, you can engage in relational repair and healing, and work toward systems-level change.

We recognize that challenging white institutional presence (Gusa, 2010) in solidarity with BIPOC colleagues and students can be difficult. You may experience criticism or pushback from other whites in your organization. Yet the urgency and the stakes transcend the temporary comfort that comes with not rocking the boat. Furthermore, the rewards of racial allyship include more authentic, meaningful, and supportive relationships with BIPOC, an expanded worldview, and the knowledge that you are making a positive difference in the fight for racial equity (Smith & Redington, 2010; Spanierman et al., 2017). Our fates are interconnected. Are you in?

References

American Psychological Association. (2019). *Psychology faculty salaries for the 2018–2019 academic year: Results from the 2019 CUPA-HR survey for four-year colleges and universities*. Author.

Anthym, M., & Tuitt, F. (2019). When the levees break: The cost of vicarious trauma, microaggressions and emotional labor for Black administrators and faculty engaging in race work at traditionally white institutions. *International Journal of Qualitative Studies in Education, 32*(9), 1072–1093. doi:10.1080/09518398.2019.1645907.

Bonilla-Silva, E. (1997). Rethinking racism: Toward a structural interpretation. *American Sociological Review, 62*(3), 465–480. https://doi.org/10.2307/2657316

Carmichael, S. (1966). *Black power address at University of California, Berkeley* [audio file]. October. www.americanrhetoric.com/speeches/stokelycarmichaelblackpower.html

Cikara, M., Botvinick, M. M., & Fiske, S. T. (2011). Us versus them: Social identity shapes neural responses to intergroup competition and harm. *Psychological Science, 22*(3), 306–313. https://doi.org/10.1177/0956797610397667

Davies, K., Tropp, L. R., Aron, A., Pettigrew, T. F., & Wright, S. C. (2011). Cross-group friendships and intergroup attitudes: A meta-analytic review. *Personality and Social Psychology Review, 15*(4), 332–351. https://doi.org/10.1177/1088868311411103

Diemer, M. A., & Blustein, D. L. (2006). Critical consciousness and career development among urban youth. *Journal of Vocational Behavior, 68*(2), 220–232. https://doi.org/10.1016/j.jvb.2005.07.001

Feagin, J. R. (2020). *The white racial frame: Centuries of racial framing and counter-framing*. Routledge.

Goodman, D. J. (2011). *Promoting diversity and social justice: Educating people from privileged groups* (2nd ed.). SAGE.

Gusa, D. L. (2010). White institutional presence: The impact of Whiteness on campus climate. *Harvard Educational Review, 80*(4), 464–490. https://doi.org/10.17763/haer.80.4.p5j483825u110002

Helms, J. E. (1995). An update of Helms's white and People of Color racial identity models. In J. G. Ponterotto, J. M. Casas, L. A. Suzuki, & C. M. Alexander (Eds.), *Handbook of multicultural counseling*. SAGE.

Jaschik, S. (2017). *A college and klan traditions*. June. www.insidehighered.com/news/2017/06/23/wesleyan-college-georgia-apologizes-decades-which-institution-embraced-ku-klux-klan

Jemal, A. (2017). Critical consciousness: A critique and critical analysis of the literature. *Urban Review, 49*(4), 602–626. doi:10.1007/s11256-017-0411-3.

Kivel, P. (2017). *Uprooting racism: How white people can work for racial justice*. New Society Publisher.

Liu, W. M., Liu, R. Z., Garrison, Y. L., Kim, J. Y. C., Chan, L., Ho, Y. C. S., & Yeung, C. W. (2019). Racial trauma, microaggressions, and becoming racially innocuous: The role of acculturation and white supremacist ideology. *American Psychologist, 74*(1), 143–155. https://doi.org/10.1037/amp0000368

Louis, D. A., Rawls, G. J., Jackson-Smith, D., Chambers, G. A., Phillips, L. L., & Louis, S. L. (2016). Listening to our voices: Experiences of Black faculty at predominantly white research universities with microaggression. *Journal of Black Studies, 47*(5), 454–474. https://doi.org/10.1177/002193471663298

Maina, I. W., Belton, T. D., Ginzberg, S., Singh, A., & Johnson, T. J. (2018). A decade of studying implicit racial/ethnic bias in healthcare providers using the implicit association test. *Social Science & Medicine, 199,* 219–229. https://doi.org/10.1016/j.socscimed.2017.05.009

Matias, J. N., Lewis, N. A., & Hope, E. C. (2022). US universities are not succeeding in diversifying faculty. *Nature Human Behaviour, 6,* 1606–1608. https://doi.org/10.1038/s41562-022-01495-4

Mongelli, F., Georgakopoulos, P., & Pato, M. T. (2020). Challenges and opportunities to meet the mental health needs of underserved and disenfranchised populations in the United States. *Focus, 18*(1), 16–24. https://doi.org/10.1176/appi.focus.20190028

Neville, H. A., Awad, G. H., Brooks, J. E., Flores, M. P., & Bluemel, J. (2013). Color-blind racial ideology: Theory, training, and measurement implications in psychology. *American Psychologist, 68*(6), 455–466. doi:10.1037/a0033282.

Showing Up for Racial Justice. (n.d.). *Our values.* https://surj.org/about/our-values/

Smith, L., & Redington, R. M. (2010). Lessons from the experiences of white antiracist activists. *Professional Psychology: Research and Practice, 41*(6), 541–549. https://doi.org/10.1037/a0021793

Spanierman, L. B., & Smith, L. (2017). Roles and responsibilities of White allies: Implications for research, teaching, and practice. *The Counseling Psychologist, 45*(5), 606–617. https://doi.org/10.1177/0011000017717712

Spanierman, L. B., Poteat, V. P., Whittaker, V. A., Schlosser, L. Z., & Arévalo Avalos, M. R. (2017). Allies for life? Lessons From white scholars of multicultural psychology. *The Counseling Psychologist, 45*(5), 618–650. https://doi.org/10.1177/0011000017719459

Stevens, F. G., Plaut, V. C., & Sanchez-Burks, J. (2008). Unlocking the benefits of diversity: All-inclusive multiculturalism and positive organizational change. *The Journal of Applied Behavioral Science, 44*(1), 116–133. https://doi.org/10.1177/0021886308314460

Watts, R. J., Williams, N. C., & Jagers, R. J. (2003). Sociopolitical development. *American Journal of Community Psychology, 31*(1–2), 185–194. https://doi.org/10.1023/a:1023091024140

Wells-Wilbon, R., Porter, R., Geyton, T., & Estreet, A. (2021). Mental health disparities. In *Encyclopedia of social work.* https://oxfordre.com/socialwork/view/10.1093/acrefore/9780199975839.001.0001/acrefore-9780199975839-e-1253

Wilder, C. S. (2013). *Ebony and ivy: Race, slavery, and the troubled history of America's universities.* Bloomsbury Publishing.

Woods-Giscombé, C. L. (2010). Superwoman schema: African American women's views on stress, strength, and health. *Qualitative Health Research, 20*(5), 668–683. https://doi.org/10.1177/1049732310361892

Yosso, T. J. (2005) Whose culture has capital? A critical race theory discussion of community cultural wealth. *Race, Ethnicity and Education, 8*(1), 69–91. https://doi.org/10.1080/1361332052000341006

Zambrana, R. E., Harvey Wingfield, A., Lapeyrouse, L. M., Davila, B. A., Hoagland, T. L., & Valdez, R. B. (2017). Blatant, subtle, and insidious: URM faculty perceptions of discriminatory practices in predominantly White institutions. *Sociological Inquiry, 87*(2), 207–232. https://doi.org/10.1111/soin.12147

Index

For Product Safety Concerns and Information please contact our EU
representative GPSR@taylorandfrancis.com
Taylor & Francis Verlag GmbH, Kaufingerstraße 24, 80331 München, Germany